BLACK FAMILIES IN THERAPY
Second Edition

BLACK FAMILIES IN THERAPY

SECOND EDITION

Understanding the African American Experience

Nancy Boyd-Franklin

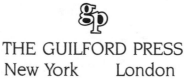

THE GUILFORD PRESS
New York   London

©2003 Nancy Boyd-Franklin
Published by The Guilford Press
A Division of Guilford Publications, Inc.
72 Spring Street, New York, NY 10012
www.guilford.com

Printed in the United States of America

This book is printed on acid-free paper.

Last digit is print number: 9 8 7 6 5 4 3 2 1

Library of Congress Cataloging-in-Publication Data
Boyd-Franklin, Nancy.
   Black families in therapy : understanding the African American
experience / Nancy Boyd-Franklin.— 2nd ed.
      p. cm.
Includes bibliographical references and index.
   ISBN 1-57230-619-X
   1. African American families—Mental health.   2. African Americans—Social
conditions.   3. Family psychotherapy.   I. Title.
RC451.5.N4B69 2003
616.89′ 156′ 08996073—dc21

                                                        2003009245

To A. J. and Mom

Thank you for your constant love and support.

About the Author

Nancy Boyd-Franklin, PhD, is a Professor in the Graduate School of Applied and Professional Psychology at Rutgers University. She is also an African American family therapist and the author or editor of several books, including the first edition of *Black Families in Therapy; Children, Families, and HIV/AIDS: Psychosocial and Psychotherapeutic Issues,* with Gloria L. Steiner and Mary G. Boland; *Reaching Out in Family Therapy: Home-Based, School, and Community Interventions,* with Brenna Hafer Bry; and *Boys Into Men: Raising Our African American Teenage Sons,* with A. J. Franklin and Pamela Toussaint.

An internationally recognized lecturer and author, Dr. Boyd-Franklin has published numerous articles on issues such as the treatment of African American families, extended family issues, spirituality and religion, home-based family therapy, group therapy for Black women, HIV and AIDS, parent and family therapeutic support groups, the multisystems model, and community empowerment.

Preface

The publication of *Black Families in Therapy* in 1989 was described as a land-mark contribution to the clinical literature. In this second edition, I have kept and updated the most important elements of the first edition, while significantly expanding into many important new areas. The last decade has brought major changes in legislation and public policy initiatives that have directly impacted the lives of many African American families. With this in mind, I have included a new chapter on public policy issues (Chapter 12) that discusses welfare reform, the Adoptions and Safe Families Act, kinship care, managed care, and affirmative action. There have also been significant demographic shifts in the African American population in recent years. Chapter 1 now includes a thorough overview of the complexity of different socioeconomic and class distinctions in African American communities, including the nonworking poor, the working poor (see also Chapter 13), and working-class, middle-class, and upper-income families (see also Chapter 15).

Black families in this country have become increasingly more diverse in recent years. I am particularly aware of the ethnic and cultural diversity that can exist in the African American community because I grew up in an African American family with both African American and Jamaican roots. My father's family is African American and moved to Harlem from North and South Carolina. My maternal grandparents both moved to Harlem from Jamaica, and my parents and I were all born in Harlem. My experiences are not unique. Unfortunately, many clinicians are unaware of the complexity of their clients' ethnic backgrounds and do not explore these issues with their African American clients, particularly in later generations. In recognition of this increasing diversity, this edition, although focusing primarily on African American families, includes in Chapter 8 a brief section on Caribbean families. Chapter 8 also includes a brief section on the issues and related treatment of biracial and multiracial children and families, another group that has been growing in recent years.

Since the literature on racism and racial identity theory has expanded significantly, Chapter 2 now includes a comprehensive exploration of the implications of a client's racial identity development on the treatment process. Chapter 5 explores gender roles in African American families and their impact on the socialization of male and female children and on adult male–female couple relationships; the concept of the "invisibility" of African American men and women; the impact of racism and sexism on couple relationships; the shortage of Black men; rising male unemployment; the decline in marriage rates among African Americans; and the complexity of couple therapy. Chapter 6, new to this edition, explores the complexity of separation, divorce, remarriage, and stepparenting in African American families. It also explores the complications that can result as a consequence of extended family involvement in these families.

One of the most groundbreaking chapters in the first edition addressed the issues of religion and spirituality in the treatment of African American families. Chapter 7 in this edition has been updated and expanded to include a discussion of such new areas as the use of spiritual metaphors and the spiritual issues related to death and dying that often present in therapy.

A number of topics not addressed in the first edition have become extremely important in recent years in African American communities. Many of these are discussed in Chapter 8, including the Afrocentric movement; Rites-of-Passage programs; the challenges related to the educational achievement of African American children, particularly males, including special education and the Ritalin controversy; HIV/AIDS; substance abuse and its burden on the older generation; violence; police brutality; and racial profiling.

The first edition focused primarily on issues for Black and White therapists in working with African American families. Chapter 9 broadens the focus of the book by expanding the discussion of the therapist's use of self and value conflicts with African American families to Latino and Asian therapists, as well as clinicians from other ethnic groups. Within the last two decades, the family therapy field has embraced many new and important theories and concepts. Chapter 10 has been expanded to include the narrative and postmodern approaches and "family therapy with one person," which can be utilized in individual therapy with African American clients.

I am truly grateful to the many readers who have given me feedback on this book over the years. This second edition represents my continuing sense of excitement in the work, as well as my ongoing belief in the empowerment of African American families and the clinicians who work with them.

Acknowledgments

I give thanks to God for the success of the first edition and for the privilege of writing this book. Throughout this process, I have had the support of many wonderful people. The first is my husband, Dr. A. J. Franklin, who shares with me a commitment to this work and who has given freely of his love, support, and considerable clinical expertise. My mother, Regina Boyd, has battled cancer for the last 3 years, but she has insisted upon reading every draft of this book and offered daily prayers for its successful completion. I would also like to thank all the members of my family and extended family for their ongoing love and support.

Throughout the publication of all my books, Hazel Staloff has been a treasure. She has done a magnificent job of providing insightful editing and coordination of the word processing of the text. It has been a pleasure to work with Jim Nageotte, Senior Editor at The Guilford Press, who has been so generous with his time, expertise, advice, and encouragement. I would also like to thank Anna Nelson, Production Editor, for her patience with me in the final production stages. My special thanks to Dr. Don-David and Judy Lusterman, who read through the entire first edition and offered invaluable insights and editorial suggestions. I would also like to thank Dr. Robert Hill for all of his contributions to this book and for his generous help throughout this process. Dr. Paulette Hines and Rosemary Allwood have always been there for me and have always given their feedback, support, and advice.

I am fortunate to have an amazing group of students in the PsyD and PhD programs at Rutgers University in the Graduate School of Applied and Professional Psychology (GSAPP), who have helped with the research for this book. I would like to thank Steven Allwood, Danielle Hawthorne, Janear Sewell, Lisa Henry, Christine Harris, Laura Fenster, Jamila Irons, Tanya Holland, and Scott Hirose for their contributions. My special thanks to Robert

Bonner, who dedicated an entire summer to researching the census material and statistics for this book. I would also like to thank all of the students in my classes who have given feedback on the first edition. My appreciation to my faculty colleagues, Drs. Shalonda Kelly and Brenna Hafer Bry, who have consistently given their friendship, help, and support in this process. I would also like to acknowledge and thank the current dean at GSAPP, Dr. Stanley Messer, and the former dean, Dr. Sandra Harris, for all of their efforts on my behalf. It is a pleasure to work with all of you at GSAPP.

Contents

III. Socioeconomic Class Issues and Diversity of Family Structures

IV. Implications for Supervision, Training, and Future Research

BLACK FAMILIES IN THERAPY
Second Edition

I

AFRICAN AMERICAN FAMILIES: THE CULTURAL AND RACIAL CONTEXT

1

Overview*

This second edition of *Black Families in Therapy* expands the vision of the first edition by providing clinicians with an even broader understanding of the cultural and racial context of African Americans. The last 40 years have brought a proliferation of material into the literature in family therapy, social work, psychology, medicine, education, and pastoral counseling on the realities facing these families. This book is an attempt to bring together that literature in one comprehensive clinical text.

Throughout the past 30 years, I have been repeatedly surprised to discover that many clinicians are totally unaware of the work of some of the preeminent researchers in this area. To further compound the problem, the student or professional seeking information on the cultural background of African Americans is now faced with the unavailability of some of the seminal books, printed in the period from 1965 to 1980, many of which received only one printing. With this in mind, I shall take the liberty once again in this edition of citing and quoting extensively from the early work of important scholars that may now be difficult to obtain.

Today, an increasing number of African American families are being referred to therapists, clinics, and community mental health centers. These families bring to therapy many issues specific to their race, cultural background, history, and response to mental health services that must be addressed. This book is intended to provide a forum for new clinicians and for therapists already experienced in the field, who are committed to including an understanding of race and ethnicity in their work with Black families. It is also intended to serve as a comprehensive text for the training of family therapists,

---

*The words "African American" and "Black" are used interchangeably throughout this book. All of the names and in some cases the identifying details have been changed in order to protect the confidentiality of the clients.

social workers, psychologists, psychiatrists and other mental health service providers, physicians, nurses, ministers, pastoral counselors, teachers, school counselors and administrators, child protective service and all other community-based family workers.

African American families constitute a distinct cultural group, but one in which there is a tremendous amount of diversity. This book will focus on these families exclusively. Clearly, there are many areas of similarity between Black families and families of other cultures. For example, there is no question that many other ethnic groups (e.g., Hispanic, Italian, Asian, etc.) have strong extended family and kinship ties, and thus may have some structural formations that correspond to those of Black families. A detailed analysis of these areas of similarity and difference, however, is beyond the scope of this book.

There is a potential in any book of this kind for stereotyping. This is a particularly sensitive issue, and I have tried very hard to avoid replacing old biases with new ones. I do believe that having a cultural framework is extremely useful in our work with clients and families. It is my hope that this book will increase the sensitivity of clinicians to the cultural variables and diversity among Black families. As a family therapist, I view this cultural material as providing the beginning hypotheses that clinicians can use as a framework in their work with African American families. I hope that these hypotheses are not viewed rigidly as applying to all Black clients, but instead are carefully assessed with each new family that enters treatment. The metaphor of the camera lens is a helpful one. It is useful to view the material presented in this book as a camera lens, which must be adjusted for each new individual or family that we treat. Throughout this book, I will stress the importance of recognizing individual differences and the unique qualities of each client and family.

DIVERSITY WITHIN
AFRICAN AMERICAN COMMUNITIES

First, it must be stressed that there is tremendous cultural diversity within and between African American communities in the United States. Hines and Boyd-Franklin (1996) discussed such sociological variations and sensitized clinicians to the cultural and racial context in which African Americans have lived and continue to live in the United States. This sensitization is an ongoing challenge. The tendency of policymakers and clinicians alike has been to categorize racial and cultural groups along stereotypical lines. This tendency is particularly prevalent with regard to African American families. Given the heterogeneity of cultural variables that are present in Black families and communities, it ought to be patently clear that there is no such entity as *the* African American family. When writing a book about African American families, one must acknowledge a certain level of racial and cultural similarity. It is possible, however, to highlight group tendencies without ignoring individual differences.

The great diversity of values, characteristics, and lifestyles that arises from such elements as geographical origins, level of acculturation, socioeconomic status, education, religious background, and age must be considered in any discussion of Black families in order to avoid stereotyping.

Between 1940 and 1950, over 1.5 million African Americans migrated from the South to the North, the Midwest, and the West Coast (Hines & Boyd-Franklin, 1996). This move from the South over 50 years ago to more urban areas of the country created many stressors for Black families and drew heavily on the "survival skills" that African Americans developed during the years of slavery and in its aftermath. It is important for the therapist to recognize and validate the relevance of this background and these skills respectfully as a means of understanding these families more fully.

There are differences between African American families from the North and those from the South. For example, a large number of Black families in the South have lived in the same community for generations. Still others have moved back to the South in large numbers in recent years. There are also important urban versus rural differences. The case examples reported here were drawn primarily from a northern urban sample of poor and middle-class families. In-depth geographical comparisons are beyond the scope of this book; indeed, further work is needed by researchers and therapists in different parts of the country in order to clarify these differences.

In addition to the African American families discussed above, there have been a number of waves of Black immigration, especially from the Caribbean, in the last century. Brice-Baker (1996) and Gopaul-McNicol (1993) describe these migration patterns in detail. (See Chapter 8 for a brief discussion of Caribbean families.) There is tremendous diversity among these families. The countries of the Caribbean were colonized by the French, the British, the Spanish, and the Dutch, all of whom brought Blacks into their colonies as slaves from Africa. The history of Blacks from the Caribbean and their immigration patterns to the United States is an area worthy of future study in the research and clinical literature.

Moreover, many Black families have come to this country within the last 40 years from the countries of Africa. There has been very little clinical literature addressing the needs of this group.

Within the last 20 years there has also been a growing and more vocal group who identify as biracial or multiracial (Root, 1996). (See Chapter 8 for a brief discussion of biracial and multiracial children and families.) Although a comprehensive discussion of this topic is beyond the scope of this book, readers are referred to the growing body of literature (Buckley & Carter, in press; Carter, 1995; Gillem, Cohn, & Throne, 2001; Root, 1992, 1996) for a more detailed discussion of this topic.

The focus of this book is primarily on Black families whose ancestors were originally brought to this country from Africa as slaves and who identify as African American.

AFRICAN AMERICANS: A DISTINCT RACIAL AND CULTURAL EXPERIENCE

The three main areas in which the experience of African Americans in this country has been unique from other ethnic groups are the African legacy, the history of slavery, and racism and discrimination.

The African Legacy

Long before Africans were brought to this country as slaves, they belonged to tribes descended from ancient civilizations on the continent of Africa. This legacy is rich in custom and mythology. A number of noted scholars have documented this heritage in great detail (Akbar, 1984; Ani, 1994; Asante, 1988, 1990; Azibo, 1996; Hilliard, Payton-Stewart, & Williams, 1990; Kambon, 1998; Karenga, 1997; Mbiti, 1990, 1992; Nobles, in press; Richards [a.k.a. Marimba Ani], 1980). In the exploration of the cultural context of African American families today, this book shall focus primarily on the concept of family kinship and collective unity (Nobles, in press) and on the role of religion and the African philosophy of life (Abimola, 1997; Ani, 1994; Mbiti, 1990, 1992; Nobles, in press).

Kinship ties make up what is perhaps one of the most enduring and important aspects of the African heritage. Nobles (in press) and Mbiti (1970, 1992) have stressed the emphasis in African culture on the "survival of the tribe" that transcended concerns for the individual, the nuclear family, or even the extended family. This ethos has persisted, and the consequent survival skills are among the most significant strengths of African American families today. Nobles (in press) quotes the following from Mbiti (1970), "In traditional life, the individual did not and could not exist alone." It is often difficult for those raised within a purely Westernized system focused on the individual and the nuclear family to understand a worldview that places the well-being of the social whole before that of its members. Mbiti (1970) states the essential tenet of the traditional African's view of him- or herself: "I am because we are; and because we are, therefore, I am" (Nobles, in press).

It is important to bear in mind that this collectivistic philosophy may still be very much in evidence in some of the African American families that we treat. Individualistic concepts so central to Western therapy—differentiation, clearly defined boundaries, separation, and individuation—may contradict the cultural values of some African American families and clients from other extended family cultures.

The other aspect of the African legacy that must be recognized by clinicians who work with African American families is the central role of religion and spiritual beliefs in many Black families. These beliefs, while "permeat[ing] every aspect of the African's life," served the further purpose of the tribe:

It was, in a very real sense, not something for the betterment of the individual, but rather something for the community of which the individual was an integral part. For the traditional African, to be human was to belong to the whole community. (Nobles, in press).

Nobles (in press) describes the essential nature of African religious experience, noting the extent of the unified quality of the African spiritual sensibility:

Curiously enough, many African languages did not have a word for religion as such. Religion was such an integral part of man's existence that it and he were inseparable. Religion accompanied the individual from conception to long after his physical death.

This belief system has survived hundreds of years of slavery and its aftermath and has influenced both the strong sense of "family" (i.e., the extended family group) and the strong religious or spiritual orientation of many African American families today. In relation to these two areas of exploration, Chapter 3 explores in detail the role of the extended family, and Chapter 7 elaborates on the role of spirituality and religion in the lives of many African Americans today. (See Chapter 8 for a discussion of Afrocentricity and the Afrocentric movement.)

The Maafa: The Impact of Slavery

African people were captured and transported from many tribal communities to this country as slaves. Maafa, a Kiswahili word meaning "great disaster," has been used by Afrocentric scholars to refer to the era of slavery (Ani, 1994; Kambon, 1998; Richards, 1980). The Maafa was a wound on the soul of African Americans that has had profound multigenerational consequences. Enslavement went beyond the physical level and had an impact on the cultural, spiritual, and mental experience of its victims as well (Asante, 1988; Richards, 1980). Many African Americans, myself included, are vividly reminded of this when we construct our genograms, or family trees, and experience the gaping holes in our family histories left by the enslavement and death of our ancestors. Kambon (1996, 1998) has described the Maafa as the African holocaust. Estimates of those who died during slavery, including those lost in crossing the ocean, range from 25 million to over 100 million (Richards, 1980).

Richards (1980) and Asante (1988) have referred to the Maafa as an attempt at cultural genocide. Not only were many Africans killed during slavery, they were also forbidden to use their African names, to speak their own languages, and to transmit their culture to their children (Allwood, 2001). The impact of this process on the lives of the slaves has been described by Akbar (1984), Ani (1994), Asante (1988), Franklin and Moss, (2000), Hines and

Boyd-Franklin (1996), and Richards (1980). The institution of slavery was disruptive by nature. This institution attempted to rob the African people of their human traits as well as their homeland. Slave masters utilized a dehumanizing process that attempted to deprive African men and women of their traditions—including family ties, language, customs, food, and their gods and spiritual rituals.

Africans were bought and sold according to the slave's market value and suitability for a particular region and/or task. Slaves were often separated from other family members because each slave was considered chattel, to be sold to the highest bidder. Life expectancies were low and mortality was high (Franklin & Moss, 2000; Hines & Boyd-Franklin, 1996) since slave masters were only required to provide slaves with the bare essentials for their survival.

Additional practices were put in place in an effort to destroy the traditional concepts of family. Slaves could not marry legally—tribal ceremonies were not allowed, nor were American religious or civil proceedings—which meant that no child born to a slave could be legally recognized as a family member. Mothers, fathers, and children could be sold away from each other, disrupting any semblance of family security or stability. Both African women and men were abused sexually—women as sexual objects for White slave masters and men as breeders to increase the labor supply (Franklin & Moss, 2000; Hines & Boyd-Franklin, 1996).

Despite such attempts to deprive slaves of their culture and human rights, African Americans sought to maintain their family's tribal customs and spiritual rituals. Human dignity survived in the face of enforced degradation. Black people created their own marriage rituals such as "jumping the broom," which acknowledged a union between a man and a woman. The process of informal adoption and kinship care (discussed in Chapter 3) had its origins in African tribal traditions and in the "taking in" of children by other slave families when their parents were sold or killed.

Spirituality survived in many forms, most saliently in an African belief in familial and tribal reunion in the afterlife. It is not accidental that the "spirituals" often contain hidden messages of escape, liberation, and rebellion. Songs such as "Wade in the Water" were used to signal an escape, with Black women as well as men taking an active role in attempts at liberation (Giddings, 1983). The African heritage of loyalty to tribe and culture can still be found in African Americans' strong orientation toward a kinship network. As a colleague and I (Hines & Boyd-Franklin, 1996) have noted, "[this] kinship network, not necessarily drawn along blood lines, remains a major mode for coping with the pressures of an oppressive society" (p. 87).

In order to lend justification to the racist practices of slavery, Africans were labeled as chattel, subhuman, and inferior. The residual effects of this labeling have continued through many generations and have had the impact of a collective posttraumatic stress disorder. This is most evident in the lingering myth of African American inferiority in U.S. society. Therapists in the mental health field encounter these issues approximately every 10–20 years when a "new" theory of genetic inferiority is introduced with regard to African Americans (Tucker, 1994). Jensen (1969, 1985), Shockley (1987), and most recently Herrnstein and Murray (1994) in *The Bell Curve,* have attempted to "prove" the myth of African American intellectual inferiority through flawed statistical analysis. This has been a part of a cycle in U.S. history, beginning with slavery, in which erroneous beliefs in inferiority and invalid pseudoscience have been used as a justification for the unequal treatment of African Americans (Gardner, 1995; Gould, 1995, 1996; Nisbett, 1995; Tucker, 1994).

The Impact of Racism and Discrimination

It is difficult to convey fully to someone who has not experienced it the insidious, pervasive, and constant impact that racism and discrimination have on the lives of African Americans. Both affect an African American from birth until death and have an impact on every aspect of family life, from childrearing practices, courtship, and marriage, to male–female roles, self-esteem, and cultural and racial identity. They also influence the way in which many African Americans relate to each other and to the outside world (Jones, 1997).

Slavery set the tone for people of African descent to be treated as inferior. Skin color was and is a badge of difference. The process of discrimination is evident at all levels of society from theories about genetic inferiority (Herrnstein & Murray, 1994; Jensen, 1969, 1985; Shockley, 1987), to segregation that existed blatantly in the South until the civil rights era in the 1960s and still occurs in subtler forms today. Continued inequities in the United States of the 21st century are manifested by the disproportionate numbers of Black people who are poor, homeless, living in substandard housing, unemployed, and school dropouts.

This process of discrimination is evident at all class levels. It does not disappear or lessen with advances in economic status, education, the neighborhood in which one lives, career, or job level. Chapter 15 reveals that African American middle- and upper-income families continue to experience different forms of discrimination despite the advances brought about in the last 40–50 years.

Multigenerational experiences with this system of racism and oppression and the special aspects of the African American racial and cultural heritage have combined to produce features that are unique and different from those that impact any other group in U.S. history. Throughout this book, a continual question will be raised for the reader as to the relative similarities and differences between African Americans and other cultural groups. Although many similarities will be noted, there are nevertheless some striking differences, arising from the effects of forced immigration on African Americans as an enslaved population. Most ethnic groups have experienced some degree of discrimination, particularly in the first and second generations of their immigration to the United States. But for African Americans of all class levels, a markedly virulent strain of racism and discrimination has persisted in a variety of forms for multiple generations over a period of 400 years. While I recognize fully the extent to which this point of view has been debated and comparisons made to other groups, it is helpful for clinicians to understand that many African Americans in the United States hold this view and that it permeates their experiences.

AFRICAN AMERICAN FAMILIES TODAY*

The African American Population Census Results

In order for clinicians to work effectively with African American families, it is important that they understand population trends and the diversity within Black communities. Preliminary analyses of the 2000 Census showed that the total population of the United States was 281.4 million people (U.S. Bureau of the Census, August 2001b). African Americans comprised 12.9% of that total, or 36.4 million people. The African American population increased faster than the total U.S. population from 1990 to 2000. In recent years, many African American families have ventured to the Southwest and the West, and African Americans are moving back to the South in large numbers, with over half (54%) of the Black population now living there, 19% in the Midwest, 18% in the Northeast, and 10% in the West (U.S. Bureau of the Census, August 2001b).

    In 2000, the U.S. Bureau of the Census reported that the African American population is younger than the White population (33% of the Black population was under age 18 vs. 24% of the White population).

    According to the U.S. Bureau of the Census, in 2000 there were 8.6 million African American families versus 53.1 million White families (U.S. Bureau of the Census, June 2001a). Less than half (48%) of all African Americans lived in married couple families as compared to 83% of the White families. Tucker and Mitchell-Kernan (1995) have attributed this decline in marriage among African Americans to economic instability, high unemployment rates for Black men, and the shortage of African American men. (See Chapter 5 for a discussion of how this affects African American male–female relationships and the impact it has on couple therapy.) In the year 2000, the percentage of single-parent households maintained by women was 47% in the African American community and 16% among Whites (U.S. Bureau of the Census, June 2001a).

    In terms of educational attainment, a large proportion of African Americans

---

*I would like to gratefully acknowledge the help and contribution of the following colleagues to the interpretation of the Census demographics and income statistics: Dr. Robert Hill, Mr. Robert Bonner, and Dr. A. J. Franklin.

18 years and older are at least high school graduates. The percentage jumped from 65.8% in 1990 to 78.5% in 2000 (U.S. Bureau of the Census, 2000). In September 2000, however, the U. S. Bureau of the Census reported a difference of 11 percentage points between the Black and the White populations 25 and older with a high school diploma (77% of Blacks vs. 88% of Whites) (U.S. Bureau of the Census, 2000). The 2000 Bureau of the Census report showed that the proportion of Whites with a bachelor's degree from college was 28%, which was almost twice the 15% of African Americans. In 2000, the patterns in terms of gender among African Americans were the opposite of those among Whites: for African Americans, more women (16%) than men (14%) had graduated from college, while for Whites, more men (31%) than women (25%) were college graduates (U.S. Bureau of the Census, 2000).

Income and Class Trends among African Americans

Table 1.1 presents the changing demographic data on income for Black and White families in 1980 as compared with 20 years later in 2000. For the purpose of this discussion, annual family income is used as the primary criterion for classifying different class strata (Hill, 1999a). The following distinctions, (based on Hill, 1999a), have been adjusted for today's economy: poor (under $15,000), working class ($15,000–49,999), middle income ($50,000–$99,999), and upper income ($100,000 and over).

African American Poor Families

Hill (1999a) divides poor African American families into two categories: the nonworking poor and the working poor. It is important for clinicians to be aware of these categorical distinctions, as they can lead to different life circumstances and realities for the clients we serve. Overall, there was a decrease in the

TABLE 1.1. Household Income by Race, 1980 and 2000 (Income in 2001 Adjusted Dollars)

Family income	Black Families		White Families	
	1980	2000	1980	2000
$100,000 and over (upper income)	1.5	6.4	6.1	14.9
$50,000–99,999 (middle income)	14.7	21.7	28.7	30.4
$15,000–49,999 (working class)	46.9	46.2	47.7	40.5
Under $15,000 (poor)	36.9	25.6	17.6	14.2
Median income (in 2000 dollars)	$21,902	$30,495	$38,017	$45,142

Source: U.S. Bureau of the Census (2002, Appendix A, Table A-1).

number of poor African American families between the years 1980 and 2000, from 36.9% to 25.6% (see Table 1.1). And yet the percentage of Black families that are poor is twice that of White families in the same time period (see Table 1.1; U.S. Bureau of the Census, 2002). It is important to note that while the number of poor Black families appears to have dropped in the decade between 1990 and 2000, from 31% of all families to 20.8%, respectively, this decline may be an artifact of welfare reform legislation (discussed in Chapter 12) and the unusual economic prosperity of the 1990s (U.S. Bureau of the Census, 2001c). (See Chapter 13 for a more thorough discussion of the treatment of poor African American families.)

The African American Nonworking Poor

Hill (1999a) used the term "nonworking poor families" to refer to the lowest income group among African American families. This same group was identified by Wilson (1987) as "the underclass." Wilson (1987) used this term to refer to individuals living in extreme poverty, predominately in inner-city areas, who have experienced long-term joblessness or are welfare-dependent. Hill (1999a) has criticized Wilson's use of "the underclass" as a static class concept, which does not allow for aspiration and change (Hill, 1999a). (See "The Underclass Controversy," below).

The African American Working Poor

Hill (1999a) described the working poor in African American communities as

> families in which at least one head of household has a regular attachment to the labor force. He/she usually works frequently, although usually at poverty-level wages. Eight out of ten (86%) of these families have one or more earners. Most working poor—both adults and youth—work at below minimum wages and more often obtain part-time jobs. They often work at unskilled or low-paying service jobs that do not provide fringe benefits. Most (74%) of these families are concentrated in central cities. (p. 75)

Weil and Finegold (2002) have noted the increase in working poor families since welfare "reform" (see Chapter 11). It is also important to note that many working poor families live very marginally and have no health insurance (Hill, 1999a; Weil & Finegold, 2002). It remains to be seen whether such families will be able to maintain even these minimal income levels in a declining economy (Hill, 1999a, 1999b; Weil & Finegold, 2002).

Many African American working poor families lived a marginal existence and struggled to survive even during the strong economy of the 1990s. The downturn in the economy, the recession after the terrorist attacks on September 11, 2001 (i.e., 9/11), and rising unemployment rates have had a significant impact on working poor families. The Association for Children of New Jersey (ACNJ; a child advocacy group in New Jersey) has emphasized the impact "welfare reform" (see Chapter 12) has had on working poor families (Association for Children of New Jersey, 2002). Although their study was limited to New Jersey residents, the trends they identified are representative of the country as a whole:

> Despite the recent strong economy and high salaries for the average New Jersey family, many working families in New Jersey are struggling just to provide the basic necessities for their children. . . . Welfare reform has increased the number of working poor, moving recipients from welfare to work in low-wage jobs. In a November 2000 study by Mathematica Policy Research, the average yearly income is $15,600 for current and former Work First New Jersey (WFNJ) clients. This is a far cry from the estimated livable wage for a family of four in New Jersey, $37,932. . . .
> Working poor families cannot sustain a crisis event, such as illness of their breadwinner or the necessity of their breadwinner to care for an ill member of the family. Many working poor families lack health insurance or the ability to take off from their jobs for periods of time. For some families, common occurrences such as their child getting a winter cold and requiring their care at home will result in the loss of their job. (Association for Children of New Jersey, 2002, p. 1).

Both the nonworking and the working poor make up a large proportion of the caseloads of many clinicians at inner-city clinics, hospitals, and agencies. It is crucial that therapists understand the realities these families face and the multisystems with which they are involved (see Chapters 11 and 13).

African American Working-Class Families

Families are characterized as "working class" when their income is between $15,000 and $49,000. In 2000, the percentage of African American families in this category was 46.2%, a decrease from 46.9% in 1980 (see Table 1.1). The percentage of White families who were working class in 2000 was less than the percentage of Black families, a trend that has been consistent for the last 20 years (see Table 1.1 above; also see U.S. Bureau of the Census, 2002). Many African Americans in working-class families work a standard 40-hour week. But many also work more than one job, yet still find themselves in a very precarious economic condition. Many of these families are living "on the edge," struggling to survive, and are especially vulnerable to a weak economy, particularly those at the lower end of the continuum. Hill (1999a) has referred to these families as the "working near poor," which he defined as

families in which one or more of the heads of households have a strong attachment to the labor force. Nine out of ten (96%) of these black families have one or
more earners. These families often work in semi-skilled occupations or hold low-
income service or white-collar jobs. Three out of four (77%) of near poor families live in central cities. (p. 75).

African American Middle-Class Families

A middle-income African American family earns between $50,000 and
$99,999. In 2000, 21.7% of African American families were in this range,
which represented a major change from 14.7% in 1980 (see Table 1.1; U.S.
Bureau of the Census, 2002). The percentages of White families in this income
category have consistently remained higher: 30.4% in 2000 versus 28.7% in
1980 (see Table 1.1). The median income for Blacks compared to Whites has
been lower by approximately the same percentage from 1980 to 2000. It is
noteworthy that it has remained consistently lower over the last 20 years. In
1980, when Black median income was $21,902 and White median income
was $38,017, Black median income was 57.6% that of Whites. In 2000, when
Black median income was $30,495 and White median income was $45,142,
Black median income was only 67.5% of that of Whites (U.S. Bureau of the
Census, 2002; see Chapter 15 for a discussion of middle-class African American families). Hill (1999a) defines middle-class African American families as

> [those] in which both household heads are in the labor force. They hold middle-
> income white collar or professional occupations, often in the government sector.
> Although four out of five (77%) of middle class families are headed by two par-
> ents, the proportion of middle class families headed by women doubled from 12
> to 23 percent from 1969 to 1989. Contrary to popular belief, three out of five
> (62%) of middle class black families live in central cities, while only two out of
> five (38%) live in suburban areas. Nevertheless, the number of middle class fami-
> lies that live in the suburbs doubled from 20 to 38 percent. (p. 76)

African American Upper-Income Families

Upper-income families are those who earn over $100,000. While the percent-
age of upper-income African American families has risen significantly in the
United States in the last 20 years from 1.5% in 1980 to 6.4% in 2000, their
numbers are still relatively small (see Table 1.1). They constituted less than half
the percentage of White families in 2000 (14.9%) in this category (U.S. Bureau
of the Census, 2002). (Chapter 15 includes a discussion of upper-income African American families.) Hill (1999a) describes these families as those in which

> both household heads are employed. They usually occupy upper income white-
> collar jobs or are executives or managers, or are professionals—often in the pri-

vate sector. Although eight out of ten (82%) upper class families comprise two parents, the proportion of upper class families headed by women rose markedly between 1969 and 1989. (p. 77)

However, Hill (1999a) further recommends caution in interpreting these results:

> Yet, we should be careful not to exaggerate the growth of the middle and upper classes among blacks because they are often not economically comparable with white middle and upper classes. . . . First, as Oliver and Shapiro (1995) and Anderson (1994) observe, most middle and upper class black families attain their status through [two] incomes and occupations, while comparable whites achieve their status through wealth and assets, which are ten times greater than blacks. (p. 77)

UNEMPLOYMENT IN THE AFRICAN AMERICAN COMMUNITY

As the section above indicated, African American families are especially vulnerable during periods of economic instability and recession. Whether African Americans are at the poorest socioeconomic level, a part of the working poor since welfare "reform," working class, middle class, or upper income, most reach their class level through income from their jobs. The saying "last hired, first fired" unfortunately still applies to African Americans at all levels of society. The unemployment rates for Blacks have consistently been approximately twice that of Whites in every decade since the 1970s (Hill, 1999a; see Table 1.2).

It is also important for therapists to recognize that unemployment statistics often do not reflect the numbers of poor African Americans who have

TABLE 1.2. Unemployment Rates in the United States for Selected Years by Race

Year	Black	White	Black/White ratio
1972	10.4%	5.1%	2.0
1980	14.3%	6.3%	2.3
1990	11.4%	4.8%	2.4
1999	8.0%	3.7%	2.2
2000	5.4%	2.6%	2.1
2001	6.3%	3.3%	1.9

Source: U.S. Bureau of Labor Statistics (2003).

been out of the labor market for so long that they are not even counted in official reports (Hill, 1999a; Wilson, 1987, 1996). These individuals and their families make up a large part of our caseloads. Many have been taken off the welfare rolls (see Chapter 12) and placed in low-level jobs. Weil and Finegold (2002) pointed out that welfare reform was enacted during a period of economic prosperity. Since the terrorist attacks of 9/11, unemployment numbers have increased and many workers have lost their jobs. Some cities have also experienced an increase in the rates of homeless individuals and families with the downturn in the economy.

The rise in unemployment rates since 9/11 is documented in Table 1.3. When compared to Table 1.2, it is clear that after unprecedented low rates of unemployment in 2000 (5.4% for Blacks vs. 2.6% for Whites), these rates have increased dramatically in the period from January to July 2002 (10.3% for Blacks vs. 5.1% for Whites). Over 10% of African Americans lost their jobs in this 1-year period. Many African American families across class and socioeconomic levels are experiencing economic hardship at this time (U.S. Bureau of Labor Statistics, 2003; see Table 1.3).

For any family, of any race, ethnic, or cultural group, unemployment is a major stressor. For many African Americans, who are often contributing to the support of extended family members, the impact of unemployment can be devastating. During these times of stress, there is often an increase in acting-out behavior and child and family referrals as families struggle to cope with such hardships.

TABLE 1.3. Unemployment Rates in the United States for Selected Months by Race

	Black	White
January–September 2001	8.3%	3.9%
October–December 2001	9.9%	4.9%
September 2001	8.8%	4.3%
October 2001	9.6%	4.7%
November 2001	9.9%	5.0%
December 2001	10.2%	5.1%
January 2002	9.8%	5.0%
February 2002	9.6%	4.9%
March 2002	10.7%	5.0%
April 2002	11.2%	5.3%
May 2002	10.2%	5.2%
June 2002	10.7%	5.2%
July 2002	9.9%	5.3%
January–July 2002	10.3%	5.1%

Source: U.S. Bureau of Labor Statistics (2003).

THE COMPLEXITY OF CLASS ISSUES
IN AFRICAN AMERICAN COMMUNITIES

Class issues are extremely complicated in the African American community. For example, an extended family might include members who live in the inner city and have a long-term history of unemployment and welfare involvement; members, who by virtue of educational opportunities, have become middle class; and members who have achieved upper-income status and live in predominately White suburban communities.

While families in other cultural groups may have a similar socioeconomic distribution, the expectation of reciprocity in African American families often leads to more interaction between extended family members at different class levels. This is an extremely important concept for clinicians to understand as it can contribute to family pressures, obligations, and tensions. On the other hand, it can also lead to positive extended family support systems. For example, family members experiencing economic problems, homelessness, or difficulty in caring for their children may be able to turn to other extended family members for support. Or, an extended family member who is perceived as "doing well" may be overwhelmed by expectations of help from less fortunate family members.

The debate over class issues in the African American community has occupied social scientists for generations. Although increasing numbers of African Americans have achieved middle- and even upper-income levels in the last 30 years (Billingsley, 1992; Hill, 1999a; Watkins, 2001), the tenuous nature of income and class status in many African American families can contribute to psychological pressures and distress, which can present in clinics as depression and anxiety in adults and in the acting-out behavior of their children.

Throughout this book, attempts will be made to look at class and race issues together as they affect African American families at different socioeconomic levels. These issues play a major part in the life experiences of many African American families, particularly those living in poverty. One prevalent myth has been that race has declining significance for African Americans who have attained middle- or upper-income levels (Wilson, 1980). In recent years, however, many researchers have documented the continuing significance of race and the ongoing experience, albeit more subtle, of racism for middle- and upper-income African American families (Cose, 1993; Hill, 1999a; Watkins, 2001). (See Chapter 15 for further discussion of these issues.) The continued impact of racism, particularly on a psychological level, contributes to a sense of disillusionment and insecurity in many African American families who have achieved economic success.

The "Underclass" Controversy

According to the Bureau of the Census, a significant number of African Americans (20.8%) live in poverty (U.S. Bureau of the Census, 2001c). In his book *The Truly Disadvantaged,* Wilson (1987) used the term "underclass" to describe African American families who have been trapped in poverty for generations and who experience little relief or upward mobility. Some individuals have been out of the labor market for so long they do not appear in unemployment statistics. Wilson (1987) argued that traditional Black inner-city neighborhoods that once had been composed of African Americans of all classes declined when the middle-class and some working-class families moved away. Furthermore, he argued that affirmative action programs gave educational and employment opportunities predominantly to African American individuals who were already middle class and did not benefit those in the "underclass" (Hill, 1999a).

Wilson's (1987) work was challenged on a number of levels. Hill (1999a) criticized Wilson's (1987) analysis, stating that it "minimized the significance of contemporary racism as a major factor in creating and maintaining the underclass in the black community" (p. 62). Hill also pointed out that "although Wilson included the long-term unemployed and poor, his inclusion of welfare recipients, school dropouts, teenage mothers, delinquents and criminals shifted most analyses and discussions of this group to the 'undeserving' poor" (Hill, 1999a, p. 62). This pejorative portrait of the very poor was used by conservative policymakers to promote legislation affecting this group (Hill, 1999a). Hill (1999a) points out that although Wilson depicted inner-city neighborhoods as "almost exclusively poor and welfare families" (p. 63), analysis of the census data reveal that "at least half of the residents of highly concentrated poverty areas are 'working class'" (Hill, 1999a, p. 63). Gans (1995), Jencks and Peterson (1991), and Steinberg (1995) provide further discussion of the issue of the Black underclass.

Despite the debate presented above, it is indisputable that a sizeable part of the African American population lives below the poverty line, and that the income disparity is increasing between this group, middle-class African Americans, and the country as a whole (Watkins, 2001). While Watkins points out that one must acknowledge the economic and political gains made by some Blacks in this country, it is very important that educational and economic opportunities be available to all members of the African American community and that racism be challenged in its varied forms at all class levels.

THE STRENGTHS OF AFRICAN AMERICAN FAMILIES

Many of our clients come to us because they are in trouble or in pain. They present with their problems and not with their strengths. Given this reality, it is extremely important that we, as service providers, adopt a strength-based approach to treatment (Boyd-Franklin, 1989; Boyd-Franklin & Bry, 2000; Logan, 2001) and be aware of the cultural and familial strengths that many of these families possess to guide our hypotheses and interventions.

For over 30 years, a number of researchers and scholars (Billingsley, 1968, 1992, 1994; Hill, 1972, 1977, 1993, 1994, 1999a; Jones, 1998a, in press; Logan, 2001; Nobles, in press; Staples & Johnson, 1993; White, 1972, 1984, in press; White & Parham, 1994) challenged the preoccupation with pathology in African American family life promulgated by writers such as Moynihan (1965), Jensen (1969) and, more recently, Herrnstein and Murray (1995), who posited a theory of African American genetic inferiority. White (in press) has pointed out that when traditional theories, which were developed for White populations, were applied to Black people, the result was often the development of theories based on "weakness-dominated" or "inferiority-oriented" conclusions. More recently, researchers have explored the strengths of well-functioning African American families (Billingsley, 1992; Gary, Beatty, Berry, & Price, 1983; Hill, 1994, 1999a; Hines & Boyd-Franklin, 1996; Lewis & Looney, 1983; Logan, 2001; McAdoo, 1981, 1996, 2002; McAdoo & McAdoo, 1985). White and Parham (1994) have called upon scholars and researchers to view the study of African American culture from a more balanced perspective.

White (in press), Hill (1972, 1993, 1999a), and McAdoo (1981, 1996, 2002) challenged Moynihan's (1965) characterization of Black families as "matriarchal." White (in press) pointed out that many Black families are viewed from a middle-class frame of reference, which assumes that a "psychologically healthy" family must consist of two parents. Since, as White stated, African American men are often not "consistently visible to the white observer," erroneous conclusions about matriarchy are often drawn. It should also be noted that the characterization of matriarchal structures as inherently deficient is itself a product of the traditional patriarchal bias. Many African American families are headed by single mothers, but it would be a serious error to view such family structures—and thus a considerable proportion of Black families—as inherently pathological. Lindblad-Goldberg and Dukes (1985) demonstrated that a competent single parent and a sufficient extended family and/or community support system can lead to healthy family functioning (see Chapter 3).

The focus on strengths in terms of African American family lifestyles began in the late 1960s. Hill (1972, 1999a) cites strong kinship bonds, strong work orientation, adaptability of family roles, high achievement orientation, and strong religious orientation as important strengths of the African American families he studied. It is important to note here that such strengths should not be read comparatively (i.e., as perceived to be stronger than in other ethnic groups/cultures) but merely as inherent within the African American cultural framework.

The first strength that has been repeatedly recognized in Black families is that of strong kinship bonds and extended family relationships. African American families have historically taken in other children and the elderly, and "doubling up" has been a common practice among these families since the days of slavery (Hill, 1972, 1977, 1993, 1999a; McAdoo, 1981, 1996, 2002).

Throughout his career, Hill (1972, 1977, 1993, 1999a) has documented the strength of informal adoption, or kinship care, practices in African American families. In his seminal work, *The Strengths of Black Families* (1972), he describes this kinship-oriented informal adoption process in detail:

> Since formal adoption agencies have historically not catered to non-whites, blacks have had to develop their own network for informal adoption of children. This informal adoption network among black families has functioned to tighten kinship bonds since many black women are reluctant to put their children up for adoption. (p. 6)

The strengths of these bonds are also attributable to the African tribal heritage of African Americans, as well as to the importance of maintaining family and community cohesion in the face of slavery and its residue (Hill, 1999a; Nobles, in press). As Hill (1972) notes, the attention to cohesion has had positive effects on the lives of Black people: "[The] tight kinship network within black families has proven itself to be an effective mechanism for providing extra emotional and economic support in the lives of thousands of children" (p. 6).

As a result of these strong kinship bonds, many African American families have become extended families in which relatives with a wide variety of blood ties have been absorbed into a coherent network of mutual emotional and economic support. This is one of the most important facts that many deficit theorists have overlooked in their statements about the "Black matriarchy" (Moynihan, 1965).

Much of the role flexibility in African American families probably developed as a response to economic necessities. Hill (1972, 1993, 1999a) pointed out that the high percentage of women and adolescents who have had to work to help support the family has forced the typical African American family to be unusually versatile in terms of assuming and fulfilling family roles. Older children stand in as parents and caretakers, mothers fill the shoes of both parents or trade traditional roles with fathers, and so on. Hill (1972, 1999a) believes that such role flexibility has been important in stabilizing African American families. Family members are apt to be more able to cope with changes in circumstances when not restricted to what is usually a sex-stereotyped, narrowly defined role. This should be viewed as a strength.

Hill's (1972, 1993, 1999a) work stressed the importance of not viewing differences between Black and White families as pathological, and the importance of aiding the many different Black family structures to function in as healthy a manner as possible. He warned against "prejudging [a family's] adequacy on the basis of moral judgments" (Hill, 1972, p. 22).

Work orientation among African American families is another area of consideration that many have thought to be misrepresented by social scientists. Unemployment statistics and welfare rolls are often cited as examples of the lack of a strong work orientation in Black families. Little consideration has been given to the ways in which the structure of the welfare system and the reality of job discrimination have contributed to this process. In truth, labeling African Americans as "chronically unemployed" is just a way of blaming the victims for the economic and social situation that has created their victimization. In response to this approach, a number of researchers have discussed the strong emphasis on work and ambition in African American families (Hill, 1972, 1993, 1999a; Lewis & Looney, 1983). These studies have pointed out that the literature has tended to overlook the stable African American families in which hard work is an important attribute. It was quite common for women in Black families to work long before this became the norm for women in the U.S. population as a whole (Billingsley, 1968, 1992; Hill, 1972, 1993, 1999a; McAdoo, 1981, 1996, 2002). Researchers have also compared working and nonworking Black single-parent mothers and have explored values including the hard work and survival strategies of this group (Lindblad-Goldberg & Dukes, 1985). Willie (1974), in his classic article entitled "The Black Family and Social Class," described the "heroic effort" on the part of many Black families to promote family survival with their hard work.

Another strength that is well documented in the lives of African Americans is that of educational or achievement orientation (Billingsley, 1992; Boyd-Franklin, 1989; Boyd-Franklin et al., 2001; Hill, 1972, 1993, 1999a; Hrabowski, Maton, & Greif, 1998; Kunjufu, 1985, 1988; McAdoo, 2002). The salience of strong achievement orientation in Black families is often unrecognized by Whites who do not see this exhibited according to their own cultural expectations.

Lewis and Looney (1983), in their study of well-functioning working-class Black families, discuss the messages these families gave their children about how they can "make it" in spite of discrimination. Education is seen as the way out of poverty for African American families, as it is for other ethnic groups. For some African American families who value education, the ability to translate this in terms of their children's schooling has not been accomplished. This is particularly true for some inner-city Black families who feel powerless to change their schools and who have been made to feel unwelcome in these institutions (Boyd-Franklin, 1989; Boyd-Franklin et al., 2001).

Many African American families are also aware of what Kunjufu (1985) has called the "fourth-grade-failure syndrome," in which African American boys are often mislabeled by school systems and are disproportionally tracked into special education systems (see Chapters 5 and 8). One of the key themes of this book is the process of empowering African American families through therapeutic interventions to make a difference in the lives and education of their children. The therapist can utilize the African American cultural strength and belief in the education of Black children to help mobilize parents to produce change (Boyd-Franklin, 1989; Boyd-Franklin et al., 2000) and also to engage African American families who may at first be resistant to the treatment process.

One final strength that is frequently overlooked in the literature is that of spirituality and religious orientation. Lewis and Looney (1983) found that a strong religious orientation was an extremely important value in the well-functioning working-class Black families they studied. Nobles (in press) and Mbiti (1990, 1992) have both documented the significance of spirituality and religion as an important legacy of the African heritage of African Americans. African Americans have been using spirituality and religion as key survival mechanisms for generations. Many researchers and scholars have discussed this process (Billingsley, 1992, 1994; Hill, 1972, 1994, 1999a; McAdoo, 1981, 1996, 2002). Because of its central cultural importance, the psychosocial support system of religion and the innate sense of spirituality in the lives of African Americans will be discussed in detail in Chapter 7.

In summary, it is the above body of literature—representing both the deficit and strength positions—that has most strongly influenced the professional and personal perceptions of family therapists, psychologists, social workers, psychiatrists, other physicians, nurses, ministers, pastoral counselors, teachers, and educators. This book focuses on the utilization of the strengths of African American families in the treatment process of family therapy, seeking to move beyond categorization to the situation-specific consideration of the functioning of African American families.

THE PROBLEMS AND CHALLENGES FACING AFRICAN AMERICAN FAMILIES TODAY

Hill (1999a) and White and Parham (1994) argue for a solution-focused approach that clearly identifies and then addresses the problems and challenges facing African American families today. As discussed above, racism and discrimination—albeit in the more subtle and covert variety that has replaced overt segregation (Jones, 1997; Hill, 1999a)—continue to be long-term challenges for African Americans of all socioeconomic levels.

Hill (1999a) and Boyd-Franklin et al. (2001) have identified a number of additional problems, including unemployment and underemployment, economic instability, the invisibility of Black men, poverty, separation, out-of-wedlock births, delinquency, crime, domestic violence, child abuse, alcoholism, poor health, AIDS, educational failure and high dropout rates, and the disproportionate number of Black children, particularly boys, placed in special education classes and on Ritalin (see Chapter 8).

Many African Americans are very concerned about the safety of their children, particularly their sons. In addition, many African American families are concerned about the high rates of violence, racial profiling, and police brutality in their communities (Boyd–Franklin et al., 2001). Tucker and Mitchell-Kernan (1995) have attributed the decline in marriage among African Americans to a number of factors, including economic instability, high unemployment among Black men, and the shortage of African American men due to homicide, incarceration, and drug use (see Chapter 5 for a more extensive discussion of how these issues impact African American gender issues, male–female relationships and couple therapy). Many of these problems and challenges are addressed in case examples throughout this book, particularly in Chapter 8.

AFRICAN AMERICAN FAMILIES' RESPONSES TO THERAPY: THE ISSUE OF "RESISTANCE"

The response of many African American families to the treatment process is one of the central concerns of this book. "Resistance" to therapy, a common reaction of African American families, is often frustrating to the clinicians working with them (Boyd-Franklin, 1989). The presence of "resistance" and its related issues needs to be considered in relation to the timing of different therapeutic interventions. Not only can these issues influence the process of joining with all family members who enter treatment, but the therapist must also be sensitive to the fact that some interventions actually evoke "resistance" to treatment.

The traditional sources of help for African American families have been extended family members, close friends, ministers, church leaders, or members of the "church family" (see Chapter 7). For many African American families, the idea of going for treatment is a new one, and often the questions asked by therapists can be perceived as intrusive. Thus, therapeutic approaches that focus on an initial extensive history intake may increase hesitancy and suspicion rather than facilitate the process of joining. These issues will be discussed in more detail throughout this book as they relate to different models of family therapy.

Many African American families perceive therapy to be the process of labeling them as "crazy," often fearing the reaction of their extended family members, friends, and community. This is compounded by the fact that Black families are often not self-referred, but are sent for treatment by schools, courts, hospitals, or social welfare agencies, frequently under considerable threat or pressure. This can contribute to their resistance in approaching and utilizing treatment. In addition, as is fairly common in many ethnic groups, parents often place a high value on privacy, teaching their children from very early ages to "keep family business within the family," or not to "air dirty laundry in public." It is often difficult for many family therapists to comprehend the extent to which therapy is considered "public" in African American communities.

The type of resistance and suspicion often manifested by African American families should not be summarily categorized as pathological or as a contraindication for successful treatment. In their seminal work *Black Rage,* Grier and Cobbs (1968) labeled this suspicion as a "healthy cultural paranoia" that many Black families have developed over generations in response to racism, oppression, and discrimination. (Given the negative associations of the term "paranoia" in the mental health field, I prefer the term "healthy cultural suspicion.") Often it takes the form of a refusal to identify with and trust persons differing from themselves in color, race, ethnicity, lifestyle, class, and values.

Hines and Boyd-Franklin (1996) point out that this suspiciousness is frequently a direct learned survival response that African American children are socialized to adopt from an early age. This extends particularly to "White institutions," as most clinics and mental health centers are perceived in Black communities. Chapter 10 discusses the ways in which this sense of suspicion can also be heightened by premature use of paradoxical prescriptions and by some of the common training techniques employed in the field, such as one-way mirrors where sessions can be observed and the use of videotape equipment.

There are two other major areas that contribute to the resistance of African American families to treatment and to their tendency to discontinue therapy if they perceive the therapist as "prying into their business," particularly before trust has been established: (1) the negative history that many Black families have had with the welfare system and other social institutions and agencies in the past; and (2) the fear of exposing secrets or myths, particularly toxic unresolved family issues.

One of the issues that has led to the resistance of many African American families toward mental health services has come from confusion about the relationship between mental health clinics and other agencies, such as welfare departments, courts, and schools (Boyd-Franklin, 1989; Boyd-Franklin & Bry, 2000; Hines & Boyd-Franklin, 1996). (See Chapter 11.) Many African American families have a long memory and a great deal of resentment about the past practices of welfare agencies that they perceived as exceedingly intrusive, such as defining what they " 'can' or 'cannot' own (e.g., telephone or television)" (Hines & Boyd-Franklin, 1996, p. 78).

In the past, the welfare system had the power to discontinue the family's financial security if the father of the children (or another man) was proven to be living in or contributing to the household, thereby placing the family in serious economic jeopardy. If the father of a child was able to contribute to the family economically, even if the parents were not living together and the amount of financial assistance was nominal, welfare support could be at risk. (Even though these practices have changed for the most part today, many African American families have a long memory for past abuses.) Coupled with the tragic unemployment rates for Black men, and last hired, first fired policies, the fragile nature of some family units and the breakup of many African American families is unsurprising.

Given the legacy discussed above, it is not surprising that many African American families are hesitant to approach clinics, hospitals, and mental health centers. African American therapists and those from other ethnic minority groups such as Latinos and Asians are often surprised to discover that they are viewed by African American families as part of these White institutions, and thus are not trusted initially. Chapter 11 discusses the ways in which therapists can join with African American families to overcome this resistance. Chapter 9 explores the therapist's use of self in this process.

Family Secrets

Another area that contributes to treatment "resistance" by African American families is the perception by many families that therapists will pry into their family secrets. There are two forms of secrets: (1) those that are kept from "outsiders" but are known by most family members and (2) those that are kept from other family members. It is helpful to discuss each of these separately.

Clearly, families of all cultures have secrets. However, because of the legacy of mistrust and racism discussed above, there are many personal issues that African American families have learned to label as "nobody's business but our own." For example, it is not unusual for a Black family entering treatment to present as a single-parent family to the intake worker when the mother has had a live-in boyfriend for over 5 years, and this person has served as a stepfather to her children. This person is frequently an important contributor in family interaction, and true structural change cannot occur until he is involved, but the nature of the relationship will not be revealed until a high degree of trust is established between the therapist and the client.

African American families are often concerned about the judgments imposed on them by outside agencies and may therefore be sensitive about discussing with an outsider such issues as the fact that children may have different fathers. Since so much of the early social science literature (e.g., Moynihan, 1965) referred to single-parent African American families on welfare as pathological, Black people are sensitive to this bias.

The type of secret that is kept from certain members within the family is the more toxic and difficult to explore. They are often unconscious, obscure, or nebulous. Often these secrets have been passed down over generations (Bowen, 1976; Nichols & Schwartz, 1998). It is not unusual to discover that family members are aware of the secrets or loaded issues that are never discussed. These secrets take many forms and often do not surface until one is very far along in the treatment process. The issue of secrecy has serious clinical implications. The following secrets are some of the most common that therapists will encounter: (1) informal adoption and secrets about true parentage; (2) fatherhood; (3) unwed pregnancy; (4) a parent who had "trouble" at an earlier age; (5) an ancestor who was mentally ill, alcoholic, or a drug abuser; (6) ancestors (particularly White ones); and (7) skin color issues. These may be secrets kept from other family members, particularly the younger generations, or they may be toxic or loaded areas in the present family system that are never discussed. (See Chapters 2 and 3 for more information on secrets.)

FUNCTIONAL AND DYSFUNCTIONAL AFRICAN AMERICAN FAMILIES

As has been described above, a tendency has arisen based on the pejorative literature to view the standard of White nuclear families as ideal and to view the variety of family structures in the African American community as pathological. One purpose of this book and a theme throughout is to help clinicians recognize the strengths in African American families, as well as their challenges and problems, and to establish models for functional extended families and single-parent families. It will also help the clinician to distinguish what is functional and what is dysfunctional in the families they treat. It would be ludicrous to assume that the extended family *always* functions as a strength in *all* African American families. It is only when we as therapists can clearly make these distinctions that we can effectively restructure families within their cultural context, and thus produce change. Chapter 3 will focus on these issues in terms of extended family functioning.

THE CONCEPT OF EMPOWERMENT AS A TREATMENT GOAL

Empowerment and therapeutic change are important treatment goals with a family regardless of its race, ethnicity, or cultural background. However, given the legacy of slavery and the history of racism experienced by African Americans in this country, they become essential components of any treatment plan for this cultural group. One of the most devastating outcomes of the legacy of slavery and oppression is the feeling of powerlessness and rage that many Black people experience (Grier & Cobbs, 1968; Franklin, in press).

Empowerment, in this context, is defined as the process whereby the therapist restructures the family to facilitate the appropriate designation and use of power within the family system and to mobilize the family's ability to successfully interact with external systems. Solomon (1976), Boyd-Franklin (1989), Boyd-Franklin and Bry (2000), and Logan (2001) have explored this concept of the empowerment of African Americans through the use of therapeutic strategies.

Throughout this book, the concept of empowering African American families is emphasized and incorporated into the treatment process. It is important to give this concept consideration because it is central to the initiation of effective therapeutic change when treating African American families. Many of these families have a multigenerational history of victimization by poverty and racism. Unlike other cultural or ethnic groups who can "blend in" or become part of the "melting pot," Black people by virtue of their skin color are visible reminders of the inequities of society. Empowerment therefore consists of helping people to gain the ability to make and implement basic life decisions in their own lives and the lives of their children.

Empowerment often involves helping parents to take back the control of their families and feel that they can effect important changes for themselves. This is very threatening to many family therapists because it often requires them to take a stand vis-à-vis a decision made by another agency, thus forcing them to abandon their stances of "neutrality" in therapy. As many of the chapters of this book will demonstrate, therapy with families in general, and with African American families in particular, is an *active therapy* that forces the therapist to examine his or her own values and political, cultural, and religious beliefs and biases, and to intervene accordingly. It is through this examination and the therapist's ability to convey respect for the families she or he treats that the therapist creates an atmosphere in which empowerment can occur. Chapter 16 of this book explores the ways in which therapists can empower themselves through supervision and training in these cultural and clinical issues.

2

Racism, Racial Identity, and Skin Color Issues

The legacy of slavery continues to have an impact on African American families today as parents try to help their children cope with racism. When racism is external to the family, it is experienced as discrimination; when racism is internalized, it manifests as a sense of shame about oneself. A philosophy of hope and an ability to believe in a better future for their children is one of the strengths and most powerful survival skills of African Americans. Sometimes a very deeply ingrained spiritual belief system (see Chapter 7) has sustained these families through generations.

These themes were encapsulated in a memorable speech that Reverend Jesse Jackson made at the Democratic National Convention on July 19, 1988—the year in which he had been a candidate for president. He spoke eloquently of the task of all African American parents who, in the last 400 years, have had to "keep hope alive" for their children and families despite slavery, racism, and discrimination.

One of the most difficult challenges for African American families, irrespective of their socioeconomic level, is striking the precarious balance between alerting their children to the existence of racism—and helping their children learn to reality-test what is in fact related to racism in their world—and encouraging them to strive to "be all that they can be." This chapter explores the external experiences of racism and discrimination, and the complicated task African American parents have in helping children cope with these issues in both their external and internal manifestations.

Another important issue in which the legacy of slavery is still evident is skin color and its relationship to family dynamics and toxic family secrets. These have a distinct and unique significance for African American families, although they may be experienced to some degree by "people of color" throughout the world. Case examples are given throughout this chapter to illustrate the clinical implications. This second edition also includes a new, extensive discussion of racial identity theory and its implications for the treatment of African American clients and their families.

EDUCATING AFRICAN AMERICAN CHILDREN ABOUT THE REALITIES OF RACISM

A parent must help a child to develop a sense of self and a feeling of pride in being African American. At the same time, children must be given enough information about the realities of racism so that they are prepared to confront them without becoming immobilized or so bitter that they are unable to function. Many African American parents make a great effort to instill in their children an awareness of their heritage and the struggles of the civil rights movement (Boyd-Franklin et al., 2001).

Some of the poor families who come to our clinics feel powerless and hopeless in the face of the double burden of racism and poverty. Empowering parents to change their interaction with a school system and to be effective with their children begins to reverse these feelings of powerlessness and hopelessness. The challenge for poor, urban, African American families is to motivate their children to believe in themselves and achieve despite the blatant racism and discrimination they may face every day. One difficulty for parents struggling to raise motivated children is older siblings who engage in negative behaviors and activities, such as drug use and truancy. It is common to hear the admonition "You have to set an example for your younger brothers and sisters" in African American homes.

The inequities of job discrimination and unemployment can have a tremendous impact on family life, particularly on the issue of motivating children. For example, while neighbors often have jobs that take them outside the community, unemployed older teenagers and adults are on the streets and highly visible. This may lead young children to wonder why they should bother to go to school and study if they will end up the same way. The situation is made more difficult when unemployment is closer to home. An African American child who grows up seeing his father and other older relatives struggling to find work but having difficulty maintaining employment gets a message more powerful than words. The disproportionate numbers of African American men and women who are unemployed often experience blows to their self-esteem that also affect their functioning as parents. The following case example illustrates this problem.

The Davises, an African American inner-city family, came for treatment after Johnny (age 12) "threw a desk at a teacher in school." When asked about this act, Johnny reported that his teacher was "prejudiced."

His mother initially came for family sessions with Johnny and his two younger siblings (ages 10 and 8). When the therapist asked when the school problems began, Mrs. Davis reported that her husband had not worked since he lost his job as a construction worker in November. There was no "winter work" and he felt he had been "cheated out" of his unemployment benefits. Mrs. Davis worked in a luncheonette but her earnings could not support the family.

The therapist asked Mr. Davis to attend a family session. The therapist had a difficult time getting him to attend. He finally agreed to come in alone to see the therapist while his children were at school and his wife was at work. Mr. Davis was a proud tall man who told the therapist that he had never been unemployed in his life and was embarrassed about his out-of-work status. He reported that the construction business was always slower at this time of year but he felt that he had been discriminated against because he and other Black men had been laid off while White workers had been kept on.

The therapist understood his pain and joined with him on how furious he must be feeling. She asked him if he knew that his son was dealing with a very similar situation in school. He had not recognized the similarities. The therapist asked the father if he would attend a family session and talk to his son about how to handle racism and still hold onto his belief in himself. Mr. Davis came to the following family session with his wife and three children. With the therapist's encouragement he talked to Johnny about his experience at school and drew parallels with his own situation. He got very involved and told his son that there were other ways to "fight back" besides throwing a desk, such as being the best he could be in his work. The son pointed out that his father "still got burnt." The father was able to tell his son that he was furious but that he was fighting back through his determination to get another job and going out every day to look for work.

In subsequent months, Mr. Davis attended a number of family sessions. He was given the task of teaching his son about life as an African American man. Paradoxically, both father and son benefited from this task. Mr. Davis became more determined to show his son that he was not giving up, and he eventually found a job. His son learned how to continue to "fight back" by doing his best at school.

Although racism and discrimination are present in U.S. society at all levels, they may be experienced differently depending on the family's socioeconomic circumstances. Black professional families living in predominantly White suburbs are often faced with subtle forms of racism, although they may also confront blatant racism—as horrific as that faced by poor families—as the following case example illustrates.

Mr. and Mrs. Simpson moved into a small suburban town that had very few African American families. They had three children, all girls, ages 5, 7, and 10. Two days after they moved in they found a burning cross on their front lawn. They sought the help of a family therapist when their two younger children began to experience a number of phobic symptoms including nightmares and fears of leaving the house. Their 7-year-old child became school-phobic.

The first session occurred 3 months after the incident. The whole family appeared and each was very depressed. The mother stated that they all were still traumatized by the event.

The therapist first legitimized the fears and the anger that the family was experiencing as a normal reaction to a very traumatic situation. The 7-year-old had become the focus of the family's concern. The therapist was able to relabel this as a family problem and focus on their need to support each other through this crisis.

In a later session, it became clear that one of the factors that had prevented the family from "pulling together" to support each other was that the decision to move had been rushed and problematic. Mr. Simpson had been relocated by his company, so the parents had not had time to research the area. Mrs. Simpson was very angry at her husband for accepting the transfer. The therapist told the parents that they would have to talk this problem out and resolve it before they could help their family through its crisis. A number of sessions were held alone with the parents to discuss the stress this transfer had created in their marriage.

In a family session during this time, Mr. Simpson was asked to discuss with his 7-year-old daughter her fears of going to school. Both parents agreed to support their daughter by taking her to school until she felt more comfortable. With the therapist's encouragement, the parents arranged a meeting with the girls and the school principal to discuss their fears. In another session, the therapist asked Mr. and Mrs. Simpson to teach their daughters about racism so that they could understand it and ask them questions. Mr. Davis commented sadly that he had never previously felt it was necessary to explain prejudice to his daughters.

In the final months of treatment, the therapist proposed that Mr. and Mrs. Simpson had felt rushed into moving and into making decisions over which they felt no control. She encouraged them to "do their homework" about other communities in their area and pointed out that they had a choice about whether or not to remain where they were. As the school semester drew to a close, both of the older girls strongly stated their desire to move. The parents agreed to move to a more integrated nearby community.

What this family experienced was blatant racism and discrimination, not in the deep South, but in the Northeast. The following case example illustrates a more subtle form of discrimination.

Ms. Jones was a hard-working African American single parent with high aspirations for her two children, Melanie, age 9, and Brian, age 7. She was a paraprofessional in the public school system and had a great deal of knowledge about the schools in her area. The family lived in a predominantly African American area in New York City. Both of her children attended their neighborhood schools for kindergarten and first grade. Her oldest child had been there for second grade. Ms. Jones became increasingly dissatisfied with the quality of their education. She heard about a program that arranged scholarships for minority children at predominantly White prep schools. Both of her children were accepted at a very prestigious school. Melanie began to experience difficulty by December of her first year. She seemed to have given up and stopped working. Ms. Jones was furious. She had worked so hard to give her children this opportunity, and now

Melanie was "blowing it." In a family session, the therapist asked Ms. Jones to talk with Melanie about what it had been like for her going to this new school.

Melanie burst into tears. She told her mother that she had never felt so alone. She was used to having lots of friends at her other school. Here she was the only African American child in her class. None of the other children invited her to do things with them. They all wore designer clothes that she didn't have. One child had told her she was "too Black to be her friend." Ms. Jones was shocked. She asked Melanie why she had not told her about this before. Melanie stated that she had tried but her mother was so angry at her for not doing well that she was afraid to speak out.

The therapist normalized Melanie's struggle as very common for African American children who enter private schools on scholarships. She relabeled Ms. Jones's anger as her intense desire for her children to have a good education. She then helped Ms. Jones and Melanie and Brian to "brainstorm" on ways to deal with this sense of isolation. Ms. Jones shared with her children what she often felt like being one of the few African American paraprofessionals in her school. These discussions continued over many weeks. With the therapist's encouragement, Ms. Jones offered to go with Melanie to her school and talk with her teacher. She obtained the phone numbers of some of the parents of children Melanie wanted to establish friendships with and made phone calls to arrange playtime outside of school. The therapist then stated that Ms. Jones shared something in common with her daughter in having to deal with being "different." The therapist asked the mother how she had dealt with this problem. Ms. Jones stated that she had always had her own friends who had known her "all her life." She then asked Melanie if she missed her neighborhood friends. Melanie tearfully responded yes. Her mother made a commitment to both children to help them maintain their own social networks outside of school.

African American parents often find themselves faced with helping to build bicultural networks for their children so that they have the support of other African American children and families when they encounter racism in other parts of their lives. The family therapist who can recognize this struggle can be a great help to African American children as well as their parents (see Chapters 8 and 15).

BUILDING SELF-ESTEEM
AND POSITIVE RACIAL IDENTITY

One of the greatest concerns of African American parents raising children in the United States today is the process of encouraging the development of self-esteem and positive racial identity. This is not an easy task since children are often exposed to negative images or caricatures of African Americans on television and in other types of mass media. Since the 1960s many African American parents have been sensitized to the need to help their children to learn about their history and to focus on positive role models.

Many African American inner-city parents, particularly single mothers, struggle with the problem of identifying positive African American role models for their children. In the course of family therapy, these mothers often express the need for supports in this area. In these situations, it is crucial that the therapist discuss both the "traditional supports" (i.e., extended family and church) and the community resources (e.g., Big Brothers, Boys' Club, Rites-of-Passage Programs [see Chapter 8], community groups, etc.) that can provide these supports. The case that follows illustrates this difficulty.

Darryl Brown (age 10) was an African American child who was referred for treatment by his school. He was described by his teacher as bright but unmotivated. He had recently been picked up by the police for vandalizing school property with a group of other boys. His mother was a very overwhelmed single parent. She was 25 years old and had three younger children (ages 7, 2, and 1). Her boyfriend had left her, and she was trying to manage alone. Her mother, who had been her main support, had died 2 years earlier. Things had begun to "fall apart" at home after that. Her mother had helped her "control" Darryl and she didn't feel that she could do it alone. The therapist joined with her around the issue of how difficult it was to provide a child with all he or she needed. She talked with her about "getting some help."

The therapist encouraged the mother to call a local male African American social worker who had started an after-school program for boys in their area. He helped them with homework and organized basketball games for them. Ms. Brown went to meet with him and agreed to send Darryl every day.

In a family session Ms. Brown discussed this with Darryl, and told him that she would go with him to help plan out his activities after school. Ms. Brown was greatly relieved at having an option. She began to take charge. The therapist encouraged her to monitor his progress and "stay in touch" with the social worker and with Darryl's school. The social worker became a very important role model for Darryl.

Ms. Brown expressed concerns about the weekend, when Darryl was "out on the streets." In a family discussion about this issue, the therapist asked if they had ever belonged to a church. Ms. Brown explained that she had belonged to one many years ago but had not attended any church in recent years. The therapist explored whether church had ever been a support for her. Ms. Brown replied that it had. The therapist suggested that it might be a help for her in raising her children and in finding activities and positive African American role models for them. Ms. Brown and Darryl agreed to "try it." In the next few months, Ms. Brown became increasingly more active in a local church and less depressed. Darryl became more engaged in youth activities. His acting-out behavior gradually stopped.

In May, Ms. Brown was in a panic. School was ending soon and the after-school program would stop for the summer. The therapist carefully explored options with her in a family session with the children. Although Ms. Brown had repeatedly stated that she had "no family left," the therapist decided to reopen this issue. She asked her where her family came from originally and learned that she still had an aunt and uncle in South Carolina. With the therapist's encouragement, she called them to ask if they would "take Darryl for a little time." To her surprise, they invited the entire family for the summer.

This family's situation illustrates the process whereby therapists can help support families in identifying positive African American role models for their children and in providing them with constructive alternatives to "the streets." This often requires that therapists be aware of both traditional networks and community resources. Adults in many African American communities who have recognized the need for wholesome activities for children have taken the initiative to organize programs in their neighborhoods and churches. Therapists working with poor and isolated African American families in particular are advised to discover these resource people. One should also keep in mind the tradition of "sending children South," an important part of the socialization of African American children for generations. It reconnects them with their family roots and often reinforces positive identification by providing alternative familial role models.

Racial Socialization

For many generations, African American parents have struggled to provide racial socialization for their children, a process that provides children with pride in their racial and cultural identity and self-esteem, and educates them about the racism that exists in this country so that they are not caught unprepared when they encounter discrimination in their lives. The challenge for African American parents has been to accomplish this complex task without making their children bitter (Boyd-Franklin et al., 2001). McAdoo (2002) referred to the process of racial socialization as one of the most important parenting tasks of African Americans. There is a growing body of research on this topic (Jones, 2003; McAdoo, 2002; Stevenson, 1993, 1998; Stevenson, Davis, & Abdul-Kabir, 2002; Stevenson & Davis, in press).

McAdoo (2002) cites a Hatchett, Cochran, and Jackson (1991) study that found that "61% of Black children received socialization messages of one type or other; only 39% were told nothing about being Black" (p. 51). McAdoo (2002) described a variety of approaches African American parents have taken with regard to the racial socialization of their children. Their approach is often closely related to their own level of racial identity (see next section). A number of books have been written expressly to help African American parents with these dilemmas (Boyd-Franklin et al., 2001; Comer & Poussaint, 1992; Gardere, 1999; Hopson & Hopson, 1990). Therapists assisting parents with the process of racial socialization are also advised to consult Boyd-Franklin et al. (2001), Hughes and Chen (1997, 1999), McAdoo (2002), and Stevenson and Davis (in press).

It is important that therapists, particularly those from other cultures and racial groups, understand this process and why it is necessary. At the height of the civil rights movement in the 1960s, many African Americans hoped that once the nation's laws conformed to its founding principles—that all were created equal—racism would disappear in the United States. Some African

American parents, particularly those who had achieved high levels of education and socioeconomic status, began to feel that there was no longer a need to prepare their children for the realities of racism. Unfortunately, this often left their children defenseless against the entrenched, but often subtle, forms of racism that continue to exist today (Jones, 2003; McAdoo, 2002; Stevenson & Davis, in press), and led to serious damage to their self-esteem. These children are often referred to us for treatment.

Racial Identity Theory

As stated throughout this book, there is a great deal of diversity in the African American community. One area of diversity, often invisible to clinicians, is related to the racial identity of African American clients. Many Black people differ in the degree to which they identify as African American. Even within the same family there can be considerable variability.

Theories of African American identity development have existed in the literature since the 1960s (Carter, 1995; Cross, 1978, 1991; Helms, 1990; Helms & Cook, 1999; Jones, 1998b, 2003; Marks, Settles, Cooke, Morgan, & Sellers, in press).

Franklin, Carter, and Grace (1993) have offered a summary of Cross's (1978) five-stage theory of African American identity development that he called "nigrescence":

> Cross (1978) hypothesizes a five-stage process of racial identity development for Black Americans that begins at a stage called *pre-encounter*, which is characterized by dependency on White society for definition and approval. Racial identity attitudes toward one's blackness are negative, and one views White culture and society as the ideal. The next stage is called *encounter*, and it is entered when one has a personal and challenging experience with Black or White society. The encounter stage is marked by feelings of confusion about the meaning and significance of race and an increasing desire to become more aligned with one's Black identity. The *immersion-emersion* stage follows the encounter experience, and it is characterized by a period of idealization of Black culture and intense negative feelings toward Whites and White culture. One is absorbed in the Black experience and completely rejects the White world. Immersion is followed by *internalization;* during the internalization stage, one has grasped the fact that both Blacks and Whites have strengths and weaknesses. In addition, one's African American identity is experienced as positive and an important and valued aspect of self. Therefore, one's world view is Afrocentric. One's attitude toward Whites is one of tolerance and respect for differences. *Internalization-commitment* is the last stage and reflects active involvement in promoting the welfare of Black people (Goss, 1991). Empirical studies (Cross, 1991) involving racial identity have found it to be associated differentially with cultural value preferences (Carter & Helms, 1987), psychological function (Carter, 1991), self-esteem (Parham & Helms, 1985a), emotional states (Parham & Helms, 1985b), cognitive styles (Helms & Parham, 1990), psychotherapy process (Carter 1990c; Pomales, Claiborn, & LaFromboise, 1986), and prefer-

ence for race, gender, and social class of therapists (Helms & Carter, 1992; Parham & Helms, 1981). What has been missing from the psychological literature is a consideration of how racial identity for Whites might influence their perceptions of African Americans and other racial/ethnic group people. (p. 470)

Advances in the Model

One of the most important advances has been Parham's application of lifespan development theory to this model (Cross, Parham, & Helms, 1998; Jones, 1998b). Parham presented a view of the intersection of the life cycle stage of the individual and the evolution of his or her racial identity:

> Within the context of normal development, racial identity is a phenomenon which is subject to continuous change during the life cycle. While the psychological nigrescence research certainly documents how a person's racial identity can change from one stage to another. . . , previous research has failed to detail how the various stages of racial identity will be accentuated at different phases of life. My model seeks to describe how the stages of racial identity are manifested at four phases of life (late adolescence, early adulthood, midlife, and late adulthood), and how each phase of life is characterized by a central underlying theme. (Parham, 1992, as cited in Jones, 1998b, p. 16)

According to Cross et al. (1999), Parham

> presupposes that the manifestation of identity during childhood is "more the reflection of parental attitudes or societal stereotypes which a youngster has incorporated, than the integrated cognitively complex, identity structures found in adults. Consequently, Parham hypothesizes it is during adolescence and early adulthood that one might first experience nigrescence, and thereafter the potential is present for the remainder of one's life." (p. 16)

In 1992, Parham also introduced another important concept he called "recycling." Prior theories of identity development were linear and seemed to imply that all African Americans progress through these stages in the same order. Parham states:

> Recycling is defined as the reinitiation into the racial identity struggle and resolution process after having gone through the identity process at an earlier stage in one's life. In essence, a person could theoretically achieve identity resolution by completing one cycle through the nigresence process (internalization), and as a result of identity confusion, recycle through the stages again. (Parham, 1992, as cited in Cross et al., 1998, p. 16)

Cross et al. (1998) point out, however, that Parham's use of "identity confusion" has less to do with confusion and more to do with midlife developmental challenges. They note, for example, that individuals who may have resolved their own racial identity struggle in young adulthood may experience recycling through this process as they have children of their own. Cross et al. (1998) argue that parents' experience of their own children's identity struggles, particularly during their adolescence, may serve as a new encounter experience for them and recycle them through the identity process.

For many African American parents, their children's encounters with racism can be as powerful and even more painful than their own and can plunge them once again into the intense anger of the immersion/emersion period (Cross et al., 1998). The case that follows illustrates this.

Joan (age 32) and Horace (age 33) Woods had each gone through their own racial identity struggles in college. Now, 10 years later, at the internalization/commitment stage of racial identity, they were recycling through the process based on their role as parents to Ayana (age 9), their only daughter. They were raising Ayana with a strong Afrocentric belief system (see Chapter 7) and a solid African American racial identity.

Their daughter came home from school one day very upset. Her teacher at an integrated elementary school had asked the children in her class what they wanted to be when they grew up. Ayana, who was attending a weekend science enrichment program for gifted youngsters at the local community college, replied a "nuclear physicist." Her teacher, a White woman, told her that she should pick something that was more realistic for a Black girl. Ayana came home devastated.

Joan and Horace were furious when Ayana told them what her teacher had said. Their daughter's encounter with racism sent them recycling back to the intense anger of the immersion/emersion stage. First, they had to reassure Ayana that she was exceptionally intelligent. Then they went to the school to confront the teacher and the principal about the way in which the school encouraged racial stereotyping and racism. This form of recycling can reoccur many times throughout a lifetime.

Race, Racial Identity Issues, and Therapy

Two leading racial identity researchers and theorists, Janet Helms and Robert Carter, have made major contributions to the understanding of race and racial identity in the therapeutic process (Carter, 1995; Helms & Cook, 1999). Carter (1995) in his book, *The Influence of Race and Racial Identity in Psychotherapy: Toward a Racially Inclusive Model*, explored these issues in treatment. In *Black and White Racial Identity*, Helms (1990) expanded her research on Black racial identity with her theory of White racial identity. Parham and Helms (1981) developed the Racial Identity Attitude Scale (RIAS), one of the most widely used empirical measures of racial identity stages. Helms and Cook (1999) have expanded and developed the theory of racial identity as it relates to the treatment process. The section below will focus primarily on issues of African American racial identity in therapy.

Racial identity is an important variable in the therapeutic process. Therapists must be careful not to apply these models in a stereotypical way and make assumptions about an African American client's racial identity that may prove to be inaccurate. The following case example illustrates the process of "learning from our mistakes."

Ms. Fox (age 39) brought her son, Andrew (age 14), for treatment following his arrest for riding in a stolen car. He had also had two prior juvenile delinquency misdemeanors related to writing graffiti on subway cars and walls. Andrew was involved in a Black peer group that Ms. Fox felt was leading him into increasingly dangerous activity.

Because of her concern about Andrew's pending court appearance, Ms. Fox made sure that he attended all of his family therapy sessions. He had no further incidents with the law and attended school regularly after his extended period of truancy.

Pending a court appearance, the therapist, a young White woman, invited her supervisor, an African American woman, to join a session to discuss the court appearance.

The supervisor attempted to praise the mother for her determination to get help for her son and their consistent attendance at therapy sessions. She made a serious error, however, by misjudging the mother's racial identity. The supervisor mistakenly assumed that Ms. Fox shared her own level of racial identity. In an effort to join with the mother, she said "Our folks don't seek help like you do."

The supervisor was taken aback by the mother's response: "Well, I'm not one of *our* folks." Realizing that she had made an error, the supervisor asked the mother more about her own background. It became clear that although Ms. Fox was aware that she was a Black woman, she was very White-identified because of her upbringing in a predominately White community. (She was in the preencounter stage of racial identity development.)

There are many lessons to be learned from this interaction. The first has to do with avoiding stereotypes. The supervisor realized that she had made a serious error and had misjudged this mother's sense of racial identity. The supervisor was having a strong countertransference reaction as an African American woman and was very upset by the mother's response. But she knew that her first meeting with this family would not be the best time to challenge the mother's racial identity definition. She struggled to acknowledge and reframe the mother's experience. Later in the session she used the reframe: "You are a *survivor*. Now we have to help your son survive." This was her attempt to convey her understanding of the mother's experience. For therapists of all races, it is important to remember that you do not have to agree with a client's position in order to try to understand it.

Racial Identity Differences within Families

It is important for therapists to remember that members of the same family may be at different stages of racial identity development. These differences may be related to the age and generation of the person; the community in which the person was raised (Black, White, or mixed); the part of the country in which he or she was raised; his or her personal experiences with African Americans, Whites, and other ethnic groups; and his or her own idiosyncratic experiences and responses. In the case above, for example, Andrew was very Black-identified and had an almost exclusively African American peer group. He had been raised in an urban, inner-city area, while his mother had been raised in a predominantly White suburban community. They often clashed because his mother perceived Andrew's African American peer group as leading him into trouble.

In later sessions, the therapist was able to help the mother and her son to talk more about the differences in their racial identity and to help the mother to at least recognize the importance of helping her son to develop a positive identity as an African American man. This was very difficult for her given her own life experiences and feelings of abandonment by African American men, such as her own father and Andrew's father.

SKIN COLOR ISSUES AND THE STRUGGLE FOR POSITIVE RACIAL IDENTITY

Skin color has presented complex, multigenerational issues for many African Americans. In recent years, a number of authors and researchers have addressed this issue (Hall, 1992; Hughes & Hertel, 1990; Jackson & Greene, 2000; Neal & Wilson, 1989; Perkins, 1996; Russell, Wilson, & Hall, 1993; Tucker, 2000). In their classic studies of racial and skin color identification, Clark and Clark (1939) found that African American children of that generation often evaluated the color black and Black people less positively than the color white and White people. This finding causes considerable concern among African American parents to this day. Many Black parents have reported the upsetting experience of hearing their child say, "I wish I were White." Such statements are understandably a source of much anxiety for these parents.

Comer and Poussaint (1992) in their guide to childcare issues for African American parents offer vignettes and examples that can be useful to therapists in helping families cope with this issue by providing a number of ways of reframing and normalizing the experience. The authors report a frequent question from African American parents: "The first time my 4-year-old raised a question about race, he said 'I'm White.' Does this mean that he doesn't like being African American?" (p. 68). The child's sense of his race is not uncommon among Black children raised in a predominantly White neighborhood or school and does not mean that he has negative feelings about African Americans. The parents' response to such a statement can make all the difference. A simple, "No, you are African American like Daddy and Mommy" (Comer & Poussaint, 1992, p. 68) is clear and can help to reinforce positive racial identification.

If the parent is clearly proud of her or his own African American identity, this will be conveyed to the child (Hopson & Hopson, 1990; McAdoo, 2002). Many African American parents take the task of developing a sense of positive racial identification very seriously. This has been the case since the 1960s, a sentiment embodied in the popular song of that era, "I'm Black and I'm Proud," by James Brown. It has led growing numbers of African Americans to embrace Afrocentric principles in their family life (see Chapter 8). The process is a continual struggle for African American parents particularly because skin color can be such a loaded, toxic issue in families. In some cases, it can determine the nature of family interaction, as discussed below.

Skin Color and Family Dynamics

The Historical Perspective: The Role of Slavery and Racism

Historically, skin color differences began to influence the lives of African Americans in this country early in the slavery era (Hughes & Hertel, 1990; Neal & Wilson, 1989; Russell et al., 1993; Tucker, 2000). Grier and Cobbs (1968) argue that the mark of slavery has never fully disappeared for African Americans because the feelings and assumptions that formed the psychological underpinnings of the slaveholding structure have yet to be purged from the national psyche. Black and White people have been profoundly affected by this legacy:

> The culture of slavery was never undone for either master or slave. The civilization that tolerated slavery dropped its slaveholding cloak but the inner feelings remained. The "peculiar institution" continues to exert its evil influence over the nation. The practice of slavery stopped over a hundred years ago but the minds of our citizens have never been freed. (Greer & Cobbs, 1968, p. 20)

Sexual exploitation on the part of White slave masters resulted in many "mulatto" or light-skinned children, who were often raised in the master's house and became house servants. They were also given many privileges that other Blacks lacked within the plantation system. Unlike the African sense of beauty where a deep black skin color and African hair and skin features are prized, the White standard of beauty was imposed on African Americans throughout the period of slavery and Reconstruction. This tradition of favoritism toward light-skinned African Americans resulted in a system in which it was often easier for light-skinned Blacks to get an education, a job, and so on. Thus, a class system was created in many African American communities based on skin color.

The "Jim Crow" laws, mandating segregation, were pervasive throughout the South before the days of integration. African Americans were blatantly discriminated against and given separate facilities ranging from parts of restaurants and lunch counters to separate restrooms. School systems were completely segregated until the Supreme Court decided in *Brown vs. the Board of Education* in 1954 to end segregation. The civil rights movement brought moral persuasion to bear and the desegregation of public facilities and schools began to be implemented. There was powerful resistance throughout this country, particularly in the South, to complying with the Supreme Court's ruling.

Some Whites referred to Blacks with derogatory terms such as "nigger," "darkie," "coon," and so on, which reflected the caste system of skin color. The following case example illustrates this issue.

Marcus King, a 68-year-old, dark-skinned, African American man who was raised in Alabama, described the following incident, which occurred when he was 7 years old. Although it had happened over 60 years previously, it was engrained forever in his memory. He and his father, a local handyman, were walking home when a crowd of four obviously drunk White men approached them. One of the men held him while the others began taunting his father, calling him "nigga" and asking what he had in his bag. They forced him down on the ground, held a knife to Marcus's neck, and threatened to cut Marcus's throat if his father did not eat dirt from the road. After some resistance his father began to eat dirt. Marcus still recalls the rage he felt and then the immense sadness he experienced when the White men finally left and his own father was too embarrassed to look him in the eye.

This kind of behavior was not unusual in the South in the early 20th century, and is a painful reminder of the rage that many African Americans still feel and experience. This type of degradation of the honor and manhood of a African American man in front of his family has left scars that are not easily repaired.

Color has many different levels of symbolism for African Americans. Many African Americans view their color proudly, as a badge of pride and honor. African American consciousness raising in the 1960s—epitomized by the slogan "Black is beautiful" and manifested by the appearance of Afro hairstyles, African styles of dress (such as the dashiki), and Blacks' reconnection with their African heritage—was designed to change the stereotypes of the past and promote positive African American identity. (See Chapter 8 for a discussion of the Afrocentric movement in African American communities.) Unfortunately, some attitudes remain negative or at best ambivalent and some African Americans still view their blackness as a "mark of oppression" (Kardiner & Ovesey, 1951).

One of the consequences of the system of slavery and the historical legacy discussed above has been that some Black families have identified with the dominant society and incorporated some of the prejudices of the majority White culture. This internalized racism can manifest itself in a preference for light skin, straight or curly hair, and White facial features (Neal & Wilson, 1989; Russell et al., 1993; Tucker, 2000). At the most extreme end of this spectrum are the few light-skinned African Americans who, in every generation, have denied their blackness and have "passed" for White. As this chapter will demonstrate, color prejudice can sometimes even divide families.

All African Americans, irrespective of their color, shade, darkness, or lightness are aware from a very early age that their blackness makes them different from mainstream White America and also from immigrant groups who were not brought here as slaves and who have thus had a different experience in becoming assimilated into mainstream U.S. culture. The struggle for a strong positive racial identity for African American children is clearly made more difficult by the realities of racism in U.S. society and internalized racism such as color prejudice. African American writers such as Alice Walker (1982) express concerns about the divisions that skin color issues have created in African American families and communities:

> The matter of color, quiet as it is kept, is still an issue among us. Color still affects our thoughts, attitudes and perceptions about beauty and intelligence, about worth and self-esteem. Yet if we are to stand together and survive as a people, we cannot allow color to become the wedge that . . . destroys us. (p. 66)

Skin Color and the Projection Process in African American Families

Bowen (1976, 1978) described a family projection process whereby a family ascribes or projects roles, expectations, and acceptance onto an individual, as well as the multigenerational transmission process whereby these roles and expectations are passed to the next generation. All families project characteristics onto their children based on their appearance. However, since skin color, hair texture, and facial features are such toxic issues in Black culture, a child's skin color can help to explain why that child has been singled out for the family projection process. The darkest or lightest child in the family may be seen as "different," and therefore targeted as the family scapegoat at an early age.

Because of the class system that evolved from the slave system, one can find a number of responses to skin color in African American families. In some families light skin color is prized and regarded as something special, while in others dark-skinned members are preferred and light skin color is seen as a constant reminder of the abuse of Black women by White men. In these situations, there can be considerable shame and guilt attached to this issue.

Because of the laws of genetics, variations in skin color within an African American family are quite common. Allen (1982) describes such variance:

> The only real law of nature is that when African American folks' genes get together, all things and all colors are possible. . . .
> None of my parents' children came out with even remotely similar skin colors or hair textures, so conceivably we could have created our own intraracial discrimination fight in the privacy of our own home. In many African American families that's where it really does all start: parents favoring the lighter ones, telling them they're pretty, giving them a stronger sense of self worth. When the experience of the darker person in this family encompasses trauma and personal rejection, it's easy to see why the position of light-skinned folks in the universal African American family is considered a favorable one. (p. 128)

Children of different fathers may be identified as looking like their fathers, and the personality characteristics attributed to those individuals may be projected onto their children. For example, it is not unusual to hear, "He looks just like his daddy, and he's no good just like him too." A child can sometimes be significantly lighter or darker than both parents, perhaps resembling an ancestor. It is quite common in African American families, because of the laws of genetics, for children of the same mother and father to vary considerably in their appearance and skin color. Skin color differences can intensify sibling rivalry. In the case of a troubled relationship between the parents, such differences can lead to questions about the paternity of a child. Since these questions are often "secrets" and are rarely addressed directly, they are even more toxic in the family.

Examples of Skin Color Issues

This section attempts to capture through vignettes the deeply painful issue that skin color can represent for some African American individuals and families. Dark-skinned African Americans may remember painful experiences as children or even as adults when they felt rejected by family members, peers, and members of their communities. Alexis de Veaux (1982) makes a number of references to this hurt and pain in describing her interactions with her aunt when she was growing up:

> Red, you instructed me, was a color I should never wear. I was absolutely "too dark" you said. "Whose little Black child are you?" you'd tease. "Who knows who you belong to." Did you know then that your teasing mirrored my own apprehension? Who did I belong to? Who does a dark-skinned child belong to in a family where lighter skin is predominant? (p. 67)

The following case example of an African American woman seen in therapy also illustrates this point.

Carla, a 40-year-old African American woman, painfully revealed her experience of having grown up in a family in which she was openly "put down" because she was darker skinned than her mother. Her mother told her that she was too dark and that she had been "born bad," implying a connection between the two. Carla had spent much of her life in a rage at her mother. Her brother, who had a lighter complexion and "curly hair," was doted on by her mother and could do no wrong. Carla described a painful memory in which her mother openly criticized her hair but refused to cut her brother's hair until he was almost 3 years old. At the time of that haircut, her mother cried openly, carefully collected his hair, and put it away in a special box, which she would frequently take out to admire in later years.

Children can sometimes be very cruel to each other and hurtful about skin color differences. Sometimes these insults come from White youngsters:

William, a dark-skinned African American man, aged 20, reported an experience in his childhood years in which he was chased home from school in a suburban, all-White neighborhood by a group of White children, calling him a "Black nigger" and daring him to fight back. Ever since those early days William had attempted to "blend in and not make waves." He wore glasses (even though they were not needed), dressed in the most nondescript fashion, and tried hard to avoid recognition at all costs.

The following example articulates another little girl's inner struggle with a situation in which the name calling came from her African American peers.

> Blackie ain't my name, I want to say. It hurts. It's painful. It's embarrassing, Momma. Livia is dark as me. Why everything Black got to be evil, everything dark got to be ugly? I say nothing. I learn the bravado of strike back. Incorporate the language of segregation: "inkspot," "your Momma come from blackest Africa," "tar baby, tar baby," "black nigga." I say it in [great] anger to others on the block. This is a skill. It is a way to hurt another deeply. We all practice it. . . . (de Veaux, 1982, p. 68)

This form of fighting back but sometimes of disguised self-hatred can often be seen in the process of "ranking out," "playing the dozens," and "dissing" in which many African American inner-city children express their feelings toward each other within the protection of a "game."

Being light-skinned in certain African American families can lead to privileges, but it can also result in unique problems and feelings of rejection. The need for identification and a sense of belonging is an important emotional issue for everyone. For many light-skinned African Americans, the dilemma of not being identified as African American can cause pain and discomfort, as in the next case.

Jean, a 20-year-old fair-skinned African American woman, reported a number of experiences in the course of her life in which people did not know she was African American. She told of periods in her early growing-up years in Bedford-Stuyvesant, a predominantly African American section of Brooklyn, in which she was frequently called "Whitey" or "Oreo" by other children on the block. She reported an experience in therapy with a White therapist in which after 2 years of treatment, she brought in pictures of her family to show her therapist. Her therapist was stunned when she realized for the first time that Jean was African American. Jean was angry and was able for the first time to talk about her feelings of not belonging and feeling different. Her own ambivalence had kept her from openly clarifying her racial identity earlier.

Mary, another light-skinned African American woman in her 40s, had been a member of an interracial work group for many years. She was furious and hurt when a White coworker, upon learning that she was Black, said, feeling that she was giving a compliment, "Oh, I never would have known you were Black." Mary described this experience as "feeling as if a knife had been driven in her heart."

In family situations, the child who is different may receive special privileges or he or she may be scapegoated or ostracized. Ironically, both of these situations can sometimes occur simultaneously.

Sam, age 14, was a light-skinned African American adolescent who was the third child in a family of six. Although there was a range of skin colors in his family, he was the lightest. From the adults in his family and extended family, he often received many special privileges and comments about how handsome he was. This special attention created an intense sibling rivalry between Sam and his brothers and sisters, who frequently scapegoated him and excluded him from their games. Sam grew up very unsure of himself and threatened when anyone acknowledged his appearance.

In the 1960s, with the emergence of the Black power movement, and the call for "Black pride," many light-skinned African Americans found themselves the object of years of collective anger by their darker peers.

This process of denigration can be especially painful when it occurs within a family. Since African American families often have a range of skin pigmentation represented within the immediate and/or extended family, it is quite possible for a number of children of the same parents to range in skin color from very fair to very dark. African American people are acutely aware of these ranges of color, many of which are not seen or experienced by those from other ethnic groups. All of these issues and the ways in which they are handled are specific to the given family and that family's attitude toward color. The paradox remains such that a light-brown-skinned woman may be considered "dark" if she is born into a very light-skinned family or "light" if her family members have darker complexions.

Secrets about Skin Color Issues and Its Treatment Implications

Any area as toxic as this one is fertile ground for the development of family myths and secrets. This is compounded by the fact that these issues are rarely discussed openly in many African American families. Given the many family "secrets" about birth, paternity, and informal adoption (see Chapter 3), a child who looks very different from the rest of his or her family or household members may have a very difficult time while growing up. Children may be favored or rejected because of lighter skin color. A child may be scapegoated as the darkest member of the family or favored because he or she resembles a dark-skinned ancestor. This is such a toxic issue for many African American families that it is often denied; such families will often resist discussion of it in the initial stages of treatment. Alternatively, many times children experience teasing not within their families but in their peer group and in the community. The following case example illustrates this point.

The Kent family was an African American single-parent unit composed of Martha Kent (age 30) and her three children: Glenn (age 13), Martha Lee (age 10), and Ronald (age 8). Ms. Kent came to our clinic seeking help for her youngest child, Ronald. He had become withdrawn, isolated, and depressed, and he had begun to act oppositional toward her. When the entire family was seen, Glenn and Martha Lee reported that Ronald was often teased by other children in the neighborhood because he was very light-skinned. (His mother, brother, and sister all had dark complexions.) Glenn stated that he had had to defend his younger brother for years from kids who called him "White boy" and "oreo," but now Glenn had entered junior high school and Ronald felt he had lost his protector.

It became clear that Glenn had served as a parent figure as well as the protector in the family. Ms. Kent presented as a very depressed woman who was "trying to go back to school" and who was supporting her children on welfare. When the therapist asked her if she was aware that this had been occurring, she shrugged her shoulders, looked very sad, and stated that she had so many burdens she really had "tuned out" Ronald's problems. The therapist helped her to speak directly with her son about his concerns and about the teasing by other kids.

Ronald, who had never known his father, was able to ask some questions about him, which his mother answered honestly. She told him that his father had not been White but had been a light-skinned Black man like him. The therapist encouraged her to ask him what she could do to help. He was clear that she should get the principal to talk to the children who were bothering him.

In subsequent sessions Ms. Kent reported that she had gone to the school with Ronald and "stood up for him." She was also able to mobilize his older sister and brother to help him learn how to defend himself. Glenn agreed to "stop by the school" periodically to make his presence felt, and Martha had offered to walk him to and from school as long as he needed that support.

In other families, the issues are within the family and are far more subtle, unconscious, and entrenched. The following case provides an example.

Karen was a 25-year-old African American woman who was being treated at an inpatient unit in the Bronx following an acute psychotic breakdown. She had become extremely paranoid and felt that family members were out to get her. In the course of her inpatient treatment, she had reported to her therapist that she had always been treated as a second-class citizen in her family because she was its darkest member. As time for discharge approached, she became increasingly agitated. Family sessions were arranged.

Karen's family consisted of her father, Mr. Morris (age 45), her mother, Mrs. Morris (age 44), and her older sisters, Beatrice (age 27) and Gladys (age 26). In the family session, Mr. Morris was peripheral to the other members. Mrs. Morris, Beatrice, and Gladys sat close together and Karen sat on the other side of the room. Karen resembled her father most in complexion and features, while Beatrice and Gladys had inherited their mother's light-brown complexion. Mrs. Morris, who acted as the family spokesperson, reported that Karen had always "given her trouble" and been a "bad seed." Her sisters reinforced this view. Mr. Morris was visibly uncomfortable and turned away and became more sullen. The therapist asked Mr. Morris if he shared their view. He said "things have always been hard on Karen." The therapist asked him to switch seats with Gladys and discuss this issue with his wife.

Mr. and Mrs. Morris were very rigid. They sat turned away from each other, and there was a charged air of hostility between them. Karen became very uncomfortable when they were asked to speak to each other, and blurted out "You have always hated me because I look like him." The therapist intervened and asked the parents what Karen meant by that. Mrs. Morris stated that her husband had never "done right by the family" and she never should have married him. When this statement was explored, it emerged that Mr. and Mrs. Morris had first met in their hometown in North Carolina. Mrs. Morris's father had owned a store. Mr. Morris had been from a poor family and had been unemployed. Her parents had objected to their relationship and to the fact that he was dark-skinned.

Mrs. Morris had become pregnant with Beatrice and had been "forced" to marry Mr. Morris. They moved north, where Mr. Morris had had many difficult years supporting the family. When Karen was born, Mrs. Morris had transferred her anger, frustration, and disappointment onto this child. Mr. Morris had withdrawn and become more and more peripheral to his family.

The therapist asked Mr. and Mrs. Morris if they thought there was any way to get past this history, and make a home for Karen. The parents talked openly for the first time about their disappointment in and anger at each other.

Mrs. Morris was helped to discuss these issues openly with Karen. She acknowledged her feelings of resentment but shared with her daughter how frustrated and overwhelmed she had felt having had three babies in 3 years. Karen was able to share with her mother how she bitterly resented the preferential treatment her sisters had received.

The channels for communication were opened. Mr. and Mrs. Morris were asked to discuss with Karen what would have to change in order for her to return home. They set rules about her return to her job and continuing in outpatient treatment. A contract was made in which the family would be seen also for outpatient family therapy after her release.

Thompson (1987) reports the following experience from her psychoanalytic treatment of an African American female patient.

Ms. B., the oldest of three children, lived most of her childhood with her divorced mother, her grandmother, her aunt, and two siblings. She came from an essentially middle-class family where skin color was part of the attribution of middle-class status. Ms. B. described herself as a favored child by her aunt and her grandmother. However, she described herself as falling from grace once she began to make friends with the neighborhood children. The following two vignettes helped us begin to understand and disentangle the morass of rejection and isolation. At about age 7, Ms. B. was playing with a neighborhood child when her aunt came outside and sent the child away, yelling at the patient that she was not to play with that child because she was too dark skinned.

Ms. B. needed to deny the perception that the child rejected by her caretakers was more like her mother in appearance than anyone else in the family. To protect herself and to preserve the idealizations of her mother, she accepted the rejection to be of herself, rather than her mother. Self-rejection further served to shield her from her mother's pain. When the patient became angry with her mother and devalued her, she raged with her for not protecting her from the aunt and grandmother. She was unable to see that her mother could not protect her because she too was a victim of the same rejection.

At about age 20, Ms. B. spent the summer in a theater company where she became friends with a young White man. She invited him to her home to meet her family. After the family visit, Ms. B. stopped being friendly with him because she felt the young man did not accept her more obviously African American mother. These vignettes allowed the patient to understand the reversal and ambivalence that characterized her relationship with her mother. She began to allow the deeply denied pain of her mother's existence to come to consciousness. During this process Ms. B. became able to understand her mother's idealization of her. Also, she was able to acknowledge the mother's wish that Ms. B. would become a vehicle for her acceptance within her own family. With the development of some empathy, the patient was able to talk with her mother and allow the mother to share information that, up until then Ms. B. had not known. Her mother had been adopted and had never felt accepted by the aunt or grandmother. It was never a legal adoption, but one in which she was delivered to this woman in early childhood. Ms. B.'s mother could not explain why she was "adopted." It was a family secret, but she hypothesized that she was the product of some extended family member's indiscretion. (pp. 400–401)

AFRICAN AMERICAN WOMEN AND THE ISSUE OF HAIR

Closely linked to the issue of skin color for many African American women is that of the texture of their hair. The history of slavery and U.S. racism led to what Greene, White, and Whitten (2000) have called "a conspicuous devaluation of African physical features and the establishment of beauty standards based on idealized depiction of White women's physical features" (p. 166). The impact of this was also felt in the idealization by White society of long straight hair. This led to a devaluation of African hair textures among some Black women (Greene et al., 2000; Jackson & Greene, 2000). Russell et al. (1993) have described terms such as "good hair" (naturally straight, wavy, or long), and "bad hair" (coarse or "kinky") (Tucker, 2000, p. 22), which were used by some members of the African American community to characterize different hair textures.

Many therapists have been surprised to discover the impact that this issue can have on the self-esteem and psychological adjustment of some of their African American female clients (Greene et al., 2000; Jackson & Greene, 2000; Tucker, 2000). Tucker (2000) stated that "Black women often experience a range of emotions regarding their hair, and a Black woman's feelings about her hair are frequently symbolic of her conscious and unconscious internalized feelings of herself, her identity, and her significant others" (p. 23).

One of the key components of the Black Pride movement in the 1960s and the Afrocentric movement today (see Chapter 8) was and is an appreciation for the beauty of African features and hair texture. Unfortunately, many of the old labels of "good" and "bad" hair have resurfaced in recent years. Greene et al. (2000) have shown that some "Black women struggle with . . . feelings about their hair, and spend a great deal of time, money and energy attempting to change it" (p. 171). In 1993, Russell et al. estimated that 75% of African American women chemically straighten or "perm" their hair (Tucker, 2000, p. 27). This percentage may be slightly lower today. Tucker (2000) and Greene et al. (2000) describe the much broader range of hairstyles in the African American community today, including permed or straightened hair, weaves or extensions woven into the hair, and, for women with more Afrocentric beliefs, a range of "natural" hairstyles that do not utilize chemicals, such as the short "Afro," braids, cornrows, twists, and dreadlocks or "locks." Ironically, one of the most popular styles today involves the braiding of natural or synthetic hair extensions into one's own hair to create often elaborate hairdos based on African styles (Greene et al., 2000). Many projections are made by both Black and White society onto Black women based on the type of hairstyle they choose, including assumptions about their level of "Black pride" or racial identity, Afrocenticity, White identification, socioeconomic level, and the like. Assumptions of this type can often be stereotypical and inaccurate.

Some African American women experience such shame about their hair texture that they do not allow others, even intimate partners, to touch their hair (hooks, 1993). This shame may be extremely difficult for some women to discuss in therapy and must be handled with sensitivity, especially in cross-racial treatment. Therapists working with African American women should understand that a great deal of an African American woman's feelings about her hair, appearance, self-esteem, and racial identity may be related to the messages given to her about her skin color, her appearance, and the way in which her mother, or other significant caregivers such as her grandmother, aunts, and older siblings, responded to her in the ritual of grooming her hair (Greene et al., 2000; hooks, 1993; Lewis, 1999; Russell et al., 1993).

The ritual of a mother (or mother figure) grooming or combing her daughter's hair is often a very symbolic one in the African American community. Greene et al. (2000) have indicated that some African American mothers are overly concerned about how their daughters' hair may be viewed by others. Tucker (2000) states that "the processes which Black women and young girls undergo in their efforts to style or 'fix' their hair can often be painful and tedious. Black female caregivers often place much time, energy and sometimes money, into the care and grooming of a young Black girl's hair" (p. 27). Greene et al. (2000) and Tucker (2000) have indicated that the amount of time and attention spent by African American mothers "working in their daughter's hair, and hair grooming is seen as an indication that a child, especially a female child, is either loved and valued or ignored and neglected by her caretakers" (Tucker, 2000, p. 27).

Therapists should be aware that African American women vary greatly in how they feel about these grooming rituals. Greene et al. (2000) state that "how an African American mother feels about herself may be reflected in her attitudes and care not only of her own hair but also in her attitudes toward and care of her daughter's hair" (p. 174). Grier and Cobbs (1968) gave some of the earliest accounts of African American women who experienced negative feelings related to the physical pain of having their hair "fixed" or the psychological pain related to negative comments about their hair texture made by mother figures. On the other hand, bell hooks (1993) has emphasized that for some African American women the hair-grooming ritual evokes fond memories of bonding with their mothers or mother figures. According to Tucker (2000), the "hair combing process that takes place between Black mother and daughter, grandmother and grandchild, aunt and niece, is internalized as an act of kindness, tenderness, and bonding that helps to form the strong ties that exist among Black females within the same family" (p. 28). Lewis (1999) describes a therapeutic ritual in which hair grooming is utilized in treatment with African American mothers and their daughters to facilitate bonding and physical demonstrations of love.

Therapists, particularly those from other racial and ethnic groups, have often noted that some young African American girls will "play" with the therapist's hair. It is important that therapists understand that this is often not a benign activity and may have a greater significance. Care should be taken in understanding and interpreting this behavior, particularly in cross-racial treatment. For some, it may be an expression of internalized racism and the wish for the long straight hair of the White therapist. In other children, it may be an expression of a desire for nurturance and attention. It is therefore very important that therapists inquire carefully about this issue and be sensitive to the implications for the child's racial identity development. This discussion can also be used to validate a young African American girl in terms of her own unique beauty and appearance.

Sensitive topics such as racism, skin color, and hair present problems for African American parents in terms of fostering a sense of pride, self-esteem, and positive racial identification in their children. These issues may arise in individual, family, or group psychotherapy with adult women as well. While it is very important that clinicians know about these issues and pursue them in treatment, Greene et al. (2000) caution therapists to handle the discussion of hair and skin color issues with sensitivity:

> Feelings about hair [and skin color] represent issues that frequently go unexplored in the treatment setting. Nevertheless, they are the repository for many intense

feelings for Black women. Therefore, while it requires exploration, the inquiry must be sensitive, skillfully conducted, and always embedded in a strong therapeutic alliance. The conflicts and issues we discuss in this chapter should not be raised casually, or out of mere curiosity or voyeurism. Clients may experience much shame in discussing experiences about hair or acknowledging the use of hair weaves, wigs, straighteners and the like. Therapists need to appreciate this reality and proceed with caution, explore their clients' feelings about sharing the material, and consider the strength of the working alliance. Timing is important. The therapist must always consider the client's fragility and determine her emotional readiness to explore this issue. (p. 188)

The next chapter will explore other aspects of family organization, particularly the extended family and kinship system.

3

Extended Family Patterns, Kinship Care, and Informal Adoption

The extended family is so essential to an understanding of the lives of many African Americans that it is presented here in detail. We, as family therapists, must expand our field of vision from the focus on a nuclear family model to the incorporation of an extended family and multisystems model if we are to treat African American families effectively. This forces us to expand our techniques to include more complex interactions, requires special sensitivity to the strengths of this type of family organization, and calls for an awareness of the distinct problems that it can present.

A number of scholars and researchers have documented the strength that extended kinship relationships provide in many African American families (Billingsley, 1968, 1992; Hill, 1972, 1993, 1999a; Hines & Boyd–Franklin, 1996; Jones, in press; Logan, 2001; McAdoo, 1981, 1996, 2002; McAdoo & McAdoo, 1985; Stack, 1974; White, in press). As clinicians and family therapists, however, it is imperative that we understand the complex interrelationships that can exist, and that we develop some cultural and clinical guidelines as to the characteristics of well-functioning extended families. This will greatly aid us in the process of assessment and treatment planning for this population. It is my belief that understanding the cultural norms for well-functioning extended families will help us to delineate problems clearly when they exist. Although the extended family has been a major source of strength for Black people, it would be a serious error to assume that it always functions as a support within a given family. As Hill (1999a) has pointed out, an emphasis on the strengths of the extended family should not obscure the fact that a particular extended family may also have some negative characteristics. This chapter explores the positive and negative issues related to effective assessment of extended family networks in African American families. In order to accomplish this goal, the chapter is divided into three sections: (1) a comprehensive description of African American extended family networks, including discussion of reciprocity in families, nuclear family households within an extended family culture, and the different forms of extended family constellations; (2) an exploration of the differences between functional and dysfunctional patterns in African American extended families; and (3) a discussion of kinship care and informal adoption in African American families, which focuses on the benefits of this process as well as its problems, secrets, and clinical implications.

AFRICAN AMERICAN EXTENDED FAMILIES AND KINSHIP NETWORKS

Many African American families function as extended families in which relatives with a variety of blood ties have been absorbed into a coherent network of mutual emotional and economic support (Billingsley, 1968, 1992; Hill, 1972, 1993, 1999a; Hines & Boyd-Franklin, 1996; Logan, 2001; McAdoo, 1981, 1996, 2002). White (in press) has pointed to "the numbers of uncles, aunties, big mamas, boyfriends, older brothers, and sisters, deacons, preachers and others who operate in and out of the Black home" (p. 3). He adds that when Black families are viewed from this perspective, one can recognize the extent to which

> a variety of adults and older children participate in the rearing of any one Black child. Furthermore, in the process of childrearing, these several adults plus older brothers and sisters make up a kind of extended family who interchange roles, jobs, and family functions in such a way that the child does not learn an extremely rigid distinction of male and female roles.

White further emphasizes that use of an extended family model can help family theorists and therapists formulate ways to employ Black family strengths, thus lessening the negative impact of a deficit view of African American family structure.

Reciprocity and the Extended Family Network

For many African American extended families, *reciprocity*—the process of helping each other and exchanging and sharing support as well as goods and services—is a central part of their lives. It has been one of the most important Black survival mechanisms. Stack (1974), in her classic anthropological research, gave some of the most in-depth descriptions of the way in which exchange and reciprocity networks operate in many Black communities. Her observations are still relevant today. She describes a number of different levels at which family members interact, including "kinship, jural, affectional and economic" factors. This reciprocity might take many different forms, from lending money to taking out "kin insurance" by taking care of a relative's child with the understanding that the same help will be returned when needed. It also takes the form of emotional support, knowing that a relative can be counted on to "share the burden" in times of trouble, and that one will offer such emotional support in return.

An important problem in the reciprocity system in some African American families is the imbalance that can sometimes result in the overburdening of one or more individuals. Therapists need to be especially aware of this potential imbalance since it is not uncommon for an individual or individuals to come to occupy an overly central and depended-upon position in the family network, such as a member who functions as the family "switchboard" through which all messages are conveyed. In these families the extended family may exist in structure, but the exchange of support is imbalanced to the extent that one member may become "burnt out." Thus it is essential that the therapist explore not only the question of whether the extended family support system exists, but also whether it functions in a supportive, reciprocal way.

Nuclear Family Households within an Extended Family Culture

It would be supporting a common misconception to represent most African American families as living continually with extended family members. In fact, a large number of African American families function along nuclear lines, as independent single-family households with either a mother, father, and children or a single parent with children.

These individuals and families, of course, vary in their degree of contact, reciprocity, and involvement with their extended family. This can depend on a number of factors, including geographic proximity and degree of emotional connectedness. These independent nuclear family households often participate actively in the process of reciprocity described previously and are active in their extended families (Hill, 1999a; Hines & Boyd-Franklin, 1996; McAdoo, 2002; White, in press).

For many African American families who live far apart geographically, it is a common practice for one or more family members to serve in the role of "family connector" who writes, phones, or otherwise communicates regularly with different extended family members. Independent nuclear households, even in different parts of the country, are thus kept in contact and updated about births, deaths, marriages, divorces, other significant events, and family gossip.

Some African American families function largely as nuclear families and see very little of their extended kin. Some have established or re-created new networks with friends or by joining a church in their community. Given, however, that the cultural norm for many Black families is at least some regular involvement with extended family members, it is important for the therapist to explore the hypothesis of "emotional cutoff" (Bowen, 1976; Nichols & Schwartz, 1998) with a family who appears to be very isolated. Emotional cutoff can occur when a family or individual severs its relationship with extended family members. It is very rare for this to appear as the "presenting problem" in African American families. Sometimes the acting out or withdrawal of a child may serve to draw a family into treatment and it is only later that the therapist becomes aware of significant losses or cutoffs from the family of origin. Such isolation can occur when individuals and families move up the class, educational, and economic status structure. Chapter 15, on African American middle-class families, discusses this issue in detail.

Different African American Extended Family Models

African American extended families exist in many different forms, with many different structures. These are not rigid or static and may undergo considerable change over time. It would be reasonable to assume that any individual Black person may have participated in a variety of family forms at different times in his or her lifetime. Living arrangements are extremely varied and often extremely changeable in African American extended families, manifesting what Minuchin (1974) and Nichols and Schwartz (1998) have described as "permeable boundaries" (Hines & Boyd-Franklin, 1996). For example, a relative may live with his or her extended family during times of trouble and move out again when he or she is "back on his feet." Therapists must recognize this permeability if they are to understand the true nature of the interactions in these families.

Many therapists have been exposed by now to the concept of an extended family among African Americans. It is significant, however, that just as many express considerable confusion about the various types of extended families. Billingsley (1968, 1992), Hill (1977, 1999a), McAdoo (1981, 1996, 2002), and White (in press) have explored different combinations of kinship relationships. Billingsley's (1968) distinctions help to clarify some of this diversity and are still relevant today (Billingsley, 1992; Hill, 1999a). He divided African American extended families into four major types: (1) subfamilies; (2) families with secondary members; (3) augmented families; and (4) "nonblood" relatives.

Subfamilies or Subsystems

Although their seminal works were written more than 25–30 years ago, Billingsley's (1968) and Hill's (1972, 1977) classic research still offers the most comprehensive description of the different types of African American families.

Billingsley (1968) viewed subfamilies as consisting of at least two or more related individuals. Hill (1977) summarizes these as follows:

(a) The "incipient" extended family, which consists of a husband–wife subfamily with no children of their own living in the household of relatives;
(b) the "simple nuclear" extended family, which consists of a husband–wife subfamily with one or more own children living in the household of a relative's family;
(c) the "attenuated" extended family, which consists of a parent and child subfamily living in the house of a relative. (p. 33)

Because of the economic realities facing many Black families, the involvement of subfamilies is extremely common. This type of extended family often confuses clinicians because they are constrained by their own narrow definition of a "home" or a "household." It is very common for this type of extended family to be spread over many households that live in the same building, next door to one another, or very close by.

The first example given by Hill (1977) is a very common structure in the initial young-adult phase of the family life cycle (Hill, 1999a; Hines & Boyd-Franklin, 1996). A young couple (who may or may not be legally married) may live in the home of the man's or woman's family of origin until they can "be on their own" financially. This is particularly common in situations in which a teenager or young woman becomes pregnant.

Over time, this initial situation can extend to a whole nuclear family unit living within a larger extended family household. Often there is more than one subfamily within the broader household. The case of the Colt family illustrates this pattern.

Mr. and Mrs. Colt had married very young and had two daughters, Angie (age 35) and Alice (age 40). Alice had become pregnant at age 17 and her son, Clarence, had been raised as part of the Colt family. Alice and Clarence had always lived within the extended family household.

The younger daughter, Angie, had left home at age 20 at the time of her first marriage. When she was divorced 3 years later, she returned "home" to her mother's house. Three years later, she began dating Manny. They married a year later and were given a floor in her mother's house. At present, Angie, Manny, and their two children (ages 5 and 2) are part of this large extended family household.

It is extremely important to ask African American families where they are living and also to ask them to describe their living arrangements. Many poor African American families are forced by their economic circumstances to "double up" in situations that create overcrowding and lack of privacy. Therefore, defining the boundaries around the spouse subsystem (Minuchin, 1974) or the subfamily becomes very difficult. The following case provides an example.

Carl Brown (age 12) was referred to our clinic for acting-out behavior in school, truancy, and fighting with other children.

Mary Brown and Earl Stetson had been living together with Ms. Brown's two young children (ages 12 and 5) for 3 years. After a fire in their apartment, they were forced to move in with Ms. Brown's mother and her two adolescent children (ages 18 and 17). This apartment had two bedrooms, a living room, a kitchen, and a bathroom. Ms. Brown and Mr. Stetson were given a small bedroom that they shared with her two children. The two teenagers had to sleep in the living room.

Both Ms. Brown and Mr. Stetson described the living arrangement as a nightmare in which they had no privacy. They could not discipline their children or raise them in terms of their own lifestyle. There was a constant bottleneck in the kitchen and in the bathroom.

Carl and the other children were all furious with each other because of the disruption in their lives. When the family was asked what the problems were, they all focused immediately on their living situation.

Secondary Members

Hill (1977) has identified a group of extended families who take in different relatives or "secondary members": (1) "minor relatives" (e.g., nieces, nephews, cousins, grandchildren, siblings under age 18); (2) "peers of the primary parents" (e.g., cousins, siblings close in age to the primary parents); (3) "elders of the primary parents" (e.g., grandparents, great-grandparents, aunts, uncles); and (4) "parents of the primary family" (p. 34). Hill (1999a) further points out that many of the dependent secondary members in African American families are grandchildren and great-grandchildren.

There are endless examples of African American extended families containing "secondary members" (Hill, 1977, 1999a). The vast majority of these family members are children (Boyd-Franklin, Steiner, & Boland, 1995; Hines & Boyd-Franklin, 1996; McAdoo, 2002; White, in press). These situations are discussed in more detail in a later section of this chapter on kinship care and informal adoption. Here, the focus is on adult "secondary members," who fall most commonly into the following three categories: (1) peers of the primary parents, (2) elders of the primary parents, and (3) parents of the primary parents. An example of this arrangement is provided by the next case.

Jo Ann was 18 when her mother died. She was the youngest of three children. Her older siblings Anna (age 28) and Calvin (age 30) lived with their own families. Anna felt that Jo Ann was too young to "live on her own," so she asked Jo Ann to live with her, her live-in boyfriend, and her two children (ages 5 and 3).

Some adults move in with extended family when they are "between jobs," "between relationships," or following a divorce. Because of the problems of job discrimination, chronic unemployment, and cost of housing, this is a common occurrence.

Jimmy (age 35) was a divorced man who had a history of long periods of unemployment. He had worked as a dishwasher, as a hospital porter, and in a grocery store but had been laid off whenever times were bad. During these times, Jimmy moved in with his sister Janice and her two teenage children. The children had long known that Uncle Jimmy was likely to show up at any time and stay with them for an indefinite period of time.

Black families are far more likely than some White families to take in elderly family members; nursing home care is usually considered only as a last resort. This is particularly true for elderly parents and grandparents, partly because of the long parenting role African American grandparents play in family systems (Billingsley, 1992; Boyd-Franklin et al., 1995; Hill, 1999a; Hines & Boyd-Franklin, 1996; McAdoo, 2002; White, in press). Leisurely retirement is rare; the African American elderly must be really physically incapacitated to warrant hospital rather than home care. What often happens is illustrated by the following case example.

Ellie (age 75) was living in Harlem on the top floor of the home of a friend. She had lived on her block for many years. Her daughter and her family had moved to the South and repeatedly begged her to join them. Ellie insisted on staying in her own home with her friends and in the neighborhood where she had lived for 50 years.
    During a visit to her daughter, Ellie suffered a stroke. Her daughter took in Ellie and she became a part of their household.

Augmented Families

A smaller but significant number of African American children are being raised in households in which they are not even related to the heads of these households (Billingsley, 1992; Hill, 1977, 1999a; Hines & Boyd-Franklin, 1996; White, in press). It is also very interesting to note that a large proportion of nonrelated individuals living with African American families are adults, including roomers, boarders, lodgers, or other long-term guests. Hill (1999a) has discussed the fact that some African Americans live with families with whom they have no biological relationship. This is a very important piece of information for a therapist who is attempting to build and/or contact a network for an adult African American patient who may have been discharged from a psychiatric hospital or who may be homeless. This "taking in" of adults and children has been a way that Black families have augmented their incomes and shared limited living space.

Nonblood Relatives

One distinction between African American and some other cultures that share the extended family pattern is the presence and importance of individuals who are not related by blood ties but who are part of the "family" in terms of involvement and function. Stack (1974) referred to these family members as "fictive kin." These "fictive kin" might include "play mamas," "play aunts," or "play uncles," godmothers and godfathers, babysitters, or neighbors (Billingsley, 1968, 1992; Hill, 1999a; Logan, 2001; McAdoo, 2002; White, in press).

I remember that as a child in my own family, I was not allowed to call adults by their first names without using the title "aunt" or "uncle." My parents' close friends were treated as part of the family. It was not until I was about 6 or 7 that I began to make clear distinctions between these "aunts" and "uncles" and my blood relatives. Godparents are often very important in African American families. My own godmother had been my mother's best friend since childhood, and she was extremely close to our family and played a very special role in my growing-up years. She provided the little extras, such as gifts that my parents could not afford.

In addition, the large proportion of nonrelated individuals living with African American families that was mentioned under the heading "augmented families"—roomers, boarders, lodgers, or other long-term guests—could also be included in this category, with the distinction that while some of these relationships are transient, individuals may live with a family for many years and eventually be accepted as part of the family. My paternal grandmother, whose family came originally from North and South Carolina, moved to Harlem and over the years frequently took in boarders. Many of these were young women from her hometown who were new to the "big city." These women became part of her "extended family" and would often come back to visit her with their own children.

Neighbors, close friends, babysitters, and former babysitters are also important extended family members in many African American families. These individuals often become "play mamas" or "play aunts" to children (White, in press).

The Role of Family Reunions in Many African American Extended Families

Family reunions have long served a function of bringing together extended kin in African American families who may not see each other regularly (Boyd-Franklin et al., 2001). There has been a resurgence of interest in this time-honored family ritual since the publication of Alex Haley's (1977) book *Roots*. Some families have constructed a "family tree" that includes special pictures and memories. Some have interviewed older "family historians" who know the background and generational connections of the family.

As in many other cultures, family reunions can take many forms and serve many different functions. Weddings and funerals provide impromptu reunions in which connections are renewed and maintained. Once a year or every few years some families gather in a central, convenient location or return to their hometowns in the South. Often for children raised in northern or western cities, these returns to the South offer a rare glimpse of the growing-up experiences of their parents and their grandparents. Although family reunions vary considerably according to family style and traditions, there are some common experiences. One is the central and unifying role of food. Everyone participates in the cooking, and platters of turkey, ham, fried chicken, candied yams, potato salad, collard greens and ham hocks, black-eyed peas and rice, and so on abound. Some families with strong religious backgrounds will focus a part of their reunion around reconnecting with their home church or "spiritual roots." Attempts are made to bring everybody home, and often money is pooled to help pay the travel expenses of those who could not otherwise attend. Many African American families with strong Afrocentric beliefs (see Chapter 8) pour a "libation" (usually water or another drink) to the ancestors, an African ritual that honors the ancestors and the older generations in the family who are now deceased.

In some African American families, these reunions do not begin until the death of a very central family member who may have served as the family's "switchboard" or "connector." Often families will then perceive a vacuum for which the ritual of the reunion begins to compensate.

In any case, these reunions are special joyous occasions that provide a very welcome emotional and spiritual refueling for all generations. They bring together the young, middle, and older generations and give all a sense of their roots and family continuity.

It is important for therapists to be aware of this ritual in African American families. In some families where geographic distance has created isolation, the ritual of a reunion can sometimes be prescribed or recommended as a therapeutic intervention to help to rebuild or strengthen family ties, particularly after a major loss.

THE QUESTION OF FUNCTIONAL VERSUS DYSFUNCTIONAL EXTENDED FAMILIES

As has been established above, the presentations of African American extended families may vary considerably. The extended family system can clearly be a source of strength and support in many African American families (Billingsley, 1968, 1992; Hill, 1972, 1999a; Hines & Boyd-Franklin, 1996; Jones, in press; Logan, 2001; McAdoo, 1981, 1996, 2002; White, in press). As family therapists, however, we must be able to distinguish between functional and dysfunctional African American extended families.

Just as there is considerable diversity among African American nuclear families, there are many different types of extended family structures. It is important for therapists to understand how these structures and roles interplay when they are functional and how they become problematic and dysfunctional when they are confused or unclear. It would be doing a great disservice to the African American families we treat if we so glorified the strengths of the extended family that we could not recognize problems when they appear. Once we have a model of what is functional, we have the beginning of a strategy for therapeutic change and restructuring.

Minuchin (1974) and Nichols and Schwartz (1998) have used the terms *enmeshed* and *disengaged* to describe a continuum of family functioning, with enmeshed being the overinvolved end of the continuum and disengaged the extreme of being cut off. Extended families also present along this continuum. In some African American families, the extended network is so enmeshed that extended family members are constantly intruding in the core family's functioning, role relationships, and boundaries (Minuchin, 1974; Hines & Boyd-Franklin, 1996), or at the least rules of participation become blurred. In other families who present with dysfunctional patterns at our clinic, extended family members are structurally present but do not get involved or interact in a supportive way. These families are more disengaged and it often takes a great deal of acting out by the identified patient to bring them in for treatment. Still other dysfunctional families are cut off entirely from extended family contacts, in a state of isolation that often contributes significantly to their presenting problems.

The Functional Extended Family: Clear Boundaries

The extended family model found among the African American population was perceived by some social scientists as somehow aberrant and dysfunctional (Moynihan, 1965; Hines & Boyd-Franklin, 1996). The strengths and positive aspects of such familial systems were lost in the shadow of the "normal" nuclear family model. However, there is growing evidence that extended families are indeed functional family models (Billingsley, 1968, 1992; Hill, 1972, 1999a; McAdoo, 1981, 1996, 2002; McAdoo & McAdoo, 1985; White, in press).

The following case example highlights the basic components that distinguish a functional extended family system from one that is having difficulties.

Joyce, a 25-year-old African American female, grew up within an extended family system that consisted of her maternal grandparents, a maternal aunt and uncle who were married, two nephews, and a younger uncle who was unmarried. All of the married family members had their own living space within the house. Joyce's parents moved into a very large room on the second floor of the home that had an adjoining bathroom. They shared the kitchen with the grandparents, who lived on the first and second floors. Off the kitchen on the first floor was a small room that was occupied by "Aunt" Joan, a close friend of the grandmother, who boarded with the family. She had a job as a live-in domestic with a White family during the week and stayed with Joyce's family on the weekends.

The family was able to have "private" places for each subfamily unit. Children had free rein of the house and interacted with and were cared for by all the adults, but it was also very clear as to who each child's parents were. Although there were kitchens in the top two apartments, the grandparents' kitchen was the hub of the house. The family table could seat 16 and often did, especially on Sundays and holidays. Joyce often played on the floor of the kitchen with her siblings and cousins while the adult women were cooking.

When Joyce was 2, her mother returned to work and her grandmother took care of her and the other children in the household. There was an interchange of babysitting, children's clothes, maternity clothing, cribs, baby carriages, and so on between the different families.

This combination of separate, private subfamilies in one extended family household and easy sharing and interchange clearly outlines the elements that make an extended family system function well. First, the boundaries were flexible but also very clear (Minuchin, 1974; Hines & Boyd-Franklin, 1996). Second, there was no confusion with regard to who were the parents or executive figures, and thus parental authority was not undermined. The meeting of emotional needs and the availability of a support system for both children and parents are also components important for the functioning of this model. Another important pattern in many African American families is that of informal adoption.

INFORMAL ADOPTION AND KINSHIP CARE
AMONG AFRICAN AMERICAN FAMILIES

The terms "informal adoption" (Hill, 1977, 1999a) and "kinship care" (Hill, 1999a; Report to Congress on Kinship Foster Care, 2000) refer to an informal social service network that has been an integral part of the African American community since the days of slavery (see Chapter 12). It began as, and still is, a process whereby adult relatives or friends of the family "took in" children and cared for them when their parents were unable to provide for their needs, whether for medical, emotional, financial, housing, or other reasons. As Hill (1977) has pointed out, "during slavery, for example, thousands of children of slave parents, who had been sold as chattel, were often reared by elderly relatives who served as a major source of stability and fortitude for many Black families" (p. 1). This informal adoption network still serves many vital functions for African American families, such as "income maintenance and day care, services to out-of-wedlock children and unwed mothers, foster care and adoption" (Hill, 1977, p. 3). Today this process has been denoted "kinship care" by the child welfare system. It has become even more common as many African American families struggle with losses due to parental drug and alcohol abuse, AIDS, and incarceration (Boyd-Franklin et al., 1995; Hill, 1999a; Hines & Boyd-Franklin, 1996; Logan, 2001).

Child welfare and social service policies have changed a great deal in recent years. Unfortunately, although many states' child welfare agencies explore extended family members as possibilities for placement, they often do not know enough about African American cultural patterns to go far enough in searching for blood and nonblood supports. African American children are still disproportionately represented in foster care; extended family members who take in children are often given little or no financial support as compared with nonfamilial foster parents; and many states are still struggling to effectively implement "kinship care" policies (Hill, 1999a; Report to Congress on Kinship Foster Care, 2002; Wilson & Chipungu, 1996). (See Chapter 12.)

The original adoption agencies were not designed to meet the needs of Black children. During segregation, Black children could not be placed through adoption agencies (Billingsley & Giovannoni, 1970). Therefore, the kinship care and informal adoption process provided an unofficial social service network for African American families and children, one that was totally unrelated to the official child welfare system (Hill, 1999a; Hines & Boyd-Franklin, 1996).

There are many different reasons why an "informal" adoption might occur in an African American family. Children born out of wedlock are often informally adopted by an older female relative. This is particularly true in situations such as teenage pregnancy where a mother is too young to care for her child alone. Her female relatives will assume some of the responsibility for raising the child. In some circumstances, where the mother is extremely young, Stack (1974) points out that she "may give the child to someone who wants the child, for example, to the child's father, a childless couple or to close friends" (pp. 65–66).

The literature provides a number of useful examples. Hill (1977, 1999a) and Hines and Boyd-Franklin (1996) have all emphasized the importance of parental divorce or separation as a factor leading to informal adoption and kinship care among African Americans. Stack (1974) gives some examples of such situations, all of which illustrate the notable flexibility of the Black extended family to cope with a variety of family structures. This kind of structural flexibility is in response to the changes in familial arrangements due to the breakup of marriage or "consensual union" (Stack, 1974). Children are frequently divided among various immediate and/or extended family members until the custodial parent (usually the mother) is able to take actual custody of them again.

The following case describes a slightly different situation.

> Soon after Flats resident Henrietta Davis returned to the Flats to take care of her own children, she told me, "My old man wanted me to leave town with him and get married. But he didn't want to take my three children. I stayed with him for about two years and my children stayed in town with my mother. Then she told me to come back and get them. I came back and stayed." (Stack, 1974, p. 65)

Hill (1977, 1999a) and Billingsley (1968, 1992) indicate that the death, illness, or hospitalization of one or more of the child's parents is another factor often leading to informal adoption. Instead of orphaned children becoming state wards, a relative or close friend of the family will "adopt" the children, as in the following case.

Mattie Cornwell had inherited from her mother and grandmother the job of being the switchboard and caretaker of her extended family. When she was in her 70s her two young great-nieces (ages 4 and 6) were orphaned. As their great-aunt and the oldest female in the family, she took the children in and raised them with her husband.

Short-Term Adoptions or Kinship Care Arrangements

The circumstances discussed above are more likely to lead to long-term informal adoption arrangements. There are, however, a number of short-term kinship care arrangements that often arise out of economic necessities, crisis situations, or childcare needs. In situations in which the parent is involved in a new relationship or marriage, the children are sometimes left with grandparents or other relatives until their mother can establish her new home (Hines & Boyd-Franklin, 1996; McAdoo, 2002). Boyd-Franklin et al. (1995) give many examples of short-term kinship care arrangements that occur when a parent with AIDS is hospitalized. These may eventually become permanent informal adoptions with the death of the parent(s). Therapists should also be aware that mothers are often forced to give up their children to the child welfare system when they seek drug or alcohol treatment. Extended family members will often take in the children in order to avoid their placement in foster care if they are contacted in time.

A mother may request that her relatives keep one of her children. An offer to keep the child of a relative has a variety of implications for both child givers and child receivers. It may be that the mother is enduring hard times and desperately wants her close kin to temporarily assume responsibility for her children. Extended family members rarely refuse such requests to keep one another's children; likewise they recognize the right of kin to request that children be raised away from their own parents (Billingsley, 1968, 1992; Hill, 1972, 1999a; Hines & Boyd-Franklin, 1996; Logan, 2001; Stack, 1974). Individuals allow extended family members to create alliances and obligations toward one another, obligations that may be called upon in the future.

Hill (1977) points out that "many children are often taken in by relatives simply because they wanted a child to raise" (p. 49). Sometimes this is prompted by a fear of being alone in old age. Other individuals and families are unable to have children of their own and may want to adopt a child. Often a teenage pregnancy or the addition of another child to a financially overburdened family may prompt an informal adoption.

Bessie (age 40) and her husband Howard (age 42) had been married for 12 years. They had been trying to have a child for many years and had gone through extensive infertility testing. They were considering adoption when they received a call from a cousin in Georgia telling them that a younger cousin was pregnant. Both of her parents worked and were unable to care for the child and they were concerned that having a baby so young would drastically alter their daughter's life. Bessie and Howard offered to adopt the child right after birth. They traveled to Georgia, picked up the child, and raised her as their own.

Short-term kinship care or informal adoption can also become an extension of already existing daycare services provided by African American extended family members in order to permit a parent to go to work, school, or a training program (Hill, 1977, 1999a; Hines & Boyd-Franklin, 1996). A similar common scenario is the result of the strong educational orientation of most Black families (Hill, 1972, 1999a; Hines & Boyd-Franklin, 1996; McAdoo, 1981, 1996, 2002; McAdoo & McAdoo, 1985). Tremendous sacrifices are often made to permit a child to go to or live closer to a good school. In some circumstances, a child will live with relatives closer to the desired school during the week and return home on the weekends.

Problems Presented by Kinship Care and Informal Adoptions

There are a number of levels on which informal adoptions can present problems in some African American families. The last part of this chapter discusses the secrets that can arise in Black families surrounding issues often related to informal adoptions. These secrets can be very harmful to family relationships and can persist for many generations.

Another level of conflict has to do with the perceptions by different family members of the duration of the kinship care or informal adoption. For example, as stated above, children are sometimes placed with a family member after a death, a hospitalization, a separation, or a divorce. Often the family member who takes in the child does so with the belief that the adoption will be permanent, or the process of adoption is left ambiguous. If, at a later point, the natural parent reclaims the child, this can present heart-wrenching problems. The following case example illustrates this common dilemma.

Karima (age 12) was referred for treatment by her guidance counselor. She had been a good student until this school year when her grades began to deteriorate rapidly and she seemed very preoccupied. Mrs. Bond, her grandmother, brought her for therapy at the school's request.

The following history emerged. Karima's mother had died when she was 3 years old. Her father, Mark Bond, who worked as a teacher and had an active social life, felt that she would be cared for best by his mother, Mrs. Bond. In the last year Mark Bond had remarried, his new wife was pregnant, and at her urging he was beginning to try to "bring his family together" by taking Karima to live with him. Mrs. Bond began to panic. She lived alone, loved her granddaughter, and was very threatened by her loss. Karima felt caught. Her loyalty was torn. She became sad and depressed and reported that she loved both her father and her grandmother.

The therapist asked for a session with Karima, her grandmother, and her father. Both Mark Bond and Mrs. Bond seemed very angry with each other and tense. They each engaged in a process of trying to get the therapist on "their side." Karima, sitting in the middle, burst into tears. The therapist asked her to come out of the middle and sit next to her. She asked the father and grandmother to talk with each other about the issue of where Karima should live and what was best for Karima. They found it very difficult to focus on this issue and continued to insult each other. Mrs. Bond accused her son of "dumping his daughter on her" when he needed to and now he was "tearing her heart out" by taking her away. Mr. Bond accused his mother of stealing his daughter's love and turning her against him.

The therapist persisted and pointed out that this battle was "tearing Karima apart." She asked if they could put their own issues aside long enough to decide what might be best for her. A number of sessions were necessary before they could successfully negotiate an arrangement in which Karima would continue to live with her grandmother during the week and go to her same school. She would visit her father on the weekends.

This case has much in common with custody battles between divorcing parents, in which the angry issues between the couple are acted out over the issue of custody of the child. In "informal" adoption situations it is more complex because the biological or natural parent often has legal guardianship in the eyes of the law. It is a very recent notion in the eyes of the court to establish the question of "psychological bonding" in these complex situations and to allow extended family members to become legal guardians.

Often family therapists can find themselves in the middle of complex custody battles surrounding informal adoption in African American families. This is often complicated by child welfare agencies attempting to clarify or formalize this process. In the following case example, the therapist was asked by the state child welfare agency to make a recommendation regarding custody. He found himself faced with an impossible, Solomon-like problem.

The Elison family was referred by their state child welfare agency for evaluation. Rashan, age 5, had been raised since he was a 1-year-old by his grandmother, Fanny Elison (age 45). She had taken in her grandchild at that point because her daughter Clessy Elison (age 25) had been neglecting him. Clessy had been a heroin addict and had often neglected the care of her child as her craving for drugs increased. She had entered a drug treatment program and claimed to be "drug-free." Clessy had been involved with Rashan inconsistently for many years. In the last 6 months, however, she had been taking him each weekend. Fanny Elison reported that her daughter frequently returned Rashan to her in a dirty and disheveled state after these weekend visits. She also claimed that Clessy's live-in boyfriend was a drug dealer who had gotten Clessy "hooked on cocaine." Clessy Elison denied this and accused her mother of trying to take her son from her.

The therapist, in the course of Rashan's evaluation, met with many different subsystems in the family. He interviewed Rashan, Clessy Elison and Rashan, and

Fanny Elison and Rashan and determined that the child was fond of both "parents" and got along well with both.

A number of sessions were scheduled with Fanny and Clessy Elison to discuss the issue further. Each managed to cancel repeatedly. Finally, with the intervention of the child welfare agency, a session was scheduled at which both appeared.

The therapist and his supervisor met with both family members. Both Fanny and Clessy Elison were obviously angry but very "cold" toward each other. They each chose seats as far from each other as they could in a small room.

Initially the grandmother accused her daughter of being on cocaine and neglecting her son. They had a number of angry arguments about her lifestyle. The therapist pushed them to talk together about Rashan and observed that in his separate sessions it was clear that he loved both of them very much. Fanny Elison told her daughter in a very emotional way that she did not want to "keep her from her son," but that she was very worried about his safety and care. Clessy was able to answer that she never felt that her mother would let her "make up" for past mistakes.

They agreed to work together to try to establish the best living arrangement for Rashan. The grandmother offered to try to help Clessy regain custody by working with her on parenting skills.

In an ideal world, the treatment might have ended on that note. However, approximately 2 weeks later, Fanny Elison appeared very angry when she arrived for the session. She raged at Clessy and told her that Rashan had reported to her that he had seen his mother take drugs in her home. Clessy angrily denied it. Fanny demanded that her daughter leave her "drug-dealing boyfriend" immediately. Clessy refused.

The therapist, who was also becoming very concerned about the presence of drugs in Clessy's life, proposed a compromise. He asked Clessy if she was willing to go into a drug counseling program. She agreed. Fanny Elison agreed that if her daughter gave up drugs she would work with her to share parenting responsibilities. Clessy went for one meeting with her counselor but dropped out of the program when she learned that she would have to be tested regularly for the presence of drugs in her system.

Clessy then dropped out of therapy. Fanny Elison continued to come for family sessions with her grandson for a number of weeks and was helped to work out a series of visitation agreements with her daughter and grandson, in the grandmother's home, that did not put his well-being in jeopardy.

This case was a very problematic one for the therapist on a number of levels. First, it forced him to face his own value issues regarding the "best interest of the child," particularly regarding the question of drugs. Second, his ideal resolution—that is, a gradual return of custody to the mother with the grandmother helping her daughter to assume appropriate parenting responsibilities—did not occur. Third, the therapist felt pressured by the child welfare agency, the court, the grandmother, and the mother to make a recommendation. He was thus torn between his goal of keeping the child in touch with both parental figures as sources of love and caring and the desire not to place him in a situation that was detrimental to him.

With his supervisor's help, the therapist was able to extricate himself from these complex demands and place the responsibility for the decision on the family. Attempts to negotiate a solution failed and the mother made her own choice to withdraw. Ultimately the court made the decision to award custody to the grandmother but to allow the mother to continue to visit her son regularly.

The therapist in such situations must work to avoid the temptation that results from the varying pulls of the family system and the child welfare or legal system to "play God." Ultimately the responsibility must be placed on the family members to set clear limits for each other and to renegotiate complex custody arrangements that may have begun as informal adoptions.

Secrets about Informal Adoption and Parentage: Clinical Implications

As a result of the informal adoption process, a member of the extended family may have raised a child whose parents were unable to do so. In some cases, this is known by all family members, including the child, and the child often sees his or her natural parents while growing up. In such families, although the child may have been told who his or her real parent is, there may be another secret kept from the child—for example, the real reason why he or she was given up or "taken in." Sometimes there may also be secrets about the parent's present lifestyle. The following case offers an example of this.

Mrs. Gifford, a 65-year-old maternal grandmother, sought treatment for her 11-year-old grandson, Kasim. In the last year, Kasim had become increasingly depressed, sad, and withdrawn. Finally, his school had suggested that Mrs. Gifford seek treatment for him. Kasim had lived with his grandmother since he was 1 year old. Prior to that time, he had lived with his mother. Mrs. Gifford had become concerned when she had visited her daughter and found that she was neglecting Kasim. Since his father had never been a part of his life and Mrs. Gifford was his closest relative, she took Kasim in and raised him herself. His mother, Ayana, had been in and out of his life over the years and lived in the same city but on the "other side of town."

In the last year, Mrs. Gifford reported that Kasim had begun to ask why he was not living with his mother and why she had left him. He wondered if he was to blame or if there had been something wrong with him. After careful inquiries by the therapist, he was able to share with his grandmother that other kids often teased him about his mother. Mrs. Gifford became visibly anxious when this issue was raised. The therapist finally arranged to see her alone and discovered that there was a "family secret" that she was afraid to share with Kasim: his mother had been a drug addict since her teenage years and had also engaged in prostitution to support her habit. Mrs. Gifford had not wanted Kasim to think badly of his mother and so she had never told him about her life. The therapist helped Mrs. Gifford to see that Kasim was at an age when a child naturally begins to inquire about his roots. She also discussed with the grandmother the fact that the "grapevine" in their part of the city was very strong, and Kasim probably had learned a great deal about his mother from the other children.

She agreed to have a session with Kasim and the therapist to discuss this issue further. In the family session, the therapist encouraged Mrs. Gifford to find out what Kasim had heard from the other children and what they teased him about. She was shocked to discover that other children had called his mother a "hooker" and a "drug addict" and that Kasim had kept this inside for some time. Both family members were carrying the burden of this secret. She was then able to ask Kasim if he had questions for her. He immediately asked why his mother had left him. Mrs. Gifford explained the circumstances and was able to help Kasim to understand that he was not with his mother because of her lifestyle and not because of any flaw in him.

In a subsequent session, the therapist asked that Kasim's mother attend together with Kasim and his grandmother. In this session, the therapist learned that in the last year Kasim's mother had begun to feel guilty about leaving him for so long and had started to see him more often. She had become anxious when Kasim had asked why he couldn't live with her and had been making vague promises to him that he could join her at some point in the future.

The therapist clarified the situation by demonstrating that this "mixed message" was harmful to Kasim. She encouraged Mrs. Gifford and Ayana to discuss the realities of her life situation and work out a regular visitation schedule for Kasim. Ayana shared her guilt with her mother openly for the first time and acknowledged that Kasim could not live with her. They agreed that he would continue to live with his grandmother but that Ayana would visit him regularly every Saturday. Ayana was then asked to discuss this openly with Kasim, who had been observing this discussion. Tearfully she told him that she loved him but that she was confusing him by telling him that he would live with her. She discussed with him the decision that he would live with his grandmother but that she would visit him every week.

Kasim cried also but appeared visibly relieved. In subsequent months, his depression lifted and he began to reengage with his friends.

This type of secret, which is in fact "known" by all the parties (and by the community), can be particularly toxic because of the energy that is involved in "protecting" the family members from this knowledge. The "grapevine," or informal communication network, in African American communities is very strong. The following case is another example of a complicated family secret concerning an "informal adoption."

George Kent was a 7-year-old African American boy who had been informally adopted by his aunt when he was 6 months old. His mother had "dropped him on her doorstep" one day and never returned. Olivia Kent, his aunt, had raised him along with her own children, Carol (age 20), Ivy (age 15), and Althea (age 12), and Carol's son, Billy (age 5). There had never been any formal discussion in the family as to George's real relationship to the other family members. George had begun to act out and fight at school and at home shortly after the family had been visited by a representative of the local child welfare department. George's mother, an alcoholic, had died in a local hospital. Prior to her death she had told her social worker about Olivia Kent and George. The child welfare worker informed Ms. Kent that George was now under the guardianship of her agency and a decision must be made as to whether he would remain with Ms. Kent.

This caused a major disruption in the family. Ms. Kent petitioned formally to adopt George but his acting-out behavior had raised questions as to the suitability of his placement in her home.

At the point at which Ms. Kent arrived with George for her first session at our clinic, it was clear that both of them were very frightened and angry about these developments. The therapist helped Ms. Kent to talk about the circumstances that had led up to this dilemma and helped her to discuss this openly with George. George then told her that he had always wondered why he looked different from her other children (he was darker skinned) and that Billy had often teased him about this. He shared that he was very frightened of having to leave.

Mrs. Kent arranged a meeting of all the members of her household with the therapist to discuss the situation. She told them the "secrets" in George's history and asked their support for keeping him. All of the family members were surprised to hear that there was any question of his remaining in their family. A meeting was arranged by the therapist with the child welfare worker and the family to clarify their desire to formally adopt George. He beamed throughout this session. The therapist subsequently wrote a number of letters for the family documenting the "bonding" that had occurred between George and his "family."

Ms. Kent was then able to discuss openly with George the fact that she could not tolerate his acting out at home or in school. He had been "spoiled" by the family and allowed to "get away with" a great deal. She set clear rules for him at home and enlisted the aid of his older "sisters" to enforce these rules. His behavior at home and in school dramatically improved.

Secrets Regarding Fatherhood

There are many issues concerning fatherhood that may become secrets in some African American families. For example, in the following case example, a child was raised by a stepfather and was never told the "secret" of his true paternity.

The Brown family was referred for treatment because their son Michael (age 13) had been acting out, was aggressive with peers in school, often talked back to his mother and father, and broke his curfew. The Brown family consisted of Mr. Brown (age 40), Mrs. Brown (age 30), Michael, and two younger siblings, Milton (age 9) and Karen (age 5). Mr. and Mrs. Brown reported that Michael had always respected them until the last year. Since then he had been "running wild," "talking back" to them, fighting at school, and so on. They felt helpless to control him. In the family sessions, Mrs. Brown was the family spokesman and the person who sat closest to Michael. Mr. Brown seemed to alternate between being peripheral and becoming involved in an angry, intrusive way with Michael. The parents clearly disagreed with each other about discipline and limits. The mother was overindulgent of Michael and overinvolved with him. Therefore, the therapist decided to put the father in charge of Michael. The family resisted this process for a number of weeks. Finally, the therapist confronted the parents about this resistance. They became uncomfortable and Mrs. Brown actually looked alarmed. The therapist, sensing that this was an issue between the parents, drew a boundary and asked the children to leave the room. Tearfully, Mrs. Brown explained that she had become pregnant with Michael as an unwed teenager at the age of 17. Her family had been embarrassed and angry at her because they had wanted her to go to college. They had hidden the "secret" of Michael's birth and had never discussed it, Shortly after his birth, Mrs. Brown met and married her current husband, who had raised Michael as his own. The other two children were his.

Mr. Brown explained that Michael had always been an issue between them. She had protected and spoiled him and had never really allowed Mr. Brown to be a "real father" to him. Both Mr. and Mrs. Brown agreed that Michael sensed that he was different from the other children. He did not look like anyone else in the family and had once angrily asked if he was adopted.

With the therapist's help, Mr. and Mrs. Brown were able to discuss how this secret had affected the way in which they had raised Michael and their inability to work together and parent him together. They finally decided to raise the issue with their son and to be clear with him that emotionally they were both his parents. The children were called back into the room and Mr. and Mrs. Brown discussed with Michael this "secret." Mr. Brown was able to share with him the fact that he had accepted him long ago as his son. Michael and the other children looked at each other often during this report. When the therapist inquired as to what was going on between them, Michael reported that a cousin, who had stayed with the family the previous summer, had implied that he was an "outsider" but had never told him the details.

In future sessions, the therapist was able to restructure the family by asking the mother to encourage Michael and Mr. Brown to spend time alone together in order to develop the relationship between them. Both parents were able to talk openly about setting clear limits for Michael without this toxic secret between them.

Another type of fatherhood secret may have to do with other children, another family, or another woman in a father's life. Like the secrets discussed above, these issues may be known on some level, but either denied or never discussed by family members. In many cases, these issues surface only when there is a family crisis or a major loss, such as a death of the father. The following case illustrates this dilemma.

Connie Jones, a 40-year-old Black woman, had come for treatment requesting help for her son Darryl, age 15. Darryl had two other siblings, Mary, age 10, and Robert, age 9. Their father had died suddenly in a car accident 6 months earlier. Darryl had been very angry and had been acting out since his death. He stayed out late at night, was truant from school, and was often angry and hostile toward his mother. Darryl had had a very problematic relationship with his father prior to his death and had taken his loss "hard." It was clear that the whole family was struggling with this loss and had never fully mourned or shared their pain.

In a family session, the father's death was discussed. Darryl reported that his father had really "done wrong by them." At the funeral, another woman had appeared with a child 2 years younger than Darryl and reported that this was his father's child. Darryl was furious. His mother reported that she had heard rumors about her husband's secret life but had never really confronted him or let the children know. Darryl was finally able to tell his mother that he had felt betrayed at having to find this out at a time like that (i.e., during the funeral). He was angry at his father and at her. Once this issue was discussed openly by Mrs. Jones with Darryl and the other children, they were able to talk openly about their hurt, their anger, and their sadness at the death of their father. The family's mourning process could then begin.

Bowen (1976) has discussed the emotional shock wave that a death can precipitate in a family. In many Black families, funerals are particularly emotionally loaded because they are a time when these kinds of secrets often surface. By helping the family to openly discuss their hurt and anger, an issue very central, painful, and harmful to family functioning was defused and they could begin to support each other through the mourning process.

The Discussion of "Secrets" in Family Therapy with African American Families

Family therapists have been known to err in one of two directions in relationship to family secrets with African American families. One type of error involves opening up these secrets prematurely before a bond of trust has been established. The other type of error has often been made by well-meaning therapists who have been exposed to the cultural issues related to "dirty laundry." Some of these therapists have therefore been afraid to open up such issues for fear of "losing the family." Clearly, the key issue here is one of timing. It is essential that the therapist join with the family well so that a bond of trust can be formed. This creates an atmosphere in which even the most difficult issue can be raised. The therapist can then make a decision as to which "secrets" need to be opened and explored. This need for a careful joining with Black families is crucial to overcoming resistance and to successful treatment.

This chapter has explored the diverse extended family patterns and the role of informal adoptions that are so central to the lives of many African American families. Within these complex kinship networks, it is extremely important that roles be both flexible and clear. Sometimes, however, these roles can become blurred or confused. The next chapter will explore in detail the issue of role relationships in African American families.

4

Role Flexibility
and Boundary Confusion

Role relationships are very complex in many African American families, particularly those with an extended kinship system. This chapter explores different aspects of those roles, including (1) role flexibility, (2) the roles of fathers in African American families, (3) mothering roles in African American families, and (4) the grandmother role. While this role flexibility is clearly a strength in many families, it can lead to role confusion and boundary problems in some of the African American families who come for treatment. The last part of this chapter explores such problems as the "nonevolved" grandmother, the three-generational family, and the parental child.

ROLE FLEXIBILITY

There is a great deal of reciprocity and role flexibility within both nuclear and extended African American families. Hill (1972, 1999a) refers to this flexibility as the "adaptability of family roles." It was his work that described this flexibility as a source of "strength and stability." Because of the economic realities faced by many African American families, role flexibility developed as a survival mechanism. In order for both parents to work, Black women have sometimes had to act as the "father" and Black men as the "mother." The previous chapter has already established that other relatives such as grandmothers, grandfathers, aunts, uncles, cousins, and so on, may assume parental roles. In addition, when all of the adults are working, children are often required to assume "parental child" roles necessary for family survival (Minuchin, 1974; Nichols & Schwartz, 1998).

This role flexibility, while clearly a strength in many African American families, can sometimes result in role confusion or situations in which one individual becomes overburdened. The next section will discuss the roles of African American men as fathers. A more comprehensive discussion of the role of Black men in U.S. society, the "invisibility syndrome," and male–female relationships will be provided in Chapter 5.

AFRICAN AMERICAN MEN AS FATHERS

There is, of course, considerable variability in the responses of African American men to fatherhood—as there is in all ethnic groups. Some live in the home and are very active in childrearing; some live in the home but are peripheral to their children's lives; some are involved in their children's lives but live outside the home. Some acknowledge their children, some do not; some provide financial support, others do not. Despite this obvious variability, historically, there has been an assumption in the social science literature that the Black man is peripheral to the lives of his children (e.g., Moynihan, 1965, is an early example of this pattern). This image is somewhat misguided since it was based on a study of Black families on welfare, an economic situation in which the role of fathers could not be acknowledged lest the family jeopardize their welfare payments.

African American fathers are perhaps the most misunderstood group within Black families. In an earlier paper, a colleague and I (Hines & Boyd-Franklin, 1996) pointed out that although there is great variability in the role of the African American man as father and husband, the fact that his identity is tied to his ability to provide for his family in notably adverse economic circumstances could easily give rise to perceptions of Black men as non-family-oriented or uncaring.

> Black males have had the highest job loss rates in the labor force. When employed, the number engaged in managerial and professional jobs is relatively small. The essence of these realities is that Black males may have to expend great time and energy trying to provide the basic survival necessities for their families. This investment of Black fathers in providing for their families has been overlooked by those who stress peripheralness, or the absence of participation and interest on the part of Black fathers in daily family activities (e.g., Moynihan, 1965). (Hines & Boyd-Franklin, 1996, p. 69)

The next section examines in more depth the African American fathers who are peripheral and the ways in which Black families have attempted to compensate for this absence and provide support for growing children. It should be noted that many scholars who have studied African American families believe that the issue of peripheralness has been vastly overstated in the literature (Billingsley, 1992; Hill, 1999a; Hines & Boyd-Franklin, 1996).

In his careful review of the social science literature on this topic, John McAdoo (1981) found that the "exploration of the Black father's role in the socialization of his children is almost non-existent in social science literature" (p. 225). There is clear evidence that many Black men are involved in an egalitarian manner in childrearing, particularly in decision-making patterns (Billingsley, 1992; Hill, 1999a; Hines & Boyd-Franklin, 1996). Childrearing engagement patterns do reveal differences based on class and socioeconomic level, with middle-class fathers in both Black and White homes more involved in childrearing (McAdoo, 2002). Many of these Black, middle-income fathers were equally involved in raising their children and making decisions about their lives. They were traditional, however, in their childrearing values. Good behavior and respect were demanded of children. Children were expected to respond immediately to their fathers and angry temper tantrums were rarely allowed. Verbal nurturance was much more likely than hugs or kisses (McAdoo, 1981, 2002).

"Peripheral" African American Fathers

One possible family pattern is that of the "peripheral" African American father, who lives in the home but is not really involved in the family's daily life (Boyd-Franklin et al., 2001). This, of course, is also quite common in other ethnic groups where fathers are absorbed in their work or other interests and spend relatively little time with their wives and children. Some Black fathers are divorced or separated from their families and are not involved with them on a regular basis. Divorce and separation rates in this country have risen sharply in the last 30 years among all ethnic groups. There are many more single-parent families in the U.S. population as a whole. Although the number of African American single-parent families has risen along with that of the rest of the country's population, as Chapter 14 will indicate, it would be a serious error for a therapist to assume that because an African American father is not living in the home that he is not involved with his children.

The Father's Extended Family

In addition to the individuals who directly "raise" an African American child, there may be a number who only interact periodically but do so in a major way. A father may have little or no direct contact with his child, but the father's extended family, particularly his parents and his sisters, may be very involved in the child's kinship network. Because many of these individuals do not live in the home, families often forget to mention this contact. For many African American children, contact with a father's family maintains a tie to their father whom they may in fact never see. In divorce situations, many African American children have their visitation with their fathers in their paternal grandparents' home (see Chapter 6). The father's family, including parents, grandparents, aunts, uncles, sisters, brothers, and so on can also be approached by clinicians to help provide kinship care when child welfare authorities have moved to terminate the parents' parental rights (see Chapter 12).

Because of the cycle of unemployment in which many Black men are trapped, they are often unable to contribute financially to their children. Although her research is almost 30 years old, Stack's (1974) descriptions of these situations, in which the father has acknowledged his child, are still accurate and relevant:

> The community expects a father's kin to help out. The Black male who does not actively become a "daddy" but acknowledges a child and offers his kin to that child in effect is validating his rights. . . . By validating his claim as a parent, the father offers the child his blood relatives and their husbands and wives as the child's kin—an inheritance so to speak. (Stack, 1974, pp. 51–52)

We, as family therapists, must understand the fundamental nature of these subtle kinship bonds if we are to work effectively with the African American families who come to our clinics. Often when we inquire about relatives or draw a genogram (see Chapter 11) with an African American family, they may first tell us more about certain blood/nonblood ties or disclose certain other ties at this juncture. One must be aware of these patterns in order to know the correct questions to ask, and thus to locate other resources for the child and the family. This concept is significant particularly for the family therapists who work in clinics, community mental health centers, hospitals, schools, and social service agencies that provide services to poor Black families. Often, if a parent is hospitalized, becomes disabled, or is unable to care for her or his children, the children are quickly removed by social service agencies before a careful study is made of the blood and nonblood significant others who may be willing to offer kinship care for the children. Many families of children have been divided in different foster homes because no inquiry was made concerning possible supports from the father's extended family. Recent public policies have tried to remedy this injustice and encourage kinship care placements. There are, however, many discrepancies between the pay given to nonfamilial foster parents and the pittance provided for private kinship families through Temporary Assistance for Needy Families (TANF; Hill, 1999a). (Many states provide no support for these families at all. See Chapter 12 for a discussion of the public policies involved.)

Male Role Models in African American Families

The involvement of many extended family members—both blood and nonblood kin—in the rearing of African American children multiplies the number of potential role models (Hines & Boyd-Franklin, 1996; McAdoo, 1996, 2002). Unfortunately, many therapists are unaware of this wide range of individuals who are a potential resource for a child or for a family in trouble. These resources may come from the father's extended family or the mother's kin network, from close male friends of the mother, or from the "Church family." Often men who are involved with the mothers of these children become "play daddies" (men who serve in the role of "daddy," who are not biologically related), and are often seen as the person who raised them. Frequently such a man brings his own extended family into the relationship, who may then become a part of a child's kinship network. The following description of a family highlights both types of kinship support.

> Take my father, he ain't my daddy, he's no father to me. I ain't got but one daddy and that's Jason. The one who raised me. My kid's daddies, that's something else, all their daddies' people really take to them—they always doing things and making a fuss about them. We help each other out and that's what kinfolks are all about. (Stack, 1974, p. 45)

The support of these individuals is often overlooked by our clinics. When I was working on my doctorate at Columbia University, I was assigned a case of a young Black male child (age 12) who was acting out and aggressive. The clinic coordinator first assigned the case to me and then changed her mind. When I questioned her as to why, she answered that "since the child had no male role models," she felt that he and his family should be assigned to a male therapist. I asked her how she knew that he had no male role models, and she replied that he was living in a single-parent family. She had made an assumption based on the family's stated structure during their initial intake presentation about the availability of male role models.

I convinced her to allow me to treat this family. During the course of treatment, a number of male role models emerged who were utilized to help a very overburdened single-parent mother with a number of male children. These Black male role models included in this case the mother's boyfriend, her younger brother (age 20) who sometimes stayed with them, and the boy's maternal grandfather.

Involvement of African American Men in Family Therapy

Men, in general, are less responsive to treatment than women. African American men bring with them much of the suspicion discussed in Chapter 1 (Hines & Boyd-Franklin, 1996), in addition to a feeling of defensiveness about how the therapist may judge them in the fathering role. Given this reality, it is important that the therapist make a special effort to engage Black men directly in the treatment process. Chapters 5 and 11 describe many creative aspects of this engagement process.

My colleague and I (Hines & Boyd-Franklin, 1996) have described this process in detail:

It is important for therapists to involve fathers and other significant adult males in family treatment, although this may be difficult when fathers hold several jobs or cannot take off from work to participate in therapy sessions. Many African American men are also reluctant to enter therapy because they associate it with distrusted mainstream organizations. Therapists should explore signs of ambivalence and respond with creativity and flexibility. A father who is regarded as unavailable may come for an evening session or attend a single, problem-focused session (e.g., Hines, Richman, Maxim, and Hays, 1989). Therapists might use phone contacts and letters to keep fathers apprised of developments in their families' treatment. Recognizing fathers' family roles can decrease sabotaging; even limited involvement may lead to individual or family structural changes. (Hines & Boyd-Franklin, 1996, p. 69)

"MOTHERING" ROLES
IN AFRICAN AMERICAN FAMILIES

There are a vast range of role expectations for African American women depending on a number of issues, including their age, class, generation, marital status, and the question of whether or not they have children. Many different aspects of such concerns are discussed in other chapters of this book—for example, self-concept and skin-color issues in Chapter 2, and male/female role relationships in Chapter 5. In this chapter, the aspects of female role issues to be addressed surround the "mother" role in Black families. For most African American women, irrespective of the above differences, family is extremely important. Many Black women have numerous models within their extended families of strong, self-reliant women who have helped to keep the family together. The majority of African American women have always worked as well as raised their children. Therefore, many African American women grow up with models of mothers, grandmothers, and aunts who have served both roles in their families. Many Black women place an extremely high value on motherhood. I have repeatedly found in my work with Black women that no matter how problematic their early years may have been or how much they value their careers, they feel strongly about the need to raise children.

Motherhood, then, is a very important part of the role image of many African American women. It is, however, a complex, compounded image. Many Black women grow up with multigenerational models of "mother." Mothering is usually not an isolated activity but is shared with others. "Multiple mothering" is so common that many African American women who raise their children far away from the extended family create substitute "mothers," "grandmothers," and "babysitters."

There are also generational concerns involved in the consideration of the mothering role. Many older African American women (age 60 and over) have the expectation that they will always mother. They know that even if they are working, the well-being of their children often requires reciprocal help with babysitting and childcare.

Teenage Pregnancy and Young Motherhood

A number of scholars have discussed the role of young motherhood in African American families (Hill, 1999a; McAdoo, 2002; McAdoo & McAdoo, 1985; Stack, 1974; Tatum, Moseley, Boyd-Franklin, & Herzog, 1995). This phenomenon has implications in a number of areas, including feelings about single parenthood. Attitudes toward the care of out-of-wedlock children are quite different in Black and White populations. Studies conducted in the rural South show that the majority of Black children born out of wedlock are cared for and raised within the extended family network (Hill, 1977, 1999a). This pattern was very much the norm in the South but has undergone some changes in northern cities where foster care agencies have placed large numbers of these children. Attempts are now being made in many states to consider extended family or kinship care placements first (see Chapter 12).

The pattern of out-of-wedlock pregnancy among African American teenagers often creates a family dynamic that can lead to role and boundary conflicts as the child grows older. Stack (1974) gives an example of this process:

> A girl who gives birth as a teen-ager frequently does not raise and nurture her first born child. While she may share the same room and household with her baby, her mother, her mother's sister, or her older sister will care for the child and become the child's "mama." This same young woman may actively become a "mama" to a second child she gives birth to a year or two later. (p. 47)

We will explore in later chapters how the boundaries and roles can become confused in such families as the teenage mother becomes an adult and wants to assume parental responsibilities for her firstborn child. This child not only has a particular significant tie to another "mama," but may also be either designated as "special" or scapegoated by his or her other siblings because of it.

The Grandmother Role in African American Families

The role of the grandmother is one of the most central ones in African American families. It can also be one of the most complex and problematic. Grandmothers are frequently very central to the economic support of Black families and play a crucial role in childcare. Many African American children raised in informal adoption situations are raised by grandparents (Hill, 1977, 1999a; Hines & Boyd-Franklin, 1996). They represent a major source of strength and security for many Black children.

One of the reasons for the complex nature of the role of grandmothers, however, has to do with the fact that in some African American families this role has never fully evolved or takes an extra generation to evolve. For example, if a young teenager becomes pregnant and has a baby, that infant is often raised as if it was a sibling of her mother. The biological grandmother often becomes "Mama" or "Big Mama" to the child and the biological mother is called by her first name as if she were a sibling of the child. The grandmother assumes the mothering role and does not experience any of the often advantageous situational characteristics of being a grandmother.

The process becomes more complex as the family matures and the child grows older. As the biological mother becomes an adult, she may want to take on the task of mothering her child. This transition is very complicated because to do this she must (1) displace her own mother, (2) change her family's perception of her as a sibling, and (3) change her child's and her mother's perception of her mothering role.

To further complicate this process, often there are multigenerational issues involved in the young mother's attempts to validate her role as mother. In many of these families, the biological mother may not have been raised by her own mother but by her grandmother (Tatum et al., 1995). Therefore her mother has never had a real chance to mother and is delighted to have the chance to "mother" her grandchild. Some grandmothers in African American families are in fact fairly young women (age 35–48) who had their own children in their teenage years and were also raised as siblings to their children, a situation that Colon (1980) has described as "the nonevolved grandmother." The role confusion that can result is a common treatment issue for many African American families and extended families.

ROLE CONFUSION IN AFRICAN AMERICAN FAMILIES AND ITS THERAPEUTIC IMPLICATIONS

While role flexibility is clearly a strength in many African American families, the extended family structure is one that is particularly vulnerable to boundary (Minuchin, 1974) and role confusion. This occurs in many different forms. The next section explores three of the most common forms of this type of confusion—the nonevolved grandmother, the three-generational family, and the parental child—as well as their therapeutic implications and interventions designed to restructure such family systems.

The Nonevolved Grandmother

The presence of a nonevolved grandmother in a family frequently results in issues of role confusion. First, this structure goes counter to the notion in mainstream U.S. society of a mother and father in charge of raising children. Second, the roles are constantly evolving and changing as individuals mature and grow. Third, the grandmother role in many African American families is particularly susceptible to role overload or burnout.

The fact that this role goes counter to many of the expectations of society has an impact on family life, particularly as a child reaches school age. Schools expect a "mother" to appear to register a child and sign important papers. This is also still true of many of our clinics and community mental health centers. Thus, in many situations, the primary caretaker, that is, the grandmother, is forced to take a backseat while the mother presents herself to the outside world. This is often very true for hospital or medical care. Pediatricians and therapists taking developmental histories often report that such "mothers" don't seem to remember their children's developmental milestones or give totally unrealistic ones. This is a very strong signal that the mother probably was not the child's primary caretaker at an early age and that she may not be the primary caretaker at this time.

In many of these extended families, the grandmother remains a major power in the family even if the mother presents herself as the primary caretaker of the child. Often it is the grandmother who really makes the important decisions in a child's life, including whether or not he or she should receive therapy.

The second aspect of this role confusion has to do with the developmental life cycle of such families. In any family, as people grow and mature, roles change. Families often experience difficulties at particular modal points or life-cycle junctures where roles may be changing (Carter & McGoldrick 1999; Hines, 1999). For example, this model may work very well when a young 14- or 15-year-old teenager has a baby. When that mother is 30 and her child is 15, she may want to take on more responsibility but may find that neither her mother nor her child will accept a redefinition of her role.

This life cycle is further complicated by the role of the "elderly" in African American families. Particularly in poor African American families, older individuals often experience an increase rather than a decrease in responsibility in later life:

> In contrast to middle-class families, this phase of the life cycle does not signify retirement or a lessening of daily responsibilities for poor African Americans. Many continue working to make ends meet in spite of poor health. Even when they do retire, it is unlikely they will have "empty nests." Instead, they are likely to be active members of expanding households and family systems, frequently providing care to grandchildren, adult children, and other elderly kin. (Hines, 1999, p. 338)

This grandmother or great-grandmother then becomes overly central and is a candidate for system overload and burnout. Often these women present at our clinics as profoundly depressed individuals, or their grandchildren begin to act out or to develop other symptoms in order to get help for this overburdened family system.

This overburdening of a central family member can have quite an effect on the lives of the entire extended family, from exacerbating the harsh exigencies of poverty to embroiling the family at all levels in a conflict of role-related issues (Hines, 1988). The relevance of this issue to the process of family therapy with Black extended families can hardly be overstated, involving as it does a phenomenon that can reverberate profoundly throughout the family structure:

> The active, daily involvement of multigenerational households magnifies the interplay of their own life phase task with the life stage concerns of other family members who can span three to four generations; thus, intergenerational conflicts have a high probability of arising. Reality demands that the aged assume meaningful roles, the therapeutic task is helping them to be useful without overfunctioning. Family therapy facilitated a shift towards new options that freed the multigenerational family to proceed with their intertwined lives without repetition of serious emotional patterns that led to triangling and dysfunction of younger family members. (Hines, 1988, p. 531)

Life-cycle demands of African American families thus are often complex and overwhelming. The therapeutic task is to help derailed families get back on track and proceed with life-cycle issues appropriate to each family member. In some extended families where these roles have never evolved, the therapist's task is to help the family construct that track and build the structures by clarifying the roles and boundaries that will allow them to grow and thus to move forward with their lives.

The Three-Generational Family

As we have seen in the three-generational family described above, frequently familial roles become blurred: the mother of a female adolescent with a baby never fully becomes a grandmother, while her daughter is never allowed to fully function as a mother to her own child. Minuchin (1974) has developed a structural approach to working with these families. The goal of this approach in these situations is to help the grandmother support her daughter in learning to be an effective parent, and to help both mother and grandmother to negotiate a new "alliance of executives" in which they begin to share parenting responsibilities. Thus, the family is restructured so that the child can be given clear signals and messages by both mother and grandmother.

In African American families, many other family members may also participate in childrearing. One child may respond to an executive system that includes mothers, fathers, stepparents, aunts, uncles, grandmothers, grandfathers, and/or older siblings. The structural approach is extremely useful in these cases because, as with the scenario created by the nonevolved grandmother, intervention can occur along direct, practical lines. Contact is made with the key members of this executive group. They can then be brought together to discuss the problem at hand and to clarify who is in charge of various family functions. In African American families that are functioning well, these boundaries are clear no matter how many adults are involved. In the families that appear at our clinics, however, role boundaries and thus the functional family structure have broken down and need to be redetermined and rebuilt. In many cases, a functional structure has never fully developed and needs to be built for the first time.

The following case example illustrates the latter process.

Clarence (age 12) was referred for treatment by the principal of the Catholic school he attended because of acting-out behavior. His grandmother, Mrs. Long, a 60-year-old African American woman, brought him for his first clinic appointment. She explained that his mother, Margaret Long (age 27), was at work. The grandmother herself worked half-time as a school aide at a local public school.

Margaret Long had given birth to her son Clarence when she was 15 years old. He was raised with her and her siblings. Her mother essentially functioned as his mother. Mrs. Long was a strong, domineering woman who held a great deal of power in her family. It was clear that both her grandson and her daughter were afraid to cross her. The therapist learned this quickly when he asked Mrs. Long to bring in her daughter for a session. Mrs. Long was adamant that this was impossible because of her work schedule. She further stated, "It's not necessary because I raised Clarence. I can tell you everything important." Clarence's relationship with his grandmother was a very difficult one. She reported with pride that she had always been strict with him at home but that he "didn't listen to anyone at school." The therapist joined and worked with the grandmother and Clarence for two sessions, coming up with a number of strategies that required Clarence to discuss his response to school officials with his grandmother.

When Clarence was placed on probation, the therapist moved quickly. He utilized the "crisis" situation in order to push the issue of the mother's participation. He told the grandmother that this was such a serious crisis that he would personally call the mother at work and make arrangements for her to attend the family meeting. When the mother appeared, it was clear that she felt very overwhelmed by her mother and very resentful of her. In fact, Margaret Long's posture in the session was a mirror of her son's. At a number of points when the grandmother became angry and shouted at Clarence, he and his mother exchanged glances and at one point rolled their eyes. Mrs. Long became furious and yelled at both. It was clear that both Clarence and his mother were being treated and responding as siblings. The therapist pointed this out to both the grandmother and the mother, stressing that this was a serious crisis for Clarence and that unless the grandmother and mother were able to work together, Clarence would continue to act out. The therapist moved Clarence out of the discussion and focused the grandmother and the mother on (1) the consequences for Clarence's behavior and (2) a strategy whereby the whole family and the therapist could meet together with the school officials. He made it very clear that they needed to work closely in that meeting if they were going to present a united front to Clarence and to the school.

The school interview was very successful and Clarence was reinstated in school with a clear understanding of the consequences if his disruptive behavior continued. After this interview, the therapist was able to get a contract with both mother and grandmother for ongoing involvement in the treatment process. He began to restructure the family by exploring ways in which the mother could work more closely with the grandmother in caring for Clarence. The grandmother was gradually able to help the mother assume more disciplinary responsibility for Clarence.

It is interesting that in this family, as in many Black families, the therapist was never able to put the mother in charge. He was, however, able to renegotiate an alliance of executives between the mother and the grandmother that allowed both to work together in parenting Clarence. As the rules and the family roles became more clear, Clarence's behavior improved significantly.

The Parental Child

In his classic work *Families and Family Therapy,* Minuchin (1974) examined the role of the "parental child," a role that is extremely common in African American families. With the advent of working mothers in the population at large and the increasing number of latchkey children in the United States today, the parental child has begun to appear more frequently in other cultural groups as well. Because of the economic instability that African American families have experienced in this country, the need for all members of the household to contribute in some way to the family's support is and always has been a very pressing reality. Therefore, with all available adults in a family working, responsibility for care of younger children often falls on the oldest child, placing that child in a parental role. In African American families, this role can be filled by a male or by a female child—this differs from the situation in Hispanic families where the role is usually taken by the oldest female child. In functional African American families where this role works well, the parent or parental figures delegate to this child certain responsibilities for the care of younger children when the parent is not at home. Here the boundaries of the child's or adolescent's responsibilities are clear and well defined: parental responsibilities are delegated and not abdicated; the parent is careful to remain "in charge" and to have the parental child report to her or him. It is important to stress that the parental child structure is most often not a family structure of choice but arises out of economic necessity.

The parental child family structure becomes dysfunctional when the parent or parents abdicate their responsibilities and place an unreasonable responsibility on the child in this position. This frequently occurs in African American single-parent families in which the mother becomes so overburdened that she begins to overrely on her "right-hand man (or woman)." The parental child may then become the "parent" to his or her own parent, so that the structure is maintained at the cost of the child's normal, age-appropriate thrust toward interaction with his or her peer group, and the mother is cut off from interaction with her other children.

The therapeutic goal in such situations to "realign the family in such a way that the parental child can still help the mother. . . . The parental child has to be returned to the sibling subgroup, though he maintains his position of leadership and junior executive power" (Minuchin, 1974, p. 98).

In summary, it is the therapeutic task to recognize and support the strength and stability that role flexibility has provided in many African American families without perpetuating the role confusion to which the extended family system is particularly vulnerable. The next chapter explores other aspects of gender roles in African American families and their implications for male–female relationships and couples in therapy.

5

African American Men and Women

Socialization and Relationships[*]

Racism and sexism have placed a burden on African American gender roles and male–female relationships that couples and families from many cultures do not experience (Boyd-Franklin & Franklin, 1998; Kelly, 2003). The United States's history of slavery has had a long-term impact on the gender roles of African American men and women who were treated like chattel under this system (see Chapter 1). Many of the gender stereotypes of inferiority prevalent in that period have persisted and continue to influence the ways in which Black men and women are viewed and treated by White society. Sadly, some of these stereotypes have also been internalized and continue to affect the couple and family relationships of some African Americans.

Gender roles in African American couples and families are often confusing to therapists from other racial and cultural groups. They make a serious error when they assume that such roles and relationships in Black families are equivalent to those in their own group. Racism has contributed to the oppression of both African American men and women in the United States (Boyd-Franklin & Franklin, 1998; Jones, 1997). Because Black men are so strongly oppressed by society and do not have the power held by their White counterparts, gender roles may differ in some African American families from that of other racial and ethnic groups (Boyd-Franklin & Franklin, 1998).

In order to give therapists a greater understanding of this complexity, this chapter is divided into two main sections. The first part explores the impact of

[*]I would like to acknowledge the contribution of several colleagues to this chapter: Rozetta Wilmore-Schaeffer, Anderson J. Franklin, and Charles E. Smith.

racism and the "invisibility syndrome" on the gender roles of African American men and women. It addresses their impact on the socialization practices in raising sons and daughters in African American families. The often conflicting and contradictory gender messages regarding male–female relationships are discussed. Current statistics on African American couples, particularly those related to the shortage of Black men and unemployment, are presented. A discussion of the influence of racism and sexism on African American male–female relationships completes the first part of the chapter. Case examples illustrate the ways in which clinicians can address the strain that racism and African American male unemployment can place on a relationship or a marriage.

The couple relationship is an extremely important subsystem in the treatment of any family. It is the nucleus of the family. Many clinicians, however, have not been trained to accord such relationships their proper importance in the treatment of African American families, particularly when the man is not married to the mother. (See Chapter 11 on the role of the "hidden boyfriend" in many single-parent families.). Unfortunately, because African American men are often treated as if they are "invisible" (Franklin, 1993, 1999, in press) by the mental health system, these dynamics are frequently overlooked by practitioners working with Black families.

The second part of this chapter explores the specific issues, problems, and needs that African American couples present in treatment. It addresses a number of questions that have an impact on the therapeutic process: What are the specific issues and concerns that prompt an African American couple to enter treatment? Do traditional techniques in couple therapy need to be modified in order to successfully address the problems presented by this population? For example, clinicians who work with this population have emphasized the difficulty therapists encounter when trying to engage African American couples in therapy. However, the factors that directly or indirectly maintain this "wall of resistance"—family-of-origin issues, the insidious effects of racism, socioeconomic realities, the dynamics of power, and so on—are often not articulated. These issues will be explored in the second part of this chapter.

THE IMPACT OF RACISM ON THE GENDER ROLES OF AFRICAN AMERICAN MEN AND WOMEN

African American Men and the "Invisibility Syndrome"

The issues of racism discussed in Chapters 1 and 2 are particularly relevant when exploring the roles of African American men in society and in their families. Many stereotypes that are a legacy of slavery and oppression are imposed on Black men (Franklin, 1992; Gary, 1981; Grier & Cobbs, 1968), including assumptions that they are "lazy," "peripheral," or "unavailable." High Black unemployment rates play into this stereotype, and cause many individuals in U.S. society to adopt a "blaming the victim" view. This perception, however, ignores the discrimination within the job market that often allows little access to jobs for poor African American men. Despite the gains of recent years, Black men are still unemployed in large numbers.

African American men have often described blatant examples of the discrimination they experience. Their mere presence may invoke fear in some White individuals. Franklin (in press) described the experience of a young, casually dressed African American man, the sight of whom so frightened two White women that they refused to get into the elevator they were waiting for as soon as he got on. In another situation, an African American vice-president of a bank, dressed in a business suit, tried to hail a cab after a meeting, and watched cab after cab pick up White passengers and ignore him. Franklin (in press) has called this the "invisibility syndrome," a paradoxical process in which African American men, because of their high visibility, are perceived with fear and distrust and are often ignored or avoided by White society. This can lead to a feeling of "invisibility." This fear, avoidance, and anger, often directed at African American men as a result of racism, can have a devastating impact on their self-esteem. It can also influence their ability to function in the workplace, as a lover or a spouse, and as a father.

African American Women: A Different Kind of Invisibility

African American women have to cope with all of the life stressors that other women face in addition to the chronic and insidious stressor of racism, which is a part of the daily lives of many African Americans (Greene, 1994; Jackson & Greene, 2000).

Racism and sexism have historically combined to produce a "double jeopardy" for African American women. These two forces have reinforced a number of stereotypes, which began during slavery and persist, particularly through media images. Greene (1994) and hooks (1981) have listed a number of these societal stereotypes in which African American women are viewed by White society as "sexually promiscuous, sexually aggressive, morally loose, independent, strong and assertive when compared to white women" (Greene, 1994, p. 16). The other major stereotype, also a demeaning part of the slavery legacy, has been the image of the Black woman as the "mammy," the substitute mother or caregiver of White children. The strength and assertiveness of African American women has been viewed as "not feminine" and pathologized by White patriarchal culture (Hill-Collins, 1991).

Racist demeaning messages about African American women's intelligence, ability, and beauty have been perpetuated through the media, hiphop and rap music and videos, schools, and, sadly, through some women's own families to the present day (Boyd-Franklin & Franklin, 1998; Greene, 1994; hooks, 1981, 1993; Jackson & Greene, 2000). Boyd-Franklin and Franklin (1998) address the ways in which society's devaluation of African American women rendered them, through different mechanisms, as "invisible" as Black men:

The femininity and beauty of Black women have historically been denied in a society that imposes White features as the standards against which all are judged. In
recent years, these standards have eased somewhat, but nevertheless the complex
interplay of skin color, hair texture, body type, and the negative messages from society (as well as internalized racism and sexism) continue to cause many African
American women a great deal of pain and anger. (p. 271)

These issues often manifest in the treatment of African American women in
individual, family, and group therapy sessions once trust has been established
with the therapist (see Chapter 2).

Popular culture, such as movies and music, have also contributed misogy-
nist messages about Black women (Beatty, 2002). Wyatt (1997) describes the
ways in which aggressive and sexual depictions of African American women
perpetuate existing stereotypes and may be used to justify violence against
them (Beatty, 2002).

The Socialization of African American Male and Female Children

Raising African American Sons

Clinicians need to be aware of how the experiences of racism and the "invisibility syndrome" discussed above have influenced the ways in which African
American families raise their male children. Many African American parents
express a great deal of fear for their children, particularly their sons, who are
often viewed as an endangered group (Boyd-Franklin et al., 2001; Kunjufu,
1985; White & Cones, 1999). This concern over basic survival issues for their
sons transcends class and socioeconomic levels.

From the time their children are very young, African American parents
are aware that they may be unfairly labeled in the school system and tracked
into special education classes. Kunjufu (1985) documented the ways in which
eager young African American males are often mislabeled as "aggressive" or
"hyperactive." He described a "fourth grade failure syndrome" in which the
combination of racism, low teacher expectations, and fear of young Black
males can influence teachers' treatment of them and lead to their school failure. Boyd-Franklin et al. (2001) have discussed ways in which parents and concerned others can be proactive in monitoring children's experiences in school.

African American parents are also conscious of the various factors that
can prevent Black males from reaching adulthood, such as racial profiling,
DWB ("driving while Black"), police brutality, discrimination, Black-on-
Black crime, and gang violence. The leading cause of death for African American males between the ages of 13 and 25 is homicide. Boyd-Franklin et al.
(2001) have described strategies therapists can use to help parents to prepare
their children for these threats to their survival. It is also important for therapists to stress the importance of positive male role models for Black male chil-

dren and to help parents, particularly single mothers, to find positive male role models in their extended families and in the community for their sons and daughters.

Raising African American Daughters

So much attention has been paid in the national media and in the Black community itself to the plight of African American males that the challenges facing Black girls are in danger of being overlooked by clinicians. Many Black families work to instill a strong sense of racial identity and pride in their boys and girls. Children of both genders are loved and valued in African American families. Racism affects both male and female children. These families are aware, however, that their male children are particularly at risk or endangered in society, as discussed above.

In an attempt to compensate for these threats against African American males from birth to old age, some African American families have socialized their sons and daughters very differently. White therapists often misunderstand the reasons for such disparate treatment, exemplified by the saying in some African American families that they "raise their daughters and love their sons." As Boyd-Franklin and Franklin (1998) have stated, this saying "does not imply that African American families do not love their daughters, but rather that they often try to compensate for the intense discrimination against Black males in society by attempting to protect them within the family" (p. 272).

However ameliorative the intention, the dissimilar parenting between sons and daughters contributes to the often sexist, victimizing, and contradictory messages that Black men and women receive and has had consequences for African American couples. "It has contributed greatly to the rage and pain that subsequent generations of African American women feel about male attitudes toward an equal partnership in a relationship" (Boyd-Franklin & Franklin, 1998, p. 272).

Education has always been strongly emphasized for girls and boys. African American parents are aware that they must be vigilant in terms of the messages that schools and the members of the peer group give to their daughters. Many African American families have raised their daughters to be fiercely loyal, interdependent with the family, independent, assertive, and strong. This can lead to conflicts with teachers, who often feel offended or threatened by the assertiveness and outspokenness that are common characteristics of African American girls. As with Black boys, Black girls often receive demeaning messages about their academic abilities from teachers and other school officials.

African American mothers and their daughters typically share a special bond that involves preparing them for womanhood and for the tasks of "surviving, coping, and succeeding in a hostile environment, while fostering family and community loyalty" (Cauce et al., 1996, p. 101). Hill-Collins (1991) has discussed the ways in which African American mothers serve as role models for their daughters and help to shape their sex-role behavior within an Afrocentric model that prioritizes the survival of the family.

Gender Messages in the Socialization Process Regarding Male–Female Relationships

The Socialization of African American Women in Terms of Gender Roles

For an African American woman, the area of male–female relationships becomes a loaded issue early in her socialization experience. A Black female adolescent absorbs a great deal of information about gender differentiation and women's roles from observation of various female role models in her life. Many African American women report that since they saw their mothers, aunts, and grandmothers as extremely competent women who both raised children and worked, they learned self-reliance and a belief in their own strengths and abilities based on the saying "God bless the child who's got her own." They were encouraged to get an education, a job, and to be able to provide for themselves and their families.

Although there is a great deal of variability in male–female role models in the Black community, the types of relationships that African American women in treatment have described based on their observations of their mothers' relationships with men fall into one of the following six categories: (1) father absent, (2) transient male relationships, (3) weak or dysfunctional father, (4) egalitarian marriage, (5) strong or authoritarian father, or (6) abusive male–female relationship. The type of male–female interaction pattern observed by the girl in her early socialization years clearly has an impact on her choice of men and her expectations for her own relationships. For example, African American women whose fathers were absent often report one of two experiences. Either their mothers avoided male relationships and became very involved in childrearing, family, work, and church activities or they became involved in a series of transient relationships with men during the early years of the young girl's life. Either situation might help convey to a young Black girl the sentiment that "Black men are no good" or that "they won't be there for you when you need them." Many African American women grow up with this expectation from an early age and have no experience of positive male–female relational role models. African American women whom I have treated who have had this type of early experience frequently report that they do not know how to have a positive relationship with a man.

A variation on this theme is a situation in some Black families in which the man may be somewhat weak or dysfunctional. This is clearly a continuum and can include many different kinds of experiences. On one end of the continuum one might encounter a weak, "hen-pecked" African American man who brings home his paycheck every week to a domineering wife. At the other end, one may encounter a man with alcoholism or drug addiction who has little or no ability to provide for his family. Because "last hired, first fired" policies are widespread in jobs with significant African American participation, it is not uncommon for many African American men to face chronic unemployment problems. Since this places the burden of providing on the mother, her daughters learn from a very early age not to depend on a man for financial support.

Many African American women were raised in two-parent homes by parents who had an egalitarian marriage pattern, that is, they shared power, decision making, and role responsibilities. These women often have a very realistic sense of the balance between communication, conflict resolution, and affection in a relationship. There are a number of variations on these roles, some of which are related to class differences. Many African American women who had grown up in poor, working-class, or newly middle-class families had mothers who worked. Their role as breadwinners gave them an important position in the family. A smaller number of women grew up in more middle-class homes and had mothers who raised the children and were primarily homemakers. Some of these women reported that their mothers were more dependent on their fathers. This type of relationship is often represented by the fifth category, that is, by a strong, authoritarian father. Many African American women raised in this situation identified with their fathers and became more aggressive and assertive. Others, however, clearly identified with their mothers and were often weak and submissive in their relationships with men. They expected domination and dismissed men who did not have this quality as "weak."

As in all ethnic groups, some African American women are raised in abusive homes in which there is a history of violent confrontations and physical and verbal abuse between the parents and often toward the children. These women are at particular risk for re-creating this pattern and becoming battered women as adults and/or becoming abusive toward their own children.

It is extremely important to know what the socialization experience of each member of the couple has been because these patterns are often re-created within the couple dynamic.

The Socialization of African American Men on Gender Roles

The legacy of racism and discrimination has had many effects on the socialization of African American men. Black mothers, acutely aware of this history, often attempt to protect their sons by giving them the message, "Be strong but not too strong or you will be cut down." The lesson of a Malcolm X or a Martin Luther King Jr. can sometimes be interpreted to mean that if you are too much of a threat to the powers that be, you will be killed.

On the other hand, one cannot underestimate the sociocultural impact of the Black "macho" role. This is particularly true in inner-city environments.

Young boys are taught that in order to survive and protect themselves on the streets they cannot show "weakness." The message to "act bad even if you're scared" is a clear one. If a young Black man "acts weak," he will be ostracized by his peer group. It is not an uncommon experience in early childhood that if a young child falls down and his mother runs to soothe him, his father and the older male members of the family will stop her and say, "Come on, boy, get up, you're okay."

Boyd-Franklin and Franklin (1998) have further addressed the need to hide any emotions that may be perceived as weakness: "Above all, many Black males learn that they must be 'cool'—that they must don a mask of utmost composure, no matter what is happening in their inner emotional worlds (Majors & Billson, 1992). These mixed messages create a 'double bind' for African American men as well" (Boyd-Franklin & Franklin, 1998, p. 272).

This becomes more complicated as a young boy enters adolescence and begins to establish his sexual identity. For some African American men who have been denied opportunities for educational and occupational advancement, the sexual arena becomes one of the few areas in life in which they can show their prowess and strength. Teenage boys are taught to "score" with women sexually. This concept, while it is certainly present in other ethnic groups, takes on a particular meaning for many young African American men because it is one of the few areas in which society allows them to "achieve."

All of these issues—the impact of racial discrimination, the fear of showing weakness, and the need to demonstrate sexual prowess—have weighty implications for intimate couple relationships between Black men and women.

Many African American men and women today have to cope on a daily basis with the impact of discrimination on their lives. It may be felt in the reality of the substandard housing in which they live or in the survival pressure of constant financial burdens. Since many Black families are at the mercy of urban school systems, mothers' and fathers' fears that their children will get trapped in a similar cycle are overwhelming. Even African American men and women who have managed to escape the oppressive grip of poverty and enter the middle class face subtle and overt forms of discrimination on their jobs and in their more integrated communities. These more subtle forms of racial bias can be just as deadly as the more overt forms. Such cumulative pressures on the psyche of Black people take their toll on couple relationships. Some African American women and men experience a sense of powerlessness in their interactions with the world that they angrily act out in their intimate relationships. Often a man or a woman who feels powerless in the outer world will make extreme attempts to control a loved one or spouse, making power and control issues major dynamics in many African American couple relationships. While these dynamics are often played out in the realms of finances, decision making, and other control issues, the therapist treating such couples must be aware of the complexity of other underlying dynamics.

The socialization factors that prevent African American men from showing weakness have clear implications for intimate couple dynamics. For example, a Black man who has been taught from an early age to control hurt and pain will have a very difficult time expressing those emotions to his mate. A Black man who has been taught that he can never admit that he has failed will have a very difficult time asking for the support of his mate in sharing the pressures of the outside world.

In couple dynamics, these underlying issues often present in treatment as a "lack of communication." It is common in most ethnic groups for women to report in couple therapy that their men can't "talk about their feelings." However, this lack of communicational ability is an extremely loaded issue for many African American couples because it runs directly counter to the often excessively defensive character of the socialization of many African American men. Black women rely on the support system of other women in their lives and are socialized to share feelings about relationships at least with each other. Some of these women have no experience of sharing feelings with a man in an intimate relationship and no positive role models for males in male–female relationships. Many African American women experience extreme frustration with this lack of expressiveness in their partners.

The impact on couple relationships of some Black males' need to demonstrate sexual prowess and power in relationships has many implications for the treatment of African American couples. It has implications for male–female relationships in general, particularly on the issue of fidelity. Some Black women have been socialized not to expect fidelity from a man. Others have encountered repeated experiences of infidelity, which can lead to the end of their relationships.

The couple therapist, in exploring the meaning of fidelity in a relationship, needs to be aware that it may have many different levels of meaning for African American couples. For example, since many Black men feel beaten down by their experiences in the White world, sexual prowess becomes a way to reassert their manhood and regain their pride. Extramarital or extrarelational affairs may have more to do with these burdens and less to do with the failure of their primary relationship. In such situations, the ability of the therapist to open up channels of communication about such emotionally charged areas as pride, vulnerability, and the pressures and demands facing each person can have a significant impact on a man's ability to gain respect for his manhood from his partner.

The Impact of Racism and Sexism on Couple Relationships

Boyd–Franklin and Franklin (1998) have addressed the ways in which complicated, contradictory, and often paradoxical gender roles can result from the interweaving of racism and sexism. They state that "a therapist must challenge obvious sexist behavior in a couple's relationship, but must also consider how racism may have contributed to the experience of a power imbalance in the home. When a man feels dehumanized, he may assert his power in sexist ways in order to compensate" (p. 273). Unfortunately, some African American women experience oppression and sexism from both White society and in their own relationships with Black men. Poussaint's (1993) observation encapsulates the uniquely devastating effect racism has had on relationships among African American men and women: "Although both Black men and women are victims in America, they are still victimizing each other. We have to stop inflicting more pain on each other by tearing each other apart" (p. 88). (Clinical case material will be used to illustrate these dilemmas in treatment later in this chapter.)

Research on African American Male–Female Relationships and Couples

A review of the literature on African American couples reveals a number of trends that are important for clinicians to understand if they are to do effective work with Black families. One of the most important is the decline in marriage rates among African Americans (Taylor, Jackson, & Chatters, 1997; Tucker & Mitchell-Kernan, 1995). Taylor, Tucker, Chatters, and Jayakody (1997) have shown that although the number of unmarried individuals has increased for both Blacks and Whites, the numbers are particularly striking for African Americans. They state:

> In 1993, 61% of black women and 58% of black men were not currently married, compared with 41% of white women and 38% of white men. Among black adults, a great proportion of the decline in marriage occurred because of a dramatic increase in the proportion of never marrieds. In 1993, 46% of black men and 39% of black women had never married. Among whites, however the increase in the proportion of unmarried adults was the result of increases in divorce and declines in remarriage. (p. 48)

A number of researchers have also noted that the marriage gap between Blacks and Whites is evident whether or not the woman has children (McLanahan & Casper, 1995; Taylor et al., 1997). McLanahan and Casper (1995) reported that White women are twice as likely as Black women to be married irrespective of their childbearing status.

Tucker and Mitchell-Kernan (1995) and Taylor et al. (1997) have identified the shortage of Black men and the high unemployment rates among African American men as the most important reasons for the decline in marriage rates and the rise in African American single-parent families.

The Shortage of Black Men

No issue is more emotionally laden in the African American community, particularly among single women, than the shortage of Black men due to an imbalance in the sex ratio in Black communities (Kelly, 2003; Kiecolt & Fossett, 1995; Orbuch, Veroff, & Hunter, 1999; Taylor et al., 1997). This imbalance has been attributed to higher mortality rates for Black men occurring across the entire life cycle (Stockard & Tucker, 2001); imprisonment, which is particularly striking in the younger age group, where "one in every three Black men in his 20s is either incarcerated, on parole, or on probation" (Stockard & Tucker, 2001, p. 143); and drug abuse among Black men in their 20s through their 50s (Kelly, 2003; Kiecolt & Fossett, 1995; Lawson & Thompson, 1994).

Stockard and Tucker (2001), after analyzing the March 2000 Current Population Survey, reported that in the 15- through 34-year-old age group, African American men number just over 5 million, while Black women number approximately 5.7 million. The African American young adult population is 46% male and 54% female (Stockard & Tucker, 2001). African American women have higher rates of graduation from college than African American men, who are increasingly dropping out of school, which only adds to high unemployment rates for Black men.

For many African American women, with and without children, the shortage of Black men is a major issue discussed in treatment. Some African American women are pessimistic about their chances of ever marrying, especially when some members of the older female generation of their families have been unable to model lasting relationships (Tucker & Mitchell-Kernan, 1995). The despair of some African American women that they may never find viable marriage partners has led them to have children alone, with a consequent increase in the number of single-parent Black families. In addition, I have seen a growing trend in my own practice of educated and professional African American women choosing to have a child on their own or to adopt one, particularly as they approach their late 30s and early 40s. Because of the shortage of African American men, some of these women have chosen to marry men who have less education and who hold blue collar jobs. Still others have formed cross-racial relationships, often with some ambivalence (Cose, 2003). (This and other clinical implications of the shortage of Black men will be discussed below in the "Common Issues" section of this chapter.)

The shortage of Black men can cause some Black women to stay in very destructive relationships. When this occurs, the therapist should never collude to use racism as an excuse for this behavior. Violence and use of power domination in a relationship can never be condoned. The following case (from Boyd-Franklin & Franklin, 1998) demonstrates the interaction among racism, sexism, and domestic violence.

Laura (age 41), a school aide, and Arthur (age 38), a janitor, were an African American couple who came into treatment after living together for a year. Laura had a child, Keena (age 9), from an earlier relationship. She had been celibate between the time of her daughter's birth and the relationship with Arthur. The initial presenting problem was Keena's misbehavior, which had begun the year before, when Arthur moved into their home.

After a few sessions focused on Keena's behavior (which improved significantly), the work became more concentrated on the couple. In a family session, Keena had expressed concern about the angry outbursts between her mother and Arthur. Laura and Arthur were seen alone for a number of sessions to work on these issues. Arthur frequently arrived late or missed sessions and eventually stopped coming entirely.

When Laura became pregnant with his child, Arthur's angry outbursts escalated, and he became violent toward her. He accused her of having become pregnant to "trap" him. Laura insisted that he leave her home. In subsequent sessions, Laura revealed that Arthur had told her early in their relationship that he had badly beaten an earlier girlfriend when she had tried to "force a child on him." She excused his behavior by telling the therapist that he was a Black man who had lived a very tough life. She also told the therapist (a Black woman) that at least he had a job and was trying. She had been alone for almost 9 years since Keena's birth and she was very aware of the shortage of Black men. The therapist explored with Laura how she was using racism and the shortage of Black men as excuses for his abuse of her. She told the therapist that she couldn't bear to be another "Black woman statistic" alone raising her kids.

Within several weeks, Arthur apologetically begged to return home. He refused to return for therapy, and Laura dropped out of treatment. The therapist, worried about the outcome for this family, contacted both of them a number of times to no avail.

After a year, Laura called the therapist in great distress to report that she had thrown Arthur out again after he threatened to beat Keena. She came in for a session with her daughter. Laura revealed a multigenerational history of battered women in her family of origin; in fact, her mother had encouraged her to return to Arthur. Concerned that Laura would go back to Arthur or fall into another abusive relationship, the therapist invited Laura to join a support group for African American women that the therapist also conducted. Laura learned in the group that she had a right to be treated with respect and that she did not need a relationship with a man to complete her life. The group members were able to acknowledge the role of racism, but challenged Laura's using it to excuse Arthur's abuse. Laura's story led the other women to explore times in which they had stayed in abusive situations and justified staying for these reasons. (Boyd-Franklin & Franklin, 1998, pp. 277–278)

As Boyd-Franklin and Franklin (1998) have stated, "This example provides us with a look at the complexity of racism and sexism in the lives of Black men and women. Laura had internalized sexist messages that this relationship was all that she deserved. This was compounded by multigenerational messages from her own mother. On the other hand, racism was used as an excuse for his treatment of her. Both racism and sexism must be addressed if the domestic violence in a relationship such as this is to end" (p. 278).

The Impact of Black Male Employment and Unemployment

The rates of employment and unemployment among African American males have greatly influenced their willingness to marry (Testa & Krogh, 1995; Tucker & Mitchell-Kernan, 1995). Testa and Krogh (1995) have shown that Black men who are employed are twice as likely to marry as those who are not employed. Many African American men are the "last hired, first fired" (Boyd-Franklin & Franklin, 1998). As a consequence, some Black men have a number of periods of unemployment or are underemployed (i.e., they are working in lower paying jobs for which they are overqualified). Because of racism, these issues are often present despite the educational level or socioeconomic status of the man.

The lower the Black male employment rate in a particular community, the higher the number of single-parent households, the lower the number of married couples with children, and the greater the percentage of single women (Sampson, 1995; Tucker & Mitchell-Kerman, 1995). Historically, African American couples have experienced economic instability since two incomes are often necessary for survival. This can cause relationship difficulties in a society that expects men to serve a provider role (Franklin, in press; Hatchett, Veroff, & Douvan, 1995). African American couples often experience relationship stress due to the added burden of racism and discrimination in hiring and firing practices (Boyd-Franklin & Franklin, 1998; Kelly, 2003; Lawson & Thompson, 1994).

THERAPY WITH AFRICAN AMERICAN COUPLES

Resistance of African American Couples to Treatment

Some hard-working African American families with upwardly mobile aspirations, regardless of their economic strata, emphasize "keeping up appearances." This is further complicated by the abundance of "family secrets" in many African American families and the efforts they have undergone in order to hide their problems from others. Many African American couples and families will wait until a situation has reached crisis proportions before they seek help. The following case example illustrates how this "need to keep up appearances" can manifest in a couple in therapy.

Susan and Joe were a young African American couple in their early 30s. They had one child. Joe had gone to law school and Susan had been a teacher prior to the birth of their son. They came in following a crisis in which Joe had threatened to hit Susan. She had panicked and had taken their child to a friend's home. Susan reported that verbal abuse had been occurring for more than 3 years but that this was the first time Joe had threatened to hit her. Joe had been unable to pass the bar exam since his graduation from law school 3 years previously. As the time for the bar exam approached each year, Joe became angry and verbally abusive.

Joe at first denied his abusive behavior and attempted to minimize the problem. He threatened to withdraw from treatment. The therapist saw him alone for a session and talked with him about his feelings about the exam, the rage that his difficulties provoked, and his fears of failure. He was later able to share some of these feelings with his wife. He told her that he was afraid she would condemn him for his "failure." He had therefore begun to criticize her constantly about her own insecurities, particularly concerning her inability to contribute to the family's finances. Whenever she attempted to defend herself, he would become enraged, accuse her of not caring about him, and threaten to hit her.

Both partners had hidden their difficulties from their extended families, their friends, and their neighbors. Susan expressed concerns that Joe's abuse of her might reflect on Joe professionally in their community, so they pretended nothing was wrong when they attended church every Sunday. They kept up this facade at their parties and family gatherings as well.

The therapist worked with this couple for many months before they were finally able to stop minimizing their difficulties and could begin to face the threat of domestic violence openly. Only then were they able to share their insecurities and fears and begin to ask for support from each other.

Initial Presentations of African American Couples

The process of couple therapy with Black people is complicated, but this is true also for members of other ethnic groups. Some African Americans have a special cultural resistance to seeking help from "outsiders." Nonetheless, today more Black couples than ever before are seeking treatment. Although generalizations are difficult to make, the following categories summarize the different ways in which these couples may present: (1) a married couple that requests traditional marriage counseling; (2) an unmarried couple that has had a long-term, live-in or "common law" relationship; (3) premarital therapy—a couple that is considering marriage but that has concerns about their relationship; (4) a couple in crisis that appears after a fight and then disappears for long periods of time; (5) a couple seeking divorce mediation; and (6) a couple that initially presents a child as the problem.

Traditional marriage counseling was the most common reason African American couples sought treatment 10 years ago. This has since changed radically; couples now present with many different types of relationships. One of the most common is that of an unmarried couple who have a long-term live-in or common-law relationship. Nonlegal "marriages" in which the couple is treated as married have always existed in Black communities. For some of these couples, the fact that they are not "legal" is a family secret. Treatment is often precipitated when one member of the couple begins to put pressure on the other member to "legalize" the relationship.

There are also generational and socioeconomic issues involved when a live-in couple presents. Among older African American couples, particularly those from low-income backgrounds, common-law relationships are not unusual. The couple may have a number of children together but have never married either for financial reasons or because one or both parties has/have been married before and never officially divorced.

These couples also tend to come to the attention of therapists when one member becomes dysfunctional. Common reasons for a partner's inability to function within the relationship include psychiatric problems, alcoholism, drug dependency, or a medical crisis. This last situation can often be very threatening to the relationship if the medical condition is serious and/or terminal and the healthy partner is accorded no legal status because of the couple's unmarried status.

The third example often involves young couples who may have lived together and are now considering marriage. These couples will appear for treatment for preventative purposes if they have had problems in their relationship. This is a relatively sophisticated use of couple therapy and is usually limited to young African American professionals.

The fourth example involves couples who often appear for treatment directly following a fight or a major argument and then disappear for long periods of time. The treatment with a couple such as this is often a series of crisis interventions.

The fifth example, divorce mediation, is now more common among Black couples for two reasons: (1) more lawyers tend to refer couples for therapy, and (2) the mediation process is a far more cost-effective method of working out differences than a court battle that could prove long and arduous.

The sixth example, the initial presentation of a child as the problem, is still one of the most common ways in which African American couples enter treatment. Many African American families are very child-focused and often enter treatment as a response to a problem that has developed in their child. Most of these cases are school-referred. Such a referral can make seeking help seem "safer" to some couples. The following case example is typical of the course of treatment.

The James family was an African American family that appeared at their community mental health center with their three children, ages 9, 4, and 2. They had been referred by the school because their oldest child, Clarence, was acting out in school and was often oppositional to his teachers. The initial family sessions utilized the techniques of structural family therapy (Minuchin, 1974) to help restructure the family by putting the parents in charge and helping them to work together in their parenting of Clarence. In this process, it became very clear that the James's marriage was in serious trouble. They often had angry arguments at home about their children, particularly Clarence, but they had never fully dealt with the difficulties between them.

As Clarence began to show improvement, the therapist raised the idea that Clarence's misbehavior had been a way of focusing his parents' attention onto himself and away from their own difficulties. They were told that while their son had shown some improvement, his behavior would clearly become a problem again unless they dealt with their issues as a couple. Although Mr. and Mrs. James would never have chosen couple therapy initially for themselves, they now had developed a trusting relationship with their therapist and were able to enter treatment as a couple.

The Role of African American Women in the Referral Process

Their suspicion of therapy in general and the intimacy of the issues between couples are both factors in the resistance of African American couples to treatment. Negative attitudes regarding therapy are common for both African American men and women. Many Black men, however, are particularly averse to seeking treatment, especially couple therapy.

While it is true for both the Black and the White populations that women seek therapy in greater numbers than men, in some White couples both parties mutually agree to seek treatment. This is generally rare among African Americans—although it is slightly more common for educated, middle-class Black couples. When therapy is sought, African American women almost universally initiate the move to do so, so the engagement of their Black male partners in the treatment process is the first major treatment issue.

Techniques for Engaging African American Men in Couple Therapy

Because of the resistance by many African American men to the treatment process, the therapist must often make a decision early on as to whether to begin therapy with the woman alone. In the treatment of African American couples, the therapist often has no choice and must be more flexible in his or her approach if couples are to be engaged. All the therapists interviewed for this chapter were clearly in agreement on this issue. A number of strategies can prove helpful in using this approach.

First, the therapist must keep in his or her mind a clear understanding that he or she is working with a dyadic system. When an African American woman first calls to ask for couple treatment, therefore, it is important to find out the nature of the problem and to try to understand it from her viewpoint. In the initial session, her understanding of her partner's willingness to come in can be explored. If she acknowledges that he is reluctant, then a more general statement to the effect that most men feel threatened at first may help to normalize the partner's initial response.

Second, it is important to discuss carefully the nature of her partner's resistance and to help her figure out how to get him to come in. For example, although it is generally a good practice to avoid giving ultimatums, there are some serious situations in which a woman feels so victimized that she feels she must leave her partner. When this is the case, it is often helpful for her to make very clear to her partner that if he does not attend treatment with her, she will leave him. This kind of statement should be avoided if at all possible because it sets up a situation in which a Black man may feel forced to come, which in turn frequently engenders further oppositional feelings in the man since he is then robbed of the power to choose his own way of dealing with problems. Once again, this sense of lost autonomy is a particularly sensitive issue for the Black man who feels his freedom of choice to be inhibited by a racist society. However, even if a male partner is forced to come, a therapist can establish a positive relationship with him and work through his initial reluctance.

Third, it is particularly helpful for the therapist to establish a time when he or she can talk to the man directly. Men in general, and African American men in particular, resent the feeling of being "summoned" to come in to a therapist's office. The woman should be asked, however, to tell her partner that the therapist will be calling. The therapist should call the man directly and not just use the woman as a messenger. During the initial phone conversation, it is important to establish first whether the man knows about the treatment. The therapist must be careful to clarify that she or he has spoken to his wife or partner and wants to understand his point of view in order to try to help. The woman should be prepared in advance for the process of attempting to engage her partner in therapy. The therapist can explain that since she or he has had the opportunity to get to know her, it will be necessary to devote a considerable amount of energy to engaging her partner and joining with him in the initial session. This kind of preparation is important so that the woman does not feel threatened in this first joint session. This balancing process is a very delicate one, and the therapist will have to work hard to overcome the man's perception that the therapist is aligned with the woman.

Fourth, for African American men who are particularly resistant, the therapist may have to rely on the man's natural curiosity as things begin to change. In these situations, a woman may have to be seen individually for as long as 6 months before the man can be engaged. Lastly, if the therapist has been seeing a Black woman individually, it is crucial that the man be given at least one individual session and sometimes more before the partners are seen together. This is needed in order to balance the scales.

This question of alignment and coalition between the therapist and one spouse is a difficult one and must be addressed openly early in the process of couple therapy.

Alice and Charles, an African American couple in their 30s, entered treatment after living together for approximately 2 years. They had been involved with each other for a total of 5 years. In the first session, it was clear that they were encountering serious communication difficulties and had very different ideas about male–female roles. For example, they would frequently argue about who should take the lead in their relationship. Charles would become very angry with Alice whenever she walked ahead of him.

The therapist asked Charles and Alice to share with each other where they had learned what to expect in a couple relationship and who they had used as role models. Alice related that she had been raised by her mother in South Carolina. She was the oldest of three children. Her father had left the family at a very early age. She reported that she had never had a "real-life" model for male–female relationships. Her mother did not date; her active involvement in her church was her only social outlet. Her own concepts of male–female relationships had been formed from novels and movies. She had no clear ideas as to how fights could be handled or arguments resolved. Hers was a fairy tale conception of male–female dynamics.

Charles had been raised in Harlem. He was the youngest of four boys. His father, who had been actively involved in the Nation of Islam, had died when Charles was 5. His older brothers adhered to his father's tradition and continued many of his values. Charles's mother was a Baptist by religion and had never left her Christian faith. There was always some tension in the family about this divergence in tradition and values and in the area of male–female role expectations. His brothers had married in the Nation of Islam and their wives had taken roles very much in the background of the male relationships. His mother, although she remained Christian, allowed Charles to be raised in the Nation of Islam. The behavior of women he learned to expect was that of deferral to a man and taking the role of the follower of the man's lead to an extreme degree. He reported that he had not been a practicing Muslim since the death of the Honorable Elijah Muhammad (founder of the Nation of Islam) but many of these ideas were still very much a part of him.

The therapist was able to point out to this couple that they had had very different expectations of male–female relationships. This difference was reframed as "normal" in relation to their backgrounds and the issue was removed from the emotional charge of the label "good" or "bad" behavior. They could then discuss these differences and renegotiate their relationship.

Some Common Issues in the Treatment of African American Couples

Socioeconomic Issues and Differences in the Treatment of Black Couples

A number of socioeconomic issues affect the treatment of African American couples. Many of these issues are related to the impact of racism and discrimination. For example, when treating White couples of different socioeconomic levels, a therapist often has a clear sense from the couple as to where they see their position in society. For many African American couples, this perception is contaminated by a number of factors. For example, as Black couples move up the socioeconomic ladder, they often find themselves caught between two worlds. They are in an increasingly privileged position vis-à-vis the Black community, but they may have received relatively little acknowledgment in White society at large. For example, Black doctors and dentists tend to have a very privileged position in the African American community, and in the past may have had predominantly Black practices. It is not unusual, however, for them to find themselves cut off from acceptance by the mainstream White practitioners of their professions.

This pattern is experienced by Black people at all socioeconomic levels and often leads to a feeling of dissatisfaction for many African American couples. In a similar vein, Black people without formal education frequently find themselves denied entry into the opportunity structure even though they have significant talents. Discrimination can be deeply felt and can thus have a significant impact on the couple relationship.

Often socioeconomic differences within Black couple relationships can be very problematic. It has been a common phenomenon for many generations in the African American community for women to have more formal education than men. There are a number of reasons for this disparity. For African American families living in the South in previous generations, for the most part there was only one type of work open to Black women: household domestic work. The menial nature of this work tended to put African American women in an extremely vulnerable position, open to many forms of employer abuse—including sexual harassment. So African American families of previous generations often educated their daughters at Black teachers' colleges in the South in order to avoid this cycle. But this effort to protect their daughters created a situation in which an African American woman often had more formal education than her male partner. As discussed above, because of the reported "shortage" of Black men today, many Black women are again choosing to marry across class lines. This can create a number of issues. The following case illustrates this conflict.

Mary and Bill were a young Black couple in their early 30s. Mary was enrolled in professional school, and Bill had completed his high school education. Bill had a somewhat erratic job history and had many "dreams" that Mary became involved in fantasizing about. During Mary's school years, Bill worked in a factory and supported her. As her formal training was nearing completion, however, Bill became increasingly more agitated and angry with her. Mary withdrew from him and began to complain, for the first time, about the discrepancy in their careers and lives. Their work in couple therapy involved a number of levels. First, the therapist needed to help them to address their expectations of each other that was established early in their relationship. Mary was able to admit that she had never really accepted Bill for himself, but had married a dream of his "potential." Bill was able to acknowledge conflicting expectations regarding their relationship. On the one hand, he liked the idea that Mary would be able to contribute a great deal to the relationship; on the other hand, he had some very traditional expectations in terms of male–female interactions. He became very frightened as Mary approached achievement of her personal career goals. Bill's own fears of failure were confronted and he was able to ask for Mary's help in achieving his goals. They were able to renegotiate their relationship and the role expectations between them. Each person was helped to accept the other for what he or she was rather than as fantasy figures.

Multigenerational Transmission Issues in African American Couples

Bowen (1976) has identified a multigenerational transmission process that exists in all families (see Chapter 3). By paying close attention to this process for African American couples, the therapist can help them to clarify the ways in which they are repeating in their own relationships issues that were left unresolved in their families of origin. In African American families, because of the frequency of "family secrets" that are highly toxic and never discussed, such clarification can be particularly important. It can lead to an ability to resolve the conflicts with their own extended family members. They can then avoid the reenactment of these difficulties in their own relationships. The following case example clarifies this pattern.

Art and Carol were an African American couple in their 40s. They had three children and had been together for about 10 years. Theirs was a very volatile relationship that although not physically abusive could quickly dissolve into loud angry verbal battles. Since they had never developed strategies for resolving conflicts, their antagonism persisted. Art, a businessman who made a reasonable salary, had not been able to fully support the family in the last 2 years because of his expensive cocaine habit.

The couple at first colluded to keep his drug dependency a secret from the therapist. Because of his erratic behavior, however, the therapist confronted the issue with the couple and thus opened it for discussion. Carol became very anxious during this session and was finally able to share that Art's behavior had frightened her because her father had been an alcoholic. This fact had been denied for many years by her family of origin. Her father had died approximately 2 years earlier at about the same time in which the couple's relationship began to deteriorate. She reported a sense of anger and helplessness at her mother for not challenging her father and at her father for being so verbally abusive toward her. As a result of these sessions, she finally confronted her mother with these issues and told her of her anger.

In subsequent sessions, she was able to confront Art. Ultimately she was able to state clearly that she would end the relationship if he did not enter a drug treatment program. Art was at first stunned by her assertiveness and became frightened at the thought of losing the relationship. He entered a program for his chemical dependency and managed to get himself off cocaine. Carol learned that she was codependent and had supported Art's drug habit by refusing to confront the issue. She was in fact an "enabler" of his addiction. This was very reminiscent of her mother's position vis-à-vis her father. They then began a long process of rebuilding their relationship on a healthier foundation.

Power Dynamics Issues in African American Couple Relationships

Power dynamics are one of the few areas of African American couple relationships that received some early attention in the literature. Over 25 years ago, Willie and Greenblatt (1978), Mack (1974), and Middleton and Putney (1970) studied the power relationships between Black spouses of varying social classes. They also compared these issues to those encountered in White families. Willie and Greenblatt (1978) found that, in general, African American families appeared to be more egalitarian than White families. This was especially true of many middle-class African American families who were more egalitarian than any other family type. Mack (1974) found social class to be a more powerful factor than race, with working-class husbands of both races having more power relative to their wives than middle-class husbands.

Power is a complicated dynamic in African American families. Although Moynihan (1965) claimed that the power structure of Black families was matriarchal and thus deviant from the rest of U.S. society, the other researchers mentioned above pointed to the frequent incidence of a more egalitarian structure in African American family life due at least in part to economic necessity. Although poor and working-class families of all ethnic groups clearly have to struggle with financial burdens, the socioeconomic stigma associated with being Black and poor is overwhelming for some families. Even as African American families approach a working-class or lower-middle-class lifestyle, the feeling often remains of what Robert Hill has termed "one paycheck away from poverty." Survival has been such a major issue in many working-class Black families that cooperation around this issue has added an egalitarian character to many male–female relationships.

The issue of power in African American couple relationships is greatly affected by the influences of racism and discrimination, particularly in relation to the misuses and abuses of power in these relationships. This experience of racism cuts across all class and educational levels for Black people. Because of this issue, the impact of the pressures of racial discrimination plays a very significant role in the treatment of Black people. Often African American individuals, couples, and families feel powerless in the face of this racism. Therefore, the issue of empowerment is a very prominent one in the treatment process.

Unemployment and the "Rage over Racism" Issue in African American
Couple Relationships

Boyd-Franklin and Franklin (1998) have indicated that "African Americans struggle with the inequities of racism even in very high occupational, educational, and socioeconomic levels. Unfortunately, the rage about this is often misdirected toward family and couple relationships" (p. 274). The following case provides an example of this process.

John (age 35) and Judy (age 36) were an African American professional couple with two children. They were both lawyers in major law firms until a year earlier when John was dismissed by his firm—a dismissal he attributed to "institutional racism." He had not found another permanent job since, but was doing *per diem* work. Judy, however, was on the "fast track" for partnership. Over the course of the last year, John and Judy had become more angry and verbally abusive with each other. During an early session of couple therapy, John called Judy "lazy, a lousy housekeeper, and an inadequate lover," while she referred to John as "no good, lazy, and useless." When John called her a "bad mother," Judy yelled that she was sick of carrying all of the financial, emotional, and parental responsibility for their home and family. She then began to sob. When the therapist asked John to pass her a tissue, Judy slapped it from his hand.

The therapist asked Judy to tell John what she was feeling. She told him she felt "damned if I do and damned if I don't." If she tried to support him, he told her she was condescending. If she tried to push him, he said she was a "castrating Black woman."

The therapist asked John to tell her how he felt. He said that sometimes he indeed felt "castrated"—by his former bosses, by Judy, and by others in their lives who "put me down." He added, "Why can't she [Judy] understand that it's hard for a Black man out here?"

Judy became angry at this and said that it was hard for her as a Black woman, too. She related a story about a social affair at which John had "put her down" in front of her colleagues at her law firm. John reported that he was sick of hearing about all her accomplishments. He stated that "they can take it from a Black woman, but they are threatened by me." He also reported another incident that occurred at the same social event: "Some woman thought I was a waiter earlier in the evening and asked me to get her coffee." The therapist explored how much of that feeling was underlying his anger and resentment of Judy. He talked about his experiences of racism and his sense that Judy just did not understand his pain.

Using the paradigm that they had introduced, the therapist (a Black female) told them this: She felt that they were both victims of racism, but that instead of uniting together to fight against it, they were tearing each other apart and letting racism win. This therapeutic reframe was designed to challenge their blaming definitions of the problem and to provide common ground for them to begin to work on their relationship issues.

The reframe was a turning point. It allowed John and Judy to distance from their rage at each other and to begin looking at the messages they had each been given by their families of origin and in their communities about Black male–female relationships. Judy talked about the stereotypical socialization messages she had been given that Black men are "no good" and "lazy." She acknowledged her fear that John would not find another job. John, in turn, acknowledged receiving the message from other men that he should never let a Black woman get "too strong." The therapist helped them to see that they had both learned destructive, victimizing messages. The two were then able to begin to talk honestly about how painful this period had been. John shared his fears more openly with Judy, and she was able to share her insecurities with him. The therapist worked with them on their ability to "hear" each other, so that they could get beyond their anger to the deeper issues of their pain and hurt.

At this particular stage of treatment, the therapist focused on "racism" as a shared oppression that might be used strategically to bring John and Judy together. This should not be interpreted as ignoring the complex interaction of racism and sexism in their relationship. The therapist was well aware that Judy was being blamed by John for her success and his misfortune. The therapist's decision to use the racism reframe at this point was a question of the timing of the therapeutic intervention. It was her belief that only after the couple was forced (or shocked) into standing back from their mutual oppression could they find the "common ground" necessary to begin addressing the problems in their relationship. Later in treatment, the therapist was able to confront John on some of his own sexist assumptions that he would be earning more money and have the more prestigious job. If this had been done prematurely, the couple would have fled treatment.

Because Judy and John already saw some of their issues as related to racism, the therapist struggled with how to acknowledge racism—which today is far more subtle than it was during segregation—while preventing its use as an excuse mechanism for personal failure. The racial paradigm can be a useful reframe in helping African American partners like John and Judy, who introduced racism into the treatment process, to distance from their rage at each other and look at the larger context. Although it is not appropriate for every African American couple, it is a beginning, so that each partner may take responsibility for his or her part in their difficulties; understand victimizing messages from childhood, which exacerbate an already painful situation; and, if possible, challenge racism from a position of empowerment. (Boyd-Franklin & Franklin, 1998, p. 276)

In their discussion of this case, Boyd-Franklin and Franklin (1998) state that "middle- and upper-middle-class African American couples who believe that their problem had become one of 'class, not race' react to incidents of racism with a sense of betrayal, disappointment, and often hopeless rage, which are then projected onto their loved ones" (p. 276). John and Judy's situation is reminiscent of the following statement by Poussaint (1993):

African-American men and women alike face a difficult test in understanding the complexities of their dilemma because the gender issues, whatever they may be, are compounded by racism and the subordinated roles of Blacks in American society. Sadly, Black men and women themselves harbor racial stereotypes about each other.

Both sexes are struggling for maturity in America where the rights of women are changing dramatically. White males, whose dominance has been based on female subjugation, must relinquish and share power with women. For Black males, who already feel subjugated by Whites, relinquishing dominance over women, especially Black women, is more problematic. (p. 89)

Boyd-Franklin and Franklin (1998) have also shown that "when some African American men feel threatened, they may assert their 'manhood' in destructive, often sexist ways, through violence and/or affairs. Or Black men may turn inward, leading to withdrawal and a profound sense of resignation or a 'Why bother?' attitude" (p. 277).

Communication Problems in African American Couples

Communication difficulties are one of the most common presenting issues in couple treatment in general. This clearly is true of African American couples as well. For Black couples, however, communication is complicated by all of the factors discussed above—particularly those in such sensitive areas as suspicion and male role validation. Therapists who have worked with African American couples report that generally part of the difficulty lies in their not knowing how to talk to one another. Because of many of the socialization issues previously discussed, it is often very difficult for Black people—especially Black men—to express their feelings directly. Because the expression of emotions is often seen as a sign of weakness by African American men, African American women often enter treatment with the complaint that their partners are emotionally unavailable. The therapist's first strategy in this type of situation is to join and connect with each person. Once he or she establishes a relationship of trust with both partners, the therapist can begin to explore what each member of the couple has brought to the relationship in terms of past experiences and expectations of each other. The therapist can then gradually begin to place emphasis on feelings. This process has to be handled especially delicately because many African American men may perceive this kind of emphasis as the therapist's alignment with the woman. It is essential that the therapist avoid this pitfall, but he or she must do so without failing to help the man see that his wife or mate is truly unhappy. Once the partners' mutual caring can be tapped, their willingness to work on change can be elicited. If the therapist in any way suspects that the man may feel that an alliance is forming between the woman and the therapist, it is important to raise this question directly so that the issue can be addressed and discussed.

Techniques for Enhancing Communication in African American Male–Female Relationships

One of the most important techniques for improving communication in African American male–female relationships involves an educational component. The therapist will often have to use the sessions to help African American couples learn strategies for relating. This is extremely important because many Black people who come for therapy report that they have grown up without experiencing role models for positive male–female relationships. Some have been raised in single-parent homes without a model for this type of interaction. Others have grown up in situations in which they have witnessed angry, hostile, verbal or physical exchanges as their only model of male–female interaction. Some African American men and women who have grown up in two-parent, intact families have initially reported a "good" relationship between their parents, but have later admitted that they had only a vague sense of their parents' "couple" interactions. Many older African American couples are very child-focused and do not, in fact, have much of a couple relationship.

Within this context, couple therapy is often the first time that some African American couples have actually learned about the dynamics of positive intimate relationships. This educational component can be introduced by the therapist in a number of ways. The first concept is that if a relationship or a marriage is to be truly fulfilling for both partners, both must learn to talk about issues. It is important to stress that this talking should include both positive and negative feelings. A very common statement from Black men and women is: "Why should I tell her (him) I love her (him), she (he) already knows that." Helping a couple to express tender as well as angry emotions is an important first step. Because of the socialization issues related to the macho interpersonal style discussed above, some African American men want their partners to be more docile, particularly in the area of sexual interaction. Misconceptions about sexuality, particularly female sexual arousal, abound. This can create major conflicts when their partners are assertive African American women. Some African American men have been taught that sexual fulfillment for a woman comes only through intercourse. It is helpful to change this perception and begin to gradually introduce different ideas into the treatment process.

Many therapists have used this educational approach very successfully with African American couples. The therapist works with couples to help them learn how to listen to one another and truly hear what each partner is feeling and saying. The role of the therapist centers on aiding couples in understanding that each member should never assume anything simply because he or she hears a particular statement from his or her partner. Each should, rather, stop and ask each other, "What do you mean by that?" Couples often make assumptions about each other's feelings and participate in a process of "mind reading," in which each makes assumptions about the partner's feelings without first testing those assumptions by inquiring as to the partner's true feelings.

The same techniques are useful in the area of sexual interaction with African American couples. Both partners can be helped to learn to say "That feels good," "I like that," or "Please do this" to each other. The therapist should work directly to address the process by which couples can themselves directly address problems in the relationship. Such statements as "I'm not happy about how our relationship has been going and I wonder if you have been feeling that way too" open the door for discussion rather than closing off communication by resorting to angry, accusatory statements. For many African American couples, this form of communication and directness in a relationship is very new and uncomfortable. It is therefore important to prepare both partners for the discomfort they may feel initially with adopting new patterns of communication. The therapist should state this early in the process but encourage the couple to try out these ideas even though they may initially seem foreign. Once they can push past the sense of newness they feel and their embarrassment aroused by these new ways of communicating, they will often feel more at ease both with the process and with each other. Role playing and enactment in sessions have been found to be very useful in helping them try out new ways of relating in the safety and support of the therapeutic scenario.

By exploring the clinical and cultural issues that must be considered in the treatment of African American couples, family and couple therapists alike can gain a better understanding of effective strategies for engaging and working with these couples in therapy. The sociocultural factors in some of the resistance issues that have been introduced are of central importance to the successful implementation of these strategies, particularly as they relate to the socialization of young Black men and women. It is hoped that this perspective will help increase the effectiveness of therapists working with this group. As more African American couples reach out to the mental health community, more intensive research in this clinical area should be forthcoming.

6

Separation, Divorce, Remarriage, and Stepparenting

Although divorce rates have dramatically increased for all ethnic and racial groups in the United States, "the divorce rate for African American women is more than double that of White or Hispanic women" (Tucker & Mitchell-Kernan, 1995, p. 12). According to Hatchett et al. (1995) "Getting married and staying married may become relatively rare events among Black Americans if current trends in family organization, and in the economic marginalization of young Black men, continue" (p. 177). This economic marginalization has been cited in a number of research studies as a major factor in the dissolution of African American marriages (Hatchett et al., 1995; Tucker & Mitchell-Kernan, 1995).

The issues of separation, divorce, remarriage, and stepparenting in the African American community are particularly complex because in some Black families, particularly those living in poverty, the partners may have had no formal marriage. Some African American couples, in which one or both partners already have children, may join in a blended family and not marry even though many of the dynamics of remarriage may exist in these families (McGoldrick & Carter, 1999; Visher & Visher, 1979, 1990). It is also a common trend for there to be no formal divorce when couples separate. Therapists should also be aware that a family in which a couple have lived together for many years and have raised children together may experience all of the pain associated with divorce when separation occurs even if there never was a formal marriage.

The following sections explore the dynamics of the troubled relationship, separation, divorce, remarriage, and stepparenting in African American families. The chapter concludes with a discussion of extended family involvement in divorced and remarried Black families.

THE TROUBLED RELATIONSHIP

Therapists have learned to anticipate a great deal of ambivalence from members of a couple about continuing their relationship when treating couples in couple or family therapy. One member typically voices the desire to continue the relationship, while the other voices the desire to divorce. The ambivalence may even shift, sometimes in seesaw fashion, between the parties, with each partner expressing a contrasting side of the ambivalence at different points in the treatment process.

This dynamic is common with couples from many different cultures. The following case example offers insight as to how clinicians might address this ambivalence with African American couples who seem to want different outcomes from treatment. It is also preferable for the couple to already be in treatment when the decision to separate occurs. The case example illustrates this process.

Darryl (age 30) and Virginia (age 29), an African American couple, had one child, Elijah (age 3½). They were referred for treatment by a close friend who was concerned about their constant fighting. They came for treatment reluctantly. In the first session, Darryl indicated that he "wanted out" of their 5-year marriage. He felt that he and Virginia were not "on the same page" and did not "share the same goals anymore." Virginia cried softly as he talked, and then expressed how much she wanted to make their marriage work. They had come for treatment because they did not want their incessant fighting to affect their son. They both stressed the verbal nature of the fights and denied that any domestic violence was occurring.

Both Darryl and Virginia indicated that they were not sure that therapy could be helpful because they wanted very different outcomes. The therapist was concerned that they would not return unless this issue was addressed. Therefore, she told them that therapy could help them whether they chose to stay together or to separate. She indicated that if they chose to stay together, they would have the opportunity to work through many of their areas of disagreement and find some resolution. If they chose to separate, they would have a much better understanding of what had gone wrong in their relationship so that they would not repeat these patterns in their future relationships. She also indicated that whether they chose to stay together or separate, they would need to consider how their relationship was affecting their son and to work together to help him. After a careful discussion of how therapy could be helpful at these different levels, the couple agreed to continue in treatment. (As indicated in Chapter 5, many African American couples are very new to the idea of therapy and often need help from the therapist to understand the process and benefits of treatment.)

SEPARATION

The treatment process with Darryl and Virginia was a very difficult one. Each member of the couple had issues in the marriage that they felt had damaged their relationship. Virginia was still very angry at Darryl about an affair that he had had during her pregnancy. Although the affair had ended when their son was born, it had planted a seed of distrust that impacted their relationship. Darryl resented what he described as Virginia's "bossiness" and the intrusiveness of her extended family members, particularly her mother and sisters, in their couple issues.

After 4 months of treatment, the couple announced that they had decided to separate. The therapist indicated that many couples who make that decision continue treatment to help their children cope with this decision. They agreed to this process, but before it could begin Darryl's lawyer advised him to speak to Virginia only through his lawyer. Virginia was furious about this situation and, in retaliation, she hired her own lawyer. The couple missed a number of treatment sessions. The therapist contacted each partner separately and encouraged them to return for at least one more session, which they both agreed to do.

In this session, the degree of anger in the room was greater than it had been since they began treatment. The therapist learned that their antagonism had increased exponentially since the involvement of the lawyers. The therapist explored with them the connection between the involvement of their lawyers and the increase in their mutual antagonism and shared that she had seen this process with many other couples. The therapist then offered them the alternative of divorce mediation, which she explained as a process whereby a couple could work with a team including a lawyer, a financial consultant, and a therapist to work out a divorce that would protect the interests of both parties and of their son. The couple agreed to try a referral for this process provided by the therapist. They also agreed to continue to work with the therapist in order to help their son through the process of their separation and divorce.

Over the next 3 months, the therapist helped the couple to discuss a number of issues concerning their son. They agreed to involve him in the treatment process and to tell him together about their decision to separate and divorce. Before their son was brought into the sessions, however, the therapist helped them to role-play what they would say to him. She also had a number of very difficult sessions in which Darryl and Virginia discussed the issues of custody and visitation. Throughout this process, the therapist repeatedly validated their desire to do what was in the best interest of their son. The couple finally agreed on a joint custody arrangement, which they had also discussed in divorce mediation, in which Elijah would live with Virginia during the school week. His father would pick him up after school on Friday afternoon and Elijah would stay with his father until Sunday evening.

In the session with Elijah, both parents demonstrated a great deal of love and concern for their son. The therapist reframed this love and emphasized it throughout the session. She then took a less active role and encouraged the parents to talk with Elijah together. They explained that they were having so many problems with each other that they had decided to separate. As they had earlier rehearsed with the therapist, they both emphasized that this decision had nothing to do with Elijah and that they both would always love him and be there for him. Initially, Elijah, a bright boy, was very confused. He was not sure what "to separate" meant. Darryl patiently explained that early in the next week he would move out of their home, but that Elijah would stay with him every weekend.

Elijah asked his parents why this was happening. The therapist had prepared them in advance for this question and they were able to answer honestly, but in language that was age-appropriate. Virginia explained to Elijah that she and his daddy had been fighting a lot lately and that they did not love each other any more. Elijah looked near tears and asked, "You don't love each other anymore?" Both parents, with the therapist's help, were able to explain this to Elijah. They also emphasized repeatedly that they both would always love him.

In future sessions, the family revisited these issues many times. In the session 3 weeks after his father moved out, Elijah repeatedly asked "why" questions. The therapist stated that other kids had often told her that when their parents separated or divorced they thought that they had done something wrong and she wondered whether Elijah had had similar thoughts. Elijah reported that some weeks earlier, he had broken his father's DVD player while playing with it. His father had been very angry and Elijah thought that this was why he had left.

His parents were very surprised by Elijah's remarks, but the therapist assured them that children often feel that they have done something to cause the separation and divorce. Darryl and then Virginia held Elijah and reassured him that the separation was not his fault. With the therapist's help, both parents were able to reassure Elijah that they loved him and would always be there for him. The parents were surprised by how many times they needed to revisit this issue with their son in subsequent months.

The therapist continued to help this couple to negotiate coparenting issues throughout the divorce process. With the help of divorce mediation, the process was completed within a year.

This case illustrates the benefits of beginning interventions prior to the separation and divorce. Unfortunately, all too often, couples do not seek help until after the divorce process. By that time, their children have often developed symptoms or behavioral problems.

DIVORCE

For families of all racial and ethnic backgrounds, divorce is often very painful and can lead to ongoing and unresolved feelings of anger and rage. For many African American couples, this can be compounded if there is a multigenerational history of failed relationships. After the divorce, if one parent becomes involved with a new partner, leading to a remarriage, this can open old wounds and reactivate hostility between the parents. A frequent presenting problem in these cases is acting-out behavior in the child. Many of these couples do not seek help and are often not self-referred. The next case example illustrates these complex problems.

David, a 14-year-old African American boy, was referred for treatment by his school following a number of suspensions due to fighting and acting-out behavior in the classroom. He was brought for treatment by his mother, Debbie Jackson, age 35, who had been divorced from his father for 8 years. His mother reported that David had been very close to his father prior to their divorce and that he had been very angry ever since. His father had left his mother for another woman with whom he had been having an affair. (The therapist later learned that this had been particularly painful for Debbie because her own father had left her family of origin in a similar way.) She also was obviously still very angry about this.

When the therapist asked when his acting-out behavior had begun, Debbie reported that it had started at the time of the divorce but that it had gotten much worse in the past year when David's father had suddenly become very inconsistent in seeing him on weekends and contributing to his support.

The therapist explored David's feelings about these issues. David announced "My father is an asshole," and then refused to talk about him further. As they discussed his fights in school, it was clear that a number of his altercations were with a boy named Duane, whom David resented because he had "stolen" his girlfriend. David went into great detail about how he resented seeing Duane and his former girlfriend together. Although David initially resisted, the therapist was able to help him to see the parallels to his situation with his father.

After a number of sessions in which the therapist joined with David and his mother and worked on basic parenting issues and establishing consequences for his misbehavior, the therapist raised the issue of contacting David's father. Both David and his mother objected. The therapist was persistent and explained that it was clinic policy to speak with and, preferably, to meet significant family members including parents who no longer lived with the child. Reluctantly, Debbie gave the therapist her ex-husband, Wilson's, telephone number. The therapist did a great deal of work with Debbie and David to solidify her therapeutic relationship with them prior to making the call. It was clear that both were still very angry at Wilson.

When David's father returned the therapist's call, she explained that his son had been referred for therapy by his school and that she was working with him. The father became angry and asked what his son had been referred for and why he had not been consulted.

The therapist explained the kinds of behavioral issues that had led to David's school suspensions, and also explained that she was consulting with Wilson now so that he could help his son. She made a special effort to join with the father and was eventually able to request a meeting to continue their discussion. The father refused to come into the office, but the therapist was finally able to get him to agree to talk again on the phone.

A month later, David had a very serious fight at school in which another child was injured. David was suspended again. The school principal called a meeting with his mother to discuss whether he should be referred for a child study team evaluation. Upon learning about this meeting in a phone call from the mother, the therapist called the school principal, introduced herself, and asked permission to attend the meeting. The principal was willing to have her attend and also indicated that David's father had been contacted.

In the session prior to the meeting, the therapist discussed with the mother the fact that David's father had been invited. The therapist was surprised to discover that Debbie was relieved that he had been called. She expressed doubt, however, that he would come. The therapist explored with her how she would feel about the therapist making a call to encourage him to attend. She agreed, and the therapist again contacted the father.

At the therapist's urging, the father attended the principal's meeting. Both he and Debbie expressed concerns about David's behavior and his repeated suspensions.

The principal indicated that another child had been injured in the last fight and his family had threatened to press charges against David. He indicated that he was considering special education classification and an alternative school placement for David. This news upset both parents greatly. The therapist asked if there was any chance that the principal would delay that decision for a couple of months in order to give therapy a chance to work. The principal was very hesitant. The therapist then turned to the parents and asked if they would both be willing to work with her to try to help David. Both parents hesitated because their relationship was very strained and they had no desire to meet regularly. At the therapist's urging, however, they agreed to try. The principal, having expressed his misgivings, then reluctantly agreed to give them until the end of the marking period (about 2½ months) before he made his decision.

The therapist scheduled the first meeting with Debbie and Wilson without David. They were still very angry at each other. Throughout the session, the therapist acknowledged their anger and talked with them about how their son desperately needed them to set their anger aside in order to help him. She also talked with them about the fact that children in these situations often act out in the hope of bringing their parents back together again. It was therefore important for both of them to clarify for him that they both loved and cared about him but that Wilson's involvement in the sessions did not mean that his parents would be getting back together.

In the next session, the parents clarified these issues for David. The therapist helped to facilitate a discussion between David and his father about his feelings about the divorce and his anger at his father for leaving him. With the therapist's help, Wilson was able to tell his son how sorry he was about the pain he had caused him. David also told his father that he was very upset and angry about the fact that his father no longer made any effort to see him. Wilson agreed to resume regular visitation.

The therapist talked with Debbie and Wilson about their new role as coparents for David. Debbie expressed how difficult it was for her to deal with David's anger and hurt at his father's broken promises. Initially Wilson was angry and defensive, but the therapist was able to help both parents see that despite the resentments of the past, they had to move forward and start over. The therapist scheduled a session alone with Debbie because she sensed her justifiable anger and was concerned that she would sabotage the process.

In future sessions, the therapist worked with the members of this family in various combinations. She saw Debbie alone with David, Wilson alone with David, Debbie and Wilson together, and all three together. She also had regular individual sessions with David in which she focused on anger management issues and his school behavior, as well as his feelings about his parents. She worked on clarifying parental expectations for his behavior and helped them to clarify clear consequences for misbehavior and fighting at home and in school.

Debbie was very concerned that she would become the only disciplinarian in David's life and that his father would be the "good-time dad." The therapist normalized this concern and indicated to Debbie and Wilson that many divorced mothers have this concern. The therapist asked Debbie what kind of support she needed from Wilson. She told him bluntly that she needed him to "back me up when I punish him." With the therapist's help, the parents were able to agree on clear consequences for misbehavior which included taking away time with his friends, his PlayStation and computer video games, and his TV viewing time.

David's behavior in school began to improve.

REMARRIAGE AND STEPPARENTING

The process of remarriage and stepparenting is difficult for families from all cultures. For African Americans and other extended family cultures, issues, relationships and triangles in stepfamilies can be extremely complex, partly because of the numbers of blood and nonblood relatives involved. Unfortunately, many families (and even some therapists) erroneously view stepfamilies as operating under the same rules and norms as first marriages. This is a serious error (McGoldrick & Carter, 1999; Visher & Visher, 1979, 1990).

One of the challenges facing all stepfamilies is the ambiguity of family roles and evolving and changing relationships. The following case example illustrates this process.

Miriam (age 30) and Joe (age 40) Simmons, an African American couple, were referred for treatment by a mutual friend. They had been married for 1 month and were having a great deal of difficulty with Joe's children from a previous marriage, Alicia (age 6) and Joe Jr. (age 16). Joe had been very close to his son prior to his relationship with Miriam, but there had been considerable tension between them since his involvement with Miriam. Since Joe's divorce from his ex-wife, Holly (age 40), 5 years earlier, he had had regular visitation with his children every weekend and had always contributed to their support. In the past year, Joe Jr. had become angrier and more argumentative with everyone, especially Miriam and Joe.

Since Miriam and Joe's wedding, his son no longer wanted to come to their home. When Joe insisted that he visit, the weekend would be very tense for everyone. During one week following a visit, Joe Jr. had an altercation with his homeroom teacher at school in which he "cursed her out." He was suspended for 1 week.

Joe and Miriam both reported that Miriam had always had a good relationship with Joe's daughter, Alicia, but that she was very upset by the arguing and tension in the home and had been wetting the bed.

Holly and Joe had had an amicable divorce. They both agreed that they had grown apart and Holly cooperated with Joe as long as he and Miriam were just dating. Holly had even been pleasant when she met Miriam at Alicia's kindergarten graduation party the year before. The wedding, however, had changed everything. Joe Jr. had refused to attend and Alicia, who was scheduled to serve as a flower girl, became upset and refused to walk down the aisle.

The therapist met first with Joe and Miriam for a number of sessions. His goal was to work with them to solidify their relationship and support for each other. He normalized their situation and helped them to understand that many, if not most, remarried families faced these kinds of challenges in the beginning of their relationship. They seemed surprised by this news. Like many remarried couples, they had hoped that their love for each other would enable the transition to be accomplished more easily. The therapist reframed for them the notion that the children's responses were normal and that their love for each other would carry them through the hard times. He also introduced hope by helping them to understand that many stepfamilies do eventually successfully connect despite difficult beginnings.

He worked with the couple on finding time for themselves. They established a night out each week when they would go out to dinner alone and show their love and support for each other. The therapist then worked with them on understanding their different conflicts and needs. Joe was able to tell Miriam that he loved her very much, but that he was torn apart by the reaction of his children. At times he wondered if they had made the right decision by getting married.

Miriam shared with Joe that she had been so hopeful when she first met the children. She had expected to be a second mother to them and had envisioned them as a happy family. She was devastated by the current turmoil and was also starting to question their decision to get married.

The therapist reframed their comments and emphasized their love for each other. He also again normalized the reactions of the children, underscoring the point that they did not indicate that their decision to marry was a bad one. Over the next three sessions, the therapist saw a pronounced change in the couple. They appeared to be closer to one another. The therapist continued to emphasize the importance of their love, their concern and support for each other, and their open communication.

As the therapist gained the trust of Miriam and Joe, he explained that reducing the children's distress would require some difficult interventions for them. He asked Miriam if she felt that she could support Joe by taking only a friendship role with the children and allowing Joe to have some time alone with each child. They agreed that Joe would call his ex-wife and arrange to meet with Joe Jr. alone for dinner. He had a heart-to-heart talk with his son for the first time in months and reassured him of his love. During their next weekend together, Joe spent some special time with his daughter at a movie.

Joe was eager now to bring his children in for a therapy session. The therapist cautioned Joe to discuss this plan first with his ex-wife and to invite her to meet the therapist. The therapist offered to call her directly and to talk with her. When Joe indicated that he had told his ex-wife about the treatment, the therapist called Holly and answered a number of her questions on the phone, and then invited her to come in for a session alone with him.

In his session with Holly, the therapist learned that she was still very angry with Joe about the divorce and the way in which he had handled his marriage to Miriam. She stated that the children were very upset and she was particularly concerned about Joe Jr., who continued to present behavior problems at home and in school. The therapist joined with her in her concern and told her that if Joe Jr.'s behavior was to change, she and his father and his new stepmother would have to work together to coparent him. Initially Holly was very upset by this. She was willing to meet with Joe and the children, but stated that she was "not ready" to include Miriam.

The therapist agreed to meet first with Holly, Joe, and the children to discuss coparenting issues. He also called Joe and Miriam and discussed his reasons for holding such a meeting. He scheduled a meeting for Joe and Miriam alone with him after the family session.

In the session with Joe, his ex-wife Holly, Joe Jr., and Alicia, the therapist asked the parents if they had been clear with their children about the circumstances of their divorce. He explained that many children feel that it is their fault. Both Joe and Holly reassured the children that the divorce was not their fault. With the therapist's help, they also said that both parents loved them and would always be there for them. They explained to the children that they were not able to live together and be married any longer because they had found themselves fighting all the time.

The therapist then asked Holly and Joe to discuss Joe Jr.'s misbehavior at school. They both expressed concern and agreed that his misbehavior couldn't continue. With the therapist's help, they discussed clear consequences for such misbehavior. They agreed that Joe Jr. would be restricted for a week from "hanging out" with his friends after school and during the weekend with his dad.

The therapist then asked Holly if she would encourage Joe Jr. to talk to his dad about his feelings. She did so. The therapist then asked her and Alicia to sit near him and to allow Joe to talk to his son.

Joe asked his son how he was feeling about "all this." Joe Jr. stated that he was still very angry at his father for "breaking up the family." Joe listened to his son, validated his anger, and reminded him that he and Holly had done all that they could to save their marriage, even going for therapy together, but it hadn't worked. He again told Joe Jr. that he loved him and would be willing to talk with him as often as he liked and answer any of his questions.

At the end of the session, with the therapist's encouragement, Joe took Alicia on his lap and asked how she was doing. She started to cry and Joe comforted her with Holly's encouragement. The therapist complimented Joe and Holly on their willingness to coparent for the sake of their children. He also stated that at some point in the future, when they were ready, he would like to have a session with them and Miriam to establish clear rules for the children. Neither Joe nor Holly were initially ready for such a meeting. He also indicated that he would need to have some meetings with Joe, Miriam, and the children in the future.

In the next session, the therapist met alone with Joe and Miriam. With the therapist's help, Joe explained to his wife what had occurred in the session with his ex-wife and the children. It was clear that Miriam had felt somewhat excluded. With the therapist's help Miriam was able to see why it was important to first resolve the issues between the parents.

In the next few months, the therapist met with different subsystems in this remarried family. He had a number of sessions alone with the children in which he addressed their sadness, their sense of abandonment, and the loyalty conflicts they experienced.

He had a number of sessions with Miriam, Joe, and the children to discuss their experiences on the weekends. He helped the children and the adults to see that they could love and care about their mother and father and also begin to love and accept Miriam.

About 4 months later, Joe Jr. was suspended for a fight at school. The therapist decided to use this incident to bring Joe, Holly, and Miriam together to discuss how this behavior should be handled. With a great deal of anxiety, all three met first with the therapist and then with the children. The therapist emphasized to the adults that it was very important that they agree on the handling of this misbehavior and its consequences. They agreed to attend meetings together at Joe Jr.'s school and to enforce his punishment, which was no TV or videos and no time "hanging out" with his friends for a week. They discussed this with Joe Jr. and told him that they all supported this agreement.

Although this was a very awkward and difficult meeting, it was a significant turning point in the treatment. Both of the children began to do better. Alicia's bedwetting disappeared. Joe Jr. had no further fights or suspensions from school. While there were still some difficult moments for all members of the family, Holly, Joe, and Miriam were able to communicate more appropriately about the children. Miriam was able to support Joe in spending regular individual time with each of the children, in addition to the family time she craved.

This case illustrates many aspects of the complex work of treating divorced and remarried families. There was a clear life-cycle difference between Joe and Miriam. As McGoldrick and Carter (1999) have indicated, couples in this position often do not fully understand each other's dilemmas. The therapist therefore made the decision to work first to solidify his relationship with Joe and Miriam and to open communication between them.

His outreach to Holly was also important. When one partner takes the children to a therapist, it is often very upsetting to the ex-spouse. By reaching out to Holly, the therapist was able to minimize the resistance and sabotage that might have occurred. The therapist worked hard to solidify the coparenting alliance between the adults, while honestly acknowledging their discomfort with this arrangement. Finally, the therapist met regularly with different subsystems in the family in order to help each family member deal with this highly complex and conflictual situation.

EXTENDED FAMILY INVOLVEMENT IN DIVORCED AND REMARRIED AFRICAN AMERICAN FAMILIES

One challenge for African American and other extended family cultures is that divorce or remarriage frequently has a major impact on the entire kinship network. While this may be true for all families, it is particularly relevant for large African American extended families where members are in close contact with one another. The more enmeshed, involved, or reciprocal the extended family relationships, the more painful the divorce. Therapists working with African American families through the divorce, remarriage, and stepparenting process should question the family carefully about its involvement with the extended family, including that of the ex-spouse. Therapists should also remember that in many poor African American families, the pain associated with separation, divorce, and remarriage can be felt even if no formal marriage or divorce has occurred.

When extended family members take different sides in the process, children often suffer. In the midst of an angry divorce, members of a couple often make very hostile statements to each other and to other family members. The painful feelings aroused by such outbursts may linger for a long time. In cases where the first spouse was highly thought of by his or her in-laws, contact may be maintained with the mother- and father-in-law and their extended family. This type of ongoing involvement is especially common when children or grandchildren are involved. While this is, in most circumstances, healthier for the child, these close relationships may make it difficult for a new spouse to enter a remarried family.

In some families, the bond between grandparents and grandchildren is solidified after a divorce. For example, following a divorce a mother and her children may move in with her parents, her grandparents, her sister, or her other extended family members. It is also common for noncustodial fathers to involve grandparents and other extended family members when their children are with them, whether through regular visitation sessions or more informal arrangements. These visits may even take place at the grandparents' or aunt's home. For many African American children, close extended family bonds help to sustain them through the pain of the divorce process.

In some instances, however, extended family involvement can be problematic. Family therapists will have to help all parties to renegotiate their new relationships. The following case illustrates this process.

Kyra, a 9-year-old African American girl, was referred by her school counselor because of severe anxiety. Appearing younger than her age, she was a fearful, clingy child with intense separation anxiety. She was brought for treatment by her mother Amanda (age 32), who seemed totally overwhelmed. Kyra and her mother lived in the home of Lily Dickerson (age 50), Amanda's mother. They had lived with Ms. Dickerson since Amanda's separation from Kyra's father, Wilson Pickney (age 32), 5 years earlier. Their divorce was a very angry one and involved a protracted battle for child support.

Kyra's father had not been involved in her life for the first year after the divorce because he resented the court order requiring him to pay more child support than he could afford. As tempers cooled, however, he had gradually begun to see Kyra more often. In the last year, he had remarried and Amanda was devastated. She became very depressed and overprotective of Kyra.

Ms. Dickerson refused to allow Wilson into her home and would often say negative things about him to Kyra. Kyra loved her father and liked her new stepmother, but she was torn apart by the loyalty conflict.

The therapist worked initially with Kyra and her mother to help Amanda to communicate more effectively with her daughter. Amanda was so distressed herself initially that she could not comfort Kyra. The therapist met with her individually for one session and with Kyra individually in the next. This assessment revealed that both mother and daughter were feeling pressured and caught in the middle.

Amanda had loved Kyra's father deeply and had been hurt, angry, and depressed when he initiated the divorce. His remarriage had further devastated her. Despite her feelings, she recognized that Kyra needed to have a relationship with her father. Amanda explained that she felt pressure from her mother, who had always been a dominant force in her life, to not allow Kyra to see her father. This had led to the ugly court battle that had overwhelmed Amanda.

Kyra's situation was similar in that she was torn between the people she loved: her mother, her father, and her grandmother. She was worried about her mother, whom she described as "very sad." During this discussion she became tearful as she talked about the divorce and how it had ruined her life. When the therapist inquired about this, Kyra reported that everyone is always angry now.

Kyra expressed her love for her father, but was torn because he had "hurt Mommy." The therapist asked whether she also felt hurt and Kyra nodded yes and sobbed. The therapist comforted her and helped her talk more about her feelings.

The therapist also discovered that, like her mother, Kyra loved but was very intimidated by her grandmother. She had been told by her grandmother that her father was "no good" so many times that she did not feel that she could discuss her father with anyone. She was very anxious about this and about her mother's depressed "sad" state.

Given the fragile state of both Amanda and Kyra, the therapist decided to work first with Kyra and her mother individually and then gradually to bring them together. She worked to help Amanda express her sadness, depression, hurt, and anger. After a month of individual sessions, the therapist scheduled a family session for Amanda and Kyra. Amanda was feeling stronger and was able to listen to her daughter and offer her some support. In that session, the therapist helped Kyra to express her loyalty conflicts more openly to her mother.

In their next individual session, the therapist observed for Amanda that both she and Kyra shared the feeling of loving but being intimidated by Ms. Dickerson. She reframed Ms. Dickerson's actions as an attempt to protect Amanda and Kyra from further pain. The therapist asked Amanda to invite her mother to attend a session. It took 2 months for Ms. Dickerson to agree.

The father was called by the therapist and he met with the therapist alone. He was so angry about not being allowed to see his daughter that he threatened to sue Amanda for custody. The therapist listened empathetically and helped him to deal with his anger. The sessions with Amanda and Kyra continued with an individual session one week and a family session the next.

When Ms. Dickerson's initial resistance was overcome, the therapist thanked her for agreeing to meet and acknowledged her concern for Amanda and Kyra. Ms. Dickerson looked very stiff and angry initially, but as the therapist acknowledged her concern, she began to relax. The therapist asked her to share her concerns with Amanda. She stated that "that man" (Kyra's father) had destroyed Amanda's and Kyra's lives and she was not going to give him any more opportunities to cause greater damage.

The therapist validated her for her fierce protection of her family and the statement of her determination. At the end of the session, the therapist met alone with Ms. Dickerson, who shared that Amanda's father had done the same thing to her (i.e., come in and out of her life) and that she was not going to let that happen to Kyra. The therapist thanked her for coming and asked if the grandmother would be willing to come back for a few more sessions to help Amanda and Kyra.

In the next session, the therapist did a genogram with Ms. Dickerson, Amanda, and Kyra. She asked them if they saw any similarities and differences between Amanda's father and Kyra's father. Ms. Dickerson immediately listed all the similarities. With the therapist's help, Amanda was able to share some of the differences she saw with her mother.

Reluctantly, Ms. Dickerson began to acknowledge the differences. The therapist reframed and again emphasized Ms. Dickerson's concern and caring for her daughter and granddaughter and her attempts to protect them from pain. She also began to emphasize the differences between Amanda's father and Kyra's father.

In the next family session, Kyra was included. The therapist helped Ms. Dickerson and Amanda see that Kyra was torn between her mother and her grandmother and wanted contact with her father. She helped them to understand how a child in her position could feel a loyalty conflict and become extremely anxious about hurting her loved ones. Both Ms. Dickerson and Amanda were surprised and upset by this realization. They did not want to see Kyra suffer in this way and both were able to tell her this clearly.

The therapist then sat next to Ms. Dickerson and suggested that they support Amanda and help her talk with Kyra about her desire to see her father. Amanda pulled Kyra close to her and began asking her about her feelings. For the first time Amanda was really able to hear her daughter without becoming overwhelmed. The therapist used praise liberally: praising Kyra for speaking up, Amanda for listening so well, and Ms. Dickerson for being there to support them.

This session was a turning point in the treatment. The therapist continued to see Amanda and Kyra individually for occasional sessions, but, more often, the sessions were family sessions involving Amanda, Ms. Dickerson, and Kyra, or just Amanda and Kyra. A month later, Kyra was allowed to see her father. Amanda was unwilling to meet with her ex-husband, but she did agree to call to arrange for a new visitation schedule. Kyra became less anxious and clingy and Amanda, at the conclusion of treatment, made the decision to get her GED (high school equivalency diploma). By then her relationship with her mother, Ms. Dickerson, was on a more equal level.

This case illustrates the way in which extended family members in African American families can contribute to the adjustment difficulties of children and adults in a divorce/remarriage process. If therapists ignore the role of these key family members, they miss an important opportunity for therapeutic intervention.

7

Religion and Spirituality
in African American Families

Spirituality and religion have historically been very central in the lives of many African Americans (Billingsley, 1992, 1994; Constantine, Lewis, Conner, & Sanchez, 2000; Hill, 1999a; Lincoln, 1999; Lincoln & Mamiya, 1990; Wimberly, 1997). Researchers have consistently found that African Americans report higher levels of religious and church involvement than the general population of the United States (Chatters, Taylor, & Lincoln, 1999; Constantine et al., 2000; Levin, Taylor, & Chatters, 1994; Smith, 1997; Taylor et al., 1996). Family therapists, in assessing the strengths and coping skills of African American families, must be sensitive to the roles that religion and spirituality play in the lives of many Black people (Constantine et al., 2000; Wimberly, 1997). These two concepts are listed separately because although many African Americans have been raised with and have internalized a sense of spirituality, not all are members of organized religions or churches. Brisbane and Womble (1985–1986) state this very clearly:

> Many Blacks who "grew up" in the church—most frequently of Baptist or African Methodist denomination—while continuing to claim a belief in God or to be religious, do not attend church. They vigorously maintain a conviction about spiritual power and unquestionably believe something or somebody greater than themselves is watching over them; and it provides relief and fulfillment. In fact, it may be as fundamental in the lives of Blacks as is religion. Organized religion and the church are viewed as means and places to express one's spiritual beliefs and to have spiritual needs fulfilled. (p. 250)

125

The mental health field has largely ignored the roles of spirituality and religious beliefs in the development of the psyche. In the treatment of African Americans, this can be a serious oversight. It can also be a major error to assume that all of our Black clients share these beliefs.

SPIRITUALITY AND THERAPY WITH AFRICAN AMERICANS

Spirituality is an essential and deeply embedded part of the African and African American psyche (Billingsley, 1992, 1994; Boyd-Franklin & Lockwood, 1999; Hill, 1999a; Knox, 1985). Mbiti (1990, 1992) and Nobles (in press) have demonstrated that this sense of spirituality has its roots in the tradition of African religions. According to Nobles,

> Religion permeated every aspect of the African's life. . . . Religion was such an integral part of man's existence that it and he were inseparable. Religion accompanied the individual from conception to long after his physical death.

Thus, rather than being a systemized set of religious beliefs or practices, the African sense of spirituality was woven into the very fabric of society and was a central characteristic of the African psyche.

Knox (1985) argues for a careful understanding and assessment of the role of spirituality in the lives of African American clients and their families. Her approach utilizes spirituality as a tool specifically for the assessment of African American alcoholics and their families, but her findings are relevant for a much broader Black population. Her work has provided insights into the ways in which spiritual beliefs have become an integral part of the survival system of Black people and how they may manifest themselves in the treatment process:

> Clues to spirituality, which suggest its use as a coping mechanism, are expressed during initial interviews. These should be explored as any other psychosocial area in the assessment process. The most commonly expressed clues by believers of spirituality are likely to consist of (1) "God will solve my problems"; (2) "God is punishing me for having sinned"; and (3) "The Church is my salvation." (p. 32)

Spiritual reframing is a very useful technique with African American families (Boyd-Franklin & Lockwood, 1999). Mitchell and Lewter (1986) point out that people who grow up in a "traditional Black community" are often equipped with a system of core beliefs (p. 2), particularly spiritual ones. One reframe that will often be heard is the notion that "God will know what your needs are and will supply them" and "He gives you no more than you can carry" (Knox, 1985, p. 2). This notion highlights the inner strength of the person and the power of his or her faith and belief system. These beliefs manifest themselves in many different forms clinically and can be utilized effectively by any family therapist who is aware of them.*

In the course of treatment, many African Americans will talk about their use of prayer to cope with life's challenges (Broman, 1996; Constantine et al., 2000). Broman (1996) found that this was particularly true for African American women, who use prayer to cope with health and mental health issues. Therapists should feel free to inquire about this use of prayer, and should even ask the client for examples of how she or he prays. I learned the importance of inquiring, rather than making assumptions, when treating a mother who was very distressed about her teenage son's drug use. She repeatedly reported in therapy that she prayed for her son. Most of her statements about him to me had been so negative that I decided to inquire about the words she used when she prayed for him. She replied, I pray "Dear Lord, please keep me from *killing* this child." Once I recovered from my surprise, I was able to reframe this by helping her to see the value of "positive prayer" (Boyd-Franklin et al., 2001, p. 60).

Belief statements such as those cited above often function as metaphorical communications of a generalized spiritual orientation. It is of utmost importance to therapeutic effectiveness that the presence of this manner of coping be recognized and incorporated into the therapeutic process. Failure to do so can jeopardize the joining process and impede progress in therapy via client resistance and/or a lowered level of trust.

Black Churches

A more concrete manifestation of the widespread spiritual orientation in African American families is the central role that the church plays in the lives of many Black people (Lincoln & Mamiya, 1990; Lincoln, 1999). The intersection between spiritual attitudes and the church can be seen in the extent to which the spirituality expressed within the church setting spills over into the experiences of everyday life (Boyd-Franklin et al., 2001; Knox, 1985). "While spirituality exists outside organized religion," Knox (1985) explains, "it finds its deepest expression and greatest influence in the Black family, in weekly, if not nightly participation in church activity" (p. 34). She continues,

> The organized church is by far the most profound instrument available to Blacks when it comes to coping with the multiplicity of problems that beset their lives.

---

*When I first began my doctoral training at Teachers College of Columbia University in 1972, I had the opportunity to work with Black children and their families at the Harlem Interfaith Counseling Service. Reverend Fred Dennard (the executive director) and Mrs. Doris Dennard (the clinical director) taught me a great deal about utilizing the spiritual strengths of Black families in therapy. Their therapeutic model, known as the "psychospiritual" approach to therapy, incorporates the basic belief systems of Black people into the treatment process.

Church members as well as nonmembers accept the spirituality embodied in the church and use the church to confront their own helpless and depressive attitudes and oppressive practices toward them by others. Therefore, knowledge of the client's church affiliation and the minister often proves to be a valuable resource to the therapist. (pp. 34–35)

Although strong religious and spiritual beliefs have always been an integral part of the lives of Black people in Africa (Hines & Boyd-Franklin, 1996; Smith, 1997), the spiritual heritage of African Americans is of combined origins. Over 40 years ago in his seminal work, Frazier (1963) first documented how Baptist and Methodist churches sent missionaries to work with Black slaves in the South. Gradually, an "invisible institution" (Frazier, 1963) developed, made up of Black preachers who interpreted the Bible for Black people. The African tradition of storytelling, based on a strong and vibrant oral tradition, melded with Christian teachings to produce a hybrid specific to the African American situation. The custom of preaching in a dramatic narrative style that is such a central part of Black church services today evolved from the Black oral tradition. Frazier states that "preaching meant dramatizing the stories of the Bible and the way of God to man. These slave preachers were noted for the imagery of their sermons" (p. 18). This imagery is still a very important part of Black church services today.

The Role of the Church Historically

The overt segregation that existed in most of the South and the covert discrimination that existed in the North both functioned to make the Black church, the sole institution that belonged entirely to the Black community, a central force in the lives of many African Americans (Hill, 1999a; Billingsley, 1994; Lincoln, 1999; Lincoln & Mamiya, 1990). Black churches became multifunctional community institutions. They often established their own schools and Bible societies, serving the varied and widespread needs of a disenfranchised population and became what Frazier (1963) described as "a refuge in a hostile white world" (p. 44). They were, and often still are, one of the few places where African American men and women could feel that they were respected for their own talents and abilities. A Black man or woman who might have a job as a janitor or domestic worker during the week could achieve status in the church as a deacon or deaconess. The community church became one of the most important sources of leadership experience and development in the African American community. Many African Americans have used their church as a major coping mechanism in handling the often overwhelming pain of racism and discrimination (Billingsley, 1994; Hill, 1999a; Lincoln, 1999; Lincoln & Mamiya, 1990). As Frazier (1963) and DuBois (1903) have shown, the churches have provided a mechanism for generations for African Americans to survive and to deal with their painful life experiences.

It is no accident, therefore, that the churches also became a focus of political activity in African American communities. This was true from the slavery days of activists such as Nat Turner and can still be seen through the significance of such religious/political leaders as Martin Luther King Jr., Malcolm X, and Jesse Jackson (Billingsley, 1994; Hill, 1999a; Lincoln, 1999; Lincoln & Mamiya, 1990).

Religious Denominations and Groups in the African American Community

Many different denominations and distinct religious groups are represented in African American communities within the United States. These include Baptist, African Methodist Episcopal, Jehovah's Witness, Church of God in Christ, Seventh Day Adventist, Pentecostal churches, Apostolic churches, Presbyterian, Lutheran, Episcopal, Roman Catholic, Nation of Islam, and numerous other Islamic sects. Other African Americans have been drawn to the practice of African religions including those of Kemet (which traces its roots to ancient Egypt), spiritual practices of the Akan of Ghana, and the Ifa religion, which originated with the Yoruba tribe in Nigeria in West Africa (see discussion below).

Of these groups, the Baptist and the African Methodist Episcopal churches account for the largest proportion of African Americans. After the Civil War, because of the racist attitudes of most White churches in the South, Black churches separated and formed their own congregations, eventually evolving into the Black Baptist churches and the African Methodist Episcopal churches that we know today.

Churches in African American communities do not always have large congregations. Many Baptist and African Methodist Episcopal ministers began as pastors of small "storefront churches" (Billingsley, 1994; Frazier, 1963). Small congregations are typical in many of a growing number of Pentecostal and Apostolic churches in Black urban communities. The ministers of such small churches can establish intimate relationships with members of their congregation. For family therapists and other mental health practitioners who are working with these families, some knowledge of the religious beliefs and practices of these groups is important. For example, some Black churches impose strict dress codes, and have rules that prohibit drinking, smoking, use of drugs, dancing, partying, and so on. This often causes generational conflicts for the children and adolescents in these families.

The Church "Family"

It is extremely important for therapists to understand the concept of the church "family" as it relates to African Americans. Many Black people refer to their church as their "church home" (Boyd-Franklin & Longwood, 1999). I will use the example of a Baptist church to illustrate this point, although there are many similarities in other denominations of Black churches. For many African American families, the Black church functions essentially as another extended family. The minister is usually a central figure in the life of the family and may be sought out by family members for pastoral counseling in times of trouble, pain, or loss. After the family and the extended family, the church is the most common source of help for many African Americans. Larger churches have two or more ministers who each may handle different functions within the church. The minister's wife often also serves a very important role; in some congregations, particularly smaller ones, she may also be sought out by church members for help and advice.

Many African American churches have a board of deacons and deaconesses who assist the pastor in carrying out the duties of the church. This is a position of status. If a family member tells you that he or she holds such a position in his or her church, this is clearly a sign of his or her leadership ability. Often deacons and deaconesses are sought out by other church members for help and counsel. African American churches have complex networks, relationships, and dynamics involving the entire church hierarchy and provide spiritual and social activities for the whole family. Sunday school and Bible study classes are offered to everyone from very young preschoolers to elderly members. Women in the church volunteer to teach Sunday school and to care for children in the nursery while their parents are attending services.

Members of the usher board seat church members on Sunday and collect the donations from the congregation. Churches often have a number of choirs, including a gospel choir, whose singing draws members into the services. There are also a number of parallel organizations for young people, including a junior usher board and junior choirs. Many successful Black professionals today received their initial training in leadership in these organizations.

Preaching is a very important part of the church service and often arouses strong emotions in the congregation. It is an oral art form among African American ministers. Their special training accounts for their unique brand of oratory, as evidenced by such powerful speakers as Martin Luther King Jr. and Jesse Jackson. Because of the strong emotions that can be aroused by powerful sermons, most churches also have a nurses' aid association, whose nurses are available if members become overwhelmed with emotion (i.e., "feel the spirit," "get happy," or "shout") during the service. Preaching conveys the messages of hope, the route to salvation, and the capacity for survival as a people.

Black churches also serve a social function. Meals are often served on Sunday after services, providing an opportunity for families to mingle socially. Many African American single-parent mothers will tell a therapist, "I raised my children in the church" or "He was brought up in the church." These mothers mean literally what they say: Black churches often function as surrogate families for isolated and overburdened single mothers. Many African American families, when moving to a new community, will immediately join a

Black church as a practical way to become connected to the community. (The ways in which some of these same strategies can be used by family therapists to help build new networks for isolated Black families are discussed later in this chapter.)

One of the most important "family" functions that a Black church serves is that of providing a large number of role models for young people, both male and female. These individuals represent resources that can be utilized when a child or an adolescent is in trouble. African American churches often provide non-church-related activities such as Boy Scouts and Girl Scouts, basketball teams, youth groups, and so on. Because of the need for services in many African American communities and deep concerns about the education of Black children, many churches have begun to provide daycare centers and schools on the premises. Therapists should be aware of these important community resources. The following case illustrates this process.

The Porters were a young Black family consisting of Mr. Porter (age 28), Mrs. Porter (age 27), Oscar (age 10), and three younger daughters (ages 6, 3, and 1). They came to our clinic seeking help for their son Oscar. Oscar was having a number of serious behavioral problems in the public school that he was attending. He had been truant on a number of days and had not been doing his homework. The school had suspended him a number of times. When the parents entered the first session it was clear that they were both overwhelmed. They reported that they had married when Mrs. Porter became pregnant with Oscar at age 17. Too young for parenthood, they had always found Oscar a "difficult child." The parents felt that things had become much worse with Oscar as the younger children were born because they could not give him the time and attention they felt he craved. Both the father and the mother worked and the children were often left with Oscar after school. Mr. and Mrs. Porter reported that they often had to shuttle the children to three different schools and babysitters in the morning. Therefore Oscar was often left to go to school by himself and would frequently not go.

This family presented as an overwhelmed sibling group with no functioning executives. The therapist, in an attempt to help support the parents in their parental function, asked them to discuss what they felt would help Oscar most. They replied that they wished that they could find a good school where they could find help with monitoring him. Mrs. Porter also expressed a need for a closer daycare center so that all of the children could be dropped off and picked up more conveniently.

The therapist knew of a small Baptist church in the community that had started a school and a daycare center. The therapist contacted Mrs. Clodhill, the minister's wife, who served as the school principal, and asked if she would help this family. The parents readily agreed to go and meet with her and were able to enroll all their children in the school and the daycare center on the church grounds. Mrs. Clodhill and Oscar's teacher then met with the parents and the therapist and worked out clear ways of monitoring his school attendance. An after-school program took the burden off of Oscar in terms of caring for his younger siblings until his parents returned home.

Mrs. Clodhill, the teacher, and the therapist all worked together to support the parents in their efforts to begin monitoring Oscar's homework more closely and to set clear limits for him.

The elderly make up a significant part of the congregation in many Black churches. The respect and caring they receive from church members helps to provide a sense of family as they grow older, particularly if their own adult children live far away. The minister will often visit an elderly person who is ill. Some churches will provide a car or van to bring in elderly members who could not otherwise attend services. These are resources of which family therapists are often unaware.

Jehovah's Witness Families

One church group that has gained in membership in African American communities is the Jehovah's Witness faith. Largely through the "pioneering" and missionary work of its members, many more African Americans have now been exposed to and joined this religious group. The Jehovah's Witnesses meet in the "Kingdom Hall," which is the focus of church activities, but it has become an educational center as well. Bible study is an important part of this religion, as is spreading the word of God by passing out pamphlets and discussing the Bible with people in their communities. Jehovah's Witnesses adhere to strict rules about dress and conduct, which can lead to generational conflict in families. Since holidays such as Christmas, Thanksgiving, and Easter are not observed by Jehovah's Witnesses, this too may lead to conflicts with other family members, who do celebrate these holidays. Children often find themselves "in the middle." Jehovah's Witness families have come into conflict with the medical profession because of their refusal to allow blood transfusions in hospitals. These families are often hesitant to seek mental health services, tending to rely more on the counsel of the elders at their Kingdom Hall and the other members of their fellowship. When they do approach mental health services, it is often in extreme cases, such as a child who is hallucinating, a suicidal adolescent, or the hospitalization of a family member.

Nation of Islam and Other Muslim Families

Within the African American community, particularly in urban areas, there are many small Islamic sects. Since the late 1960s and 1970s, the Nation of Islam has gained a considerable following. Based on the teachings of the Honorable Elijah Muhammad, and enjoying growth thanks to the charismatic preaching and teaching of Malcolm X, it is now under the leadership of Minister Louis Farrakhan (Lincoln, 1996). For many years now, the Nation of Islam has had very active prison ministries. These ministries have redeemed many young African American men who were involved in a life of crime or drugs and have made them into productive members of their communities. Malcolm X himself was one of the most notable prison converts. This religious group is particularly important to discuss with regard to practicing therapy because of the issues that often arise in African American families due to conflicts regarding religious practices or conversions of family members from Christian to Muslim religions.

Edwards (1968) and Lincoln (1996) have compared the beliefs of Nation of Islam families with those of African American Christian families. These differences in belief and practice between the Nation of Islam and Christian denominations often produces major problems for Black people who have converted to the Nation of Islam and their families of origin. The following excerpt summarizes the differences Edwards (1968) found, particularly in the beliefs about male and female role issues:

> A number of situations determined the break between the Muslim spouses and their relatives. In those cases where the parents and in-laws of the Muslim spouse lived within the area, "uniting with" the Nation of Islam was contrary to the wishes of these relations. This assumes added significance since the majority of these parents and in-laws belonged to Christian churches. Also of significance in the break between Muslim spouses and their parents was the inflexibility of the Muslim spouses in their adherence to the behavioral codes of the Nation of Islam. It was found that conscientious Muslims did not smoke, drink or curse, nor did they tolerate these prohibited indulgences within their homes. Since many of the Muslims' relatives did in fact indulge in these habits, a situation of mutual intolerance and estrangement soon followed. Of relevance here also were the reactions of the parents and in-laws to the Muslims, particularly as these reactions focused upon the behavior and activities of the Muslim female spouse. Muslim females never straightened their hair or wore make-up of any kind. The resulting appearance of the female was often a point of criticism and mockery from relatives, particularly it seemed from the female spouse's mother. (pp. 380–381)

Edwards's work is illustrative of the kinds of multigenerational conflict that can result in an African American family when a member or a part of the extended family converts to the Nation of Islam or another Islamic sect. The following case example demonstrates how a family therapist utilized such knowledge in her work with such a family.

Amena, a 30-year-old divorced Black woman, entered our clinic requesting help for her son, Abdullah, age 10. They had been referred by Abdullah's school after he was suspended because of his involvement in a fight with other boys. Amena reported that she had been raised in a Baptist home but that she and her husband had converted to the Nation of Islam when Abdullah was 3 years old. Amena had never had a good relationship with her family, particularly her mother, and this already tenuous relationship had been exacerbated by her conversion. Her mother was very active in her Baptist church, and Amena's father, who was deceased, had been a deacon. Her mother accused her of taking her grandson away from the family and the church. She particularly objected to Amena's having changed her own name from "Vivian" and Abdullah's from "Kerry." During her marriage, Amena relied on her husband to keep her family at bay. She saw very little of her relatives for most of the years of her marriage. In the last year, when Abdullah was 9 years old, Amena and her husband divorced. Amena had no job and was forced to move back into her mother's home. Abdullah's father did not visit him or contribute to his support.

The year prior to seeking treatment had been a very difficult one for the entire family. Amena found a job and enrolled in a training program and was forced to leave her son in her mother's care a good deal of the time. Amena and her mother would battle about everything from her choice of clothes for herself and Abdullah to her choice of names. Abdullah was very torn between his mother and his grandmother and would often withdraw and cry. His grandmother persisted in calling him "Kerry" in spite of Amena's objections. Finally, a number of children at school had begun teasing Abdullah about his name and his clothing. His fights at school were obviously a distress signal for the pain he was experiencing in his family.

The therapist saw Amena and Abdullah together in the first session and quickly realized that the grandmother was a crucial person in this family structure. With Amena's permission, the therapist called the grandmother and asked her to attend the next session. In that session, it was clear that the hostility between Amena and her mother was very intense. They engaged in a number of loud, angry shouting exchanges. As they yelled at each other, Abdullah seemed to shrink in size and began anxiously biting his nails. The therapist stopped the argument between Amena and her mother and focused their attention on what their fighting was doing to Abdullah. He began to cry at this point, joined quickly by Amena and her mother. The therapist then reframed Amena and her mother's tears as signs that they obviously had a lot of love and caring for Abdullah but that their fighting was tearing him apart. They agreed to work together in family therapy to help Abdullah. In future sessions, Amena was able tearfully to tell her mother how hurt and angry she had been when her mother criticized her appearance, her choice of religion, and her lifestyle. Her mother was eventually able to share her own hurt and sadness as she perceived Amena as pulling away from her and from the church beliefs of her youth. In a later session, the grandmother was able to acknowledge that her greatest fear had been the loss of her daughter and grandson.

The therapist was able to help the grandmother see that she was losing them both by this attack. The therapist was also able to help Amena and her mother negotiate a truce in their relationship so they could work together in raising Abdullah and stop giving him contradictory messages. The grandmother was able to support Amena in going together with her daughter and Abdullah to discuss his behavior with the school authorities and to help stop the teasing that he was experiencing in school.

Abdullah was helped to express clearly to his mother and grandmother the bind that their fighting had created for him. His behavior improved dramatically at home and in school. His two parental figures were able to put aside their differences and work together on his behalf.

AFRICAN RELIGIONS PRACTICED
BY AFRICAN AMERICANS

A small but growing number of African Americans, eager to embrace their African heritage, have been drawn to the practice of African religions, particularly those of ancient Egypt (Kemet; Amen, 1990; Budge, 1991), the Ifa religion of Nigeria (Abimola, 1997), and the Akan religion from Ghana. One of the spiritual practices embraced by some African Americans is the Ifa religion, which originated with the Yoruba tribe in Nigeria in West Africa. (Abimola, 1997).

African slaves brought Ifa and other Yoruba religions to many countries. Abimola (1997) claims that "they are currently practiced by millions of people in Argentina, Brazil, Columbia, Cuba [where it is known as Santeria], Haiti, Mexico, Trinidad, Tobago, Venezuela and the U.S.A." (p. 25). Wande Abimola (1997) helped to start the International Conference of Orisa Tradition and Culture in 1981. Its membership includes representatives from many of the countries mentioned above, as well as large numbers in Nigeria. The Congress has met in many countries, including Nigeria (twice), Brazil (twice), and San Francisco (Abimola, 1997).

The Yoruba had developed a very sophisticated civilization, one on a par with that of ancient Athens, Greece (Neimark, 1993). Those who practice Ifa believe that the creation of humanity occurred in the sacred city of Ile Ife, near the city of Lagos in Nigeria (Neimark, 1993). There are three main components to the Ifa religion. Orisa worship (spirit possession in which the spirits speak through a sacred person), ancestor worship, and divination (Abimola, 1997; Neimark, 1993). Neimark (1993) describes these as follows:

> The orisa are energy that, for the most part, represent aspects of nature. Osun (pronounced O-SHUN) represents sweet waters, love, money, conception; Sango (Zhan-GO) represents thunder and lightening, strategy, and he is the warrior; Esu (pronounced A-shew), messenger to Oludumare (the single God), owner of roads and opportunities, owner of ase (spiritual energy); Yemonja/Olukun (pronounced Yeh-MO-zha/O-lu-KUN), the ocean, mother, provider of wealth; Obatala (pronounced O-BA-ta-la), the head, clarity, arbiter of justice; Oya (pronounced Oi-YA!), marketplace, tornadoes, change of fortune, she is the female warrior; Ogun, owner of all metals, fierce warrior, honor, and integrity. Ifa also teaches that each of us has a single orisa energy that is predominant within us. We call this our guardian orisa. . . . Ancestor worship is a formalized structure for connecting with the accumulated knowledge, wisdom, and power of our dead blood relatives. . . . The energy and wisdom of our deceased blood relatives is uniquely connected with and available to us. . . . In Ifa, we believe that our destinies or life patterns are established prior to our births into this world, and that through information obtained through divination, it is

possible to know something about our futures and the outcomes of all of our undertakings. (pp. 14–15)

Divination is practiced by the Ifa as a way of connecting with the wisdom of the divinities (who are called Orisa) and the ancestors. Rituals are performed by Ifa diviners called *babalawo* (male diviner) or *iyanifa* (female diviner) (Abimola, 1997). Palm nuts or cowry shells are thrown and they produce eight symbols called *odus*. These are then read by the *babalawo* to explain and help to solve the problem that the person is experiencing (Neimark, 1993). Unlike those who espouse Western philosophy and psychology, the Ifa believe in the integration of the mind and the spirit into one harmonious whole (Neimark, 1993).

The Ifa believe that sacrifice is a critical element in human well-being (Neimark, 1993). These sacrifices may include money, food, palm oil, and so on. One highly controversial element of some who practice Ifa belief systems is the importance of animal sacrifice, particularly when the problem is a very severe one, or is a matter of life and death (Abimola, 1997; Neimark, 1993). The issue of animal sacrifice often leads to intense countertransference responses in clinicians. It has also led to criticism by animal rights supporters and others in this country (Neimark, 1993).

Death leads to *Ikole Orun,* or heaven, which is a human being's permanent home. The Ifa also believe in reincarnation or rebirth within the family (Neimark, 1993). Neimark (1993) has shown how this has been reflected in the choice of certain names for children: "The Yoruba names *Babatunde* (Father returns), *Yetunde* (Mother returns), *Jabatunji* (Father wakes once again), and *Sotunde* (the wise man returns) all offer vivid literal evidence about the Ifa concept of familial or bloodline rebirth" (p. 45).

It is important for therapists to be aware of the possible influence of African religions on some of their African American clients. For some, the practice of Ifa has become an important way to integrate Afrocentric principles (see Chapters 1 and 8) into their lives. Some have also chosen to study and go through the training process and initiation as Ifa priests and priestesses.

Therapists should also recognize that African Americans who practice African religions will often consult their spiritual leaders for help with psychological dilemmas in the way that others might consult a psychotherapist. (This is similar to the way in which some Latino clients may consult an *espiritista* [in *espiritismo*] or a *santero* [in the Santeria religion from Cuba, which is also derived from Ifa beliefs].)

Clinicians should also be aware that in some African American families in which one member of the couple practices the teachings of one of the African religions discussed above and the other is Christian, this difference may lead to major conflicts. Often these conflicts over religious beliefs are tolerated early in the relationship or marriage, but can become very problematic when childrearing becomes a factor.

IMPLICATIONS FOR FAMILY THERAPY

Spiritual Issues of Death and Dying in Therapy

One of the times in the life cycle when African American families may be referred for therapy is after the death of a significant family member. If this person was central to the family, his or her surviving family members may present with health issues, behavior problems, or mental health issues such as depression. In order to provide effective treatment for these families, it is important for therapists to have some knowledge of different African American beliefs and rituals concerning the death of a loved one. Boyd-Franklin and Lockwood (1999, pp. 97–99) have described these issues:

> For members of all cultures and religious groups, death and dying is a time when spiritual beliefs and rituals are utilized (Walsh & McGoldrick, 1991). This has been particularly true for African Americans given their historical vulnerability to sudden and often violent death. Within the African tradition, life and death are seen as part of a cycle of existence (Nobles, 1980; Mbiti, 1970). Because of the African philosophy of collective unity rather than individualism, times of loss bring the entire family, extended family, friends, members of the church family, and community together to mourn. Funerals are one of the most important rites of passage in the African American community and are often held many days after the death in order to allow extended family members who live at a distance to attend (Boyd-Franklin et al., 1995). Funerals in Black churches are frequently cathartic and very emotional experiences. In fact, many Black churches have a nursing corps to help mourners who faint or develop medical symptoms during the service.
>
> The belief in a life after death is also a strong component of the African American tradition. Funeral services are often called a "Homegoing" or "Celebration of the Life," or a "Homecoming." Music is an active part of all Black church services and expresses these deeply held beliefs. Before and after the service and the burial, family and friends bring food and gather at the home of the deceased. These occasions offer spiritual fellowship, support, shared grief and mourning, as well the joy of a lifetime of memories.
>
> It is striking, however, that after this brief period of mourning, family members are expected to "get on with life," "be strong," and "wipe away the tears." In contrast to the public spiritual catharsis of the church service, the period of mourning is often a very personal, private spiritual time. Because of the pressure to move on, there are often issues of unresolved mourning in African American families, particularly when a series of losses occur in rapid succession. African Americans experiencing this kind of pain will frequently express it in spiritual terms, such as "a pain in the soul." In many African American families when a much loved family member is lost, a vacuum in the connectedness of family relationships may be experienced. This is particularly true when the deceased held the family together and served as a "switchboard" (Boyd-Franklin, 1989).
>
> When this type of significant loss has occurred, family members are particularly vulnerable to depression, psychosomatic complaints and—in children and adolescents—acting-out or conduct-disordered behavior. The following case

[from Boyd-Franklin & Lockwood, pp. 98–99] illustrates how a therapist incorporated spirituality in helping the members of an African American family begin the healing process after multiple deaths and losses.

Jamar, a 14 year old African American male, was brought for therapy by his aunt, Laverne Smith, on the recommendation of his school guidance counselor. In the last year, Jamar's school performance had declined drastically and he was now in danger of failing. His aunt was also concerned because he had been picked up by the police in an incident that was termed "gang violence."

The therapist learned that Jamar's behavioral problems had begun when his mother died from AIDS the previous year. Approximately three months later, his maternal grandmother—who had raised him, his four brothers and sisters, and cared for his mother when she was terminal—died of a heart attack. Jamar's aunt reported that he was devastated and withdrew from the family after these losses. In her words, he "went to the streets." Prior to this, Jamar had been a parental child and had helped to care for his mother and his younger siblings (ages 11, 9, 5, and 4). His aunt now had custody of all the children but was overwhelmed, particularly by Jamar's behavior. When asked how she coped, Ms. Smith replied that she "prayed to the Lord . . . from him comes my strength."

The therapist inquired about the family's spiritual and religious beliefs. Ms. Smith replied that the family's "church home" was a large, active Baptist church in the community. She reported that Jamar had been very involved, including participation in the choir and membership on the junior usher board, but had "fallen away from the church" since the deaths of his mother and grandmother. When the therapist attempted to explore these issues with Jamar, he became silent.

In a session about three months into therapy, after the therapist had visited the school with Jamar and his aunt and was able to help them develop a plan for addressing his school problems, the therapist met with Jamar alone and again explored his feelings about his losses. He told the therapist that he had been "very angry with God" for taking his mother and his grandmother and that he had turned away from the church and his family. His therapist empathized with his loss and helped him to see that his anger was a normal part of the grieving process. For the next few months, he was seen individually with bimonthly family meetings with his aunt and occasionally with his siblings. His individual sessions were very productive. He gradually opened up and talked more about his anger and how he felt that it was "eating him up."

In one session the therapist explored Jamar's anger at his mother and grandmother for dying and leaving him. An "empty chair" technique was used to allow him to express out loud his anger, sadness, and love to his mother and grandmother. As the anniversary of his mother's death approached, the empty chair was used and he expressed his anger, sadness, and hurt to God. After both sessions, he burst into tears.

In one family session, with his therapist's help, he told his aunt and brothers and sisters what he had been experiencing. Many reported that they had been feeling these mixed feelings also but had told no one. The therapist helped to normalize the feelings of anger, sadness, loss, and love. It was clear that there was a great deal of unresolved mourning in the family. Jamar, in an important moment of insight, shared with his aunt that that was why he had pulled away from his family and the church and was "running the streets."

The therapist suggested that the entire family might benefit from a ritual of mourning during this anniversary period. With the therapist's help, they designed a "memorial service." The aunt suggested inviting their minister and some members of their "church family." As the guest list of people important to the family grew, Jamar reluctantly agreed to have the service at the church. He picked the music and his mother and grandmother's favorite hymns, which he asked a cousin to sing. The therapist attended. The minister led the service, and each family member said something about their memories of the loved ones: Jamar talked about how he had felt many feelings of love, anger, and loss. When the hymn "Precious Lord" was sung, there was not a dry eye in the congregation.

This ritual, with Jamar and other family members' active involvement and with the therapist's participation, was very significant for the entire family. Jamar became less angry. Subsequent sessions focused on "healing." His aunt reported that he was home more and was studying again. His grades began to improve. Although Jamar still does not attend church, he reports that he has "made his peace with God" (Boyd-Franklin & Lockwood, pp. 97–99).

As Boyd-Franklin and Lockwood (1999) have shown, "This case illustrates many of the multigenerational issues concerning religion and spirituality in African American families. Jamar's 'anger at God' and his rebellion against the family's religious beliefs are typical of many adolescents. The case also demonstrates the ways in which spirituality can be used as a therapeutic tool to help heal unresolved grief and mourning" (Boyd-Franklin & Lockwood, 1999, p. 99).

Therapists Who Ignore Religious Issues with African American Families

As we have seen, African American families sometimes frame issues in religious terms (Smith, 1997). If the therapist does not understand this process, a value conflict can sometimes erupt in which the family ends up disengaging from treatment. The following case example illustrates this point.

Kevin, a 14-year-old Black adolescent, was referred to a community mental health center because he was hearing voices and seeing evil spirits. The family consisted of Mrs. Clark, Kevin's mother (age 40), his father, Mr. Clark (age 41), and his sister Janice (age 17). They were seen by a resident in training who asked the entire family to come in for a number of family sessions. In the second session, the entire family attended and the daughter voiced the family's dilemma. She felt that the therapist was only dealing with Kevin on the "natural side" and not on the "spiritual side." She went on to explain that she felt that the therapist was dealing only with Kevin's mind and not with his "soul and his spirit." She stated that she felt that his problems had begun when he had stopped attending church. The therapist, instead of using this as an opportunity to pursue and explore the family's belief system, closed the door immediately. She stated, "You're right, we don't deal with the spiritual or religious aspects here." When the sister pursued her point of view, the therapist was even more adamant. She stated that "we are a mental health center and our orientation is psychological and psychiatric, not the spiritual, not the religious." She suggested that she could not provide that kind of service, and that it "could be provided probably by some kind of minister or religious person but not us." The family left treatment and did not return. (Hines, 1987, personal communication)

The family members just described undoubtedly left treatment with a sense that the therapist was not sensitive to nor inclined to value their way of thinking. With African American families such as this one, it is usually counterproductive to dismiss their definition of the problem as related to religion. Often religious issues are used as a metaphor by Black families and may be their way of testing to see if the therapist respects their beliefs. It is important in these situations to pursue such family signals and to encourage family members to explain their points of view. In this example it would have been important for the therapist to explore whether the mother, the father, and the son agreed with the sister's perspective on the situation. The therapist also missed an opportunity to explore the power issues in the family more closely by exploring the sister's comment that her brother's problems had begun when he had stopped attending church. In fact, this was a very religious African American family in which Kevin's refusal to attend services had created a major conflict. He felt trapped by their strong beliefs and saw no way to differentiate between himself and his family except through his psychosis. This would have been an opportunity for the therapist to explore the strategies that this family had used to try to reinvolve their son in the church network. The family thus would have been given the opportunity to recognize their concern for their son. The therapist then would have had the opportunity to help them to give him some of the "space" necessary for a growing adolescent. The therapist might have normalized this need for individuation and reframed it for the family by telling them that it was clear that they had instilled strong spiritual and religious values in their son and that many teenagers go through a period of questioning their family's values before accepting certain values as their own.

For some very religious African American families, church attendance and adherence to a religious code is enforced with such rigidity that adolescents choose this most restrictive area in which to rebel. The therapist would have even had the option of involving the minister to help the family cope with this transitional stage in their son's life. Unfortunately, by refusing to discuss this issue further and by ignoring the family's repeated attempts to bring up this issue, the therapist closed the door to productive work with this distressed family.

Conflicts between Therapy and Religion

Many African Americans will seek pastoral counseling through their churches (Wimberly, 1997). Therapy, however, is often seen as very secular. Therapists should also be aware that some very religious African American clients may view therapy as "antispiritual" and that this may cause conflicts for some of these clients about being in therapy (Boyd-Franklin & Lockwood, 1999). Throughout its history, the mental health field has often pathologized religious or spiritual individuals (Bergin & Jensen, 1990). Because of this history and the secularity of treatment modalities, very religious clients (and their ministers) may be suspicious of therapy and may be concerned that the therapist will not respect their religious beliefs (Boyd-Franklin & Lockwood, 1999). In these situations, it is very important that the therapist encourage the client and his or her family to discuss their concerns. In some cases, this can result in the family feeling more trust toward the therapist and choosing to continue in treatment. Sometimes, getting the family's permission to consult their minister can help with this process of joining. In other situations, some very religious African American families have requested a referral to a Christian therapist. If this occurs, the clinician should respect their request and help to expedite the referral.

Once the family therapist is aware of the significance of religious values and the resource that churches can provide in the lives of Black people, he or she can utilize this knowledge in a number of productive ways. The last section of this chapter describes some of the ways in which a minister and a church network can be put to effective use in the treatment process, especially in times of family crises when a support system is needed.

Utilizing Ministers and Other Church Members

The minister or pastor of a church has the potential to be a valuable resource, particularly in situations where he has already served as pastoral counselor for family members and knows them well. At the very least, with the family's permission, a minister who has served in this role should be contacted for information about his or her involvement. It has always been amazing to me that mental health practitioners will routinely obtain a release of information form in order to contact other clinics, hospitals, or therapists who have worked with our clients but will not investigate help that the family may have sought from a minister, deacon, deaconess, or other church member.

A minister may be involved in the therapeutic process in many different ways. Once a release form has been signed, he or she might be asked for information about the family, or to encourage them to seek or follow through on treatment. In special circumstances, he or she might even be asked to serve as a consultant or a cotherapist. The following case illustrates this type of involvement.

Anthony Hill, a 27-year-old Black man, was brought to the emergency room by the police and was admitted to the inpatient unit of a large state hospital in the Bronx. He had threatened to attack his wife because he was obsessed with thoughts that she was cheating on him. He was very withdrawn in the ward and isolated himself from other patients. Attempts to arrange family sessions with his wife and/or his parents who lived in an apartment in the same building had not

been successful. Our staff on the inpatient service had learned to pay close attention to the visitors a patient received during his hospitalization. Anthony's father
had visited a number of times, accompanied by what the staff described as a "very
distinguished older gentleman in a suit." The therapist stayed for visiting hours and
met with the father and discovered that the gentleman who accompanied him was
their minister from the Church of God in Christ. Both were very concerned
about Anthony. The therapist stressed the importance of getting the family involved in order to help Anthony and hasten his discharge. She asked the minister's
help in arranging such a session and asked if he would participate. He explained
that the family was very frightened by the hospitalization and that he would be
willing to bring them in.

In the session that followed, Anthony, his wife, Mary, his father, his mother,
and his minister were present. It quickly became clear that this was a very enmeshed extended family in which the parents frequently intruded into the lives of
Anthony and his wife. In addition, Anthony's church family consisted of the minister and small tightly knit congregation of their storefront church. The minister had
been used as a confidant by all family members and had been inducted by the family into its system dynamics. When the therapist asked Anthony and his wife to
discuss the circumstances that had brought him to the hospital, his mother intruded a number of times. The therapist blocked her intrusion and this time asked
the minister if he would help the couple to discuss this issue between themselves.
With the minister's help, Anthony and Mary painfully recounted the fact that
Mary had been mugged and raped. Anthony had reacted with rage and had
blamed Mary for this assault. He even accused her of having invited the sexual assault. Mary burst into tears. The therapist asked the minister to speak directly to
Anthony about this. The minister was able to help Anthony see that sometimes
bad things happen to good people, that people do not necessarily provoke the
things that happen to them. He also helped Anthony to recognize his wife's pain
and led both of them in a prayer for strength to survive this devastating experience.
In subsequent sessions, the minister and the therapist worked with the couple
alone (without the parents) to further support the development of some measure
of autonomy for them.

The minister and his family are often central members of a community
and an important aspect of many extended family networks. Just as families can
become "enmeshed" (Minuchin, 1974), so too can church families, as can be
seen by the entangled relations of the minister and family in the case example
above.

Utilizing Church Help in Times of Crisis

Church networks can be a very valuable resource for a family in crisis. Often
they can mobilize quickly and offer aid to a family without the bureaucratic
process of many social service agencies. The following case illustrates this process.

The Reid family, which consisted of Mrs. Reid and her three teenage daughters, was being seen in family therapy at our community mental health center. An arsonist had set a fire in their building and the family had lost all their possessions. No one was injured but the entire family was badly shaken by the experience. The family found themselves homeless. After spending one night in a city shelter, the mother became very frightened for her children's safety. She then contacted the minister of her church, who mobilized the church network. The minister and his wife arranged for a temporary home for the mother and her daughters in the house of a member of the congregation. Church members immediately donated food, clothing, and necessary household articles, and eventually helped her to find a new apartment.

Helping Isolated Families Create Church Networks

Some of the African American families who enter our clinics, agencies, and mental health centers are very socially isolated and emotionally cut off from their extended families (Bowen, 1976). These families often present with the most overburdened, multiproblem situations. Some of the most dysfunctional families are those who have no network. In Chapters 3 and 4, I have already discussed ways to help such families resolve the cutoff from their own extended families. Sometimes, however, this is not possible, and the family faces the difficult task of building an entirely new social support system. For families who have had a religious orientation or a church connection in the past, helping them locate and identify a new church network can be a very significant intervention. This is particularly true for single parents who may be struggling to raise children alone. Discharged hospital patients who have no connections to family can also benefit from this process.

A word of caution: this intervention is not for everyone. It should be made only if it appears syntonic with the family's belief system and earlier experiences.

Some of the most important historical and psychosocial experiences of African Americans and their families are strongly rooted in religious and spiritual backgrounds and experiences. The cases presented in this chapter highlight problems and dilemmas that frequently confront the therapist who works with African American families.

8

Additional Important Topics
in African American Communities

This chapter addresses a number of additional topics and issues that are important to the African American community of which therapists should be aware. The first part discusses the concept of Afrocentricity and the Afrocentric movement in the African American community. This first part includes a discussion of African Rites-of-Passage programs, which can be utilized in addition to therapy for some of our adolescent male and female clients. The second part explores the diversity in the Black community through a brief discussion of the issues presented by Caribbean and biracial families.

The third part explores a number of challenges and problems facing African American communities today, including the education of African American children, the disproportionate placement of Black male children in special education classes, ADHD and the Ritalin controversy, substance abuse, AIDS, violence, racial profiling, and police brutality.

AFROCENTRICITY AND
THE AFROCENTRIC MOVEMENT

The Afrocentric movement has been a process by which many African Americans have reclaimed the cultural strengths of their African heritage while offering them a positive alternative to the negative messages and stereotypes perpetrated by the dominant European American society. Afrocentricity has been a growing movement among African Americans since the late 1960s. According to Allwood (2001),

Afrocentricity involves the desire to keep Africa, its culture and worldview, central to all analysis relevant to people of African descent. According to Afrocentric theory, African Americans have too often allowed others to define their reality using the Euro-American norms. Afrocentricity represents the drive for self-determination using the norms of African culture as the standard. (p. 2)

For the last 40 years, there has been an ever-growing Afrocentric movement within the mental health field, but many therapists are unaware of it. Led by Afrocentric psychologists such as Nobles (in press), Akbar (1984), Kambon (1998), Azibo (1996), and Hilliard, Payton-Stewart, and Williams (1990), this movement has developed African-centered paradigms (Kambon, 1998) for understanding the psychological and mental health of African Americans. These Afrocentric psychologists have challenged the prevailing Eurocentric field of psychology, which often labels and diagnoses people of African descent in pejorative terms. They have argued that many African Americans in the 400 years since the beginning of the *Maafa* (slavery; see Chapter 1) have been, as Jackson-Lowman (1998) has described, "conceptually incarcerated by definitions of identity grounded in Western/Eurocentric thinking, with disastrous consequences for our mental health and well-being" (p. 58).

Afrocentric historians have challenged the European-centered view of history and have written about ancient African civilizations in Egypt (Kemet), Ghana, Mali, Axum, Oyo, Ife, Dahomay, Ashanti, and Great Zimbabwe, which were thriving civilizations while Europe was still in the Dark Ages (Asante, 1988, 1990; Diop, 1974; Karenga, 1997; Van Sertima, 1976). These Afrocentric historians have argued that the African worldview and African history have been so distorted in U.S. schools that many African Americans do not know their history prior to the *Maafa* (see Chapter 1). Their writings have prompted many African American parents to teach their children about African and African American history in an attempt to counter the destructive messages of the past.

Since many African American families incorporate the principles of Afrocentricity into their own lives and childrearing practices, it is important for therapists to have a clear understanding of this movement. It is also important for them to recognize that individuals and families may incorporate these ideas to different degrees. Afrocentricity has impacted contemporary African American culture in many ways (Allwood, 2001).

Therapists should be aware that African American families vary considerably in their degree of Afrocentricity and in their involvement in Afrocentric practices. While many African Americans have studied the major Afrocentric writers, who are scholars in the fields of African studies, history, anthropology, and psychology, such as Akbar (1984), Ani (1994), Asante (1988), Azibo (1996), Diop (1974), Hilliard, Payton-Stewart, and Williams (1990), Kambon (1998), Karenga (1997), Nobles (in press), and Welsing (1991), an even larger number of African Americans have incorporated African dress, art, and rituals into their family life. Many have taken African names for themselves and given them to their children. One example of the influence of the Afrocentric movement in the African American community is the increasing popularity of the holiday of Kwanzaa created by Maulana Karenga in 1966 (Karenga, 1997).

Kwanzaa, which takes place each year from December 26 to January 1, incorporates aspects of the harvest celebration from many African cultures (Karenga, 1997). This cultural celebration is based on the *Nguzu Saba,* or the Seven Principles, which include *Umoja* (Unity), *Kujichagulia* (Self-Determination), *Ujima* (Collective Work and Responsibility), *Ujamaa* (Cooperative Economics), *Nia* (Purpose), *Kuumba* (Creativity), and *Imani* (Faith) (Karenga, 1998).

According to Karenga (1997), Kwanzaa is a special time for

> gathering together family and friends to honor spiritual values (the Creator and Creation); a commemoration of ancestors who have died; and an opportunity to commit oneself once again to the spiritual and cultural values of "life, truth, justice, sisterhood, brotherhood, respect . . . for the human person, for elders and for nature." (cited in Boyd–Franklin et al., 2001, p. 43)

African American family therapists, Hines and Sutton (1997), published *Sankofa: A Violence Prevention and Life Skills Curriculum* based on Afrocentric principles. Another area in which Afrocentric thinking has had a major impact on African American youth and families has been in the development of church- and community-based programs founded on African principles, such as "Rites–of–Passage" programs (Boyd–Franklin et al., 2001; Harvey, 2001; Harvey & Rauch, 1997; Harvey & Hill, in press; Hill, 1992; Warfield–Coppock, 1992).

Rites-of-Passage Programs

Rites–of–Passage programs have become very popular in many African American communities as a way of developing a positive African American identity in young male and female adolescents (Boyd–Franklin et al., 2001; Harvey, 2001; Harvey & Hill, in press; Hill, 1992; Kunjufu, 1985; Warfield–Coppock, 1992).

Rites–of–Passage programs are based on rituals used by many African tribes to help to socialize youngsters in their transition from childhood to adulthood. Rites–of–Passage programs incorporating different socialization rituals for boys and girls are based on Afrocentric principles such as those of the *Nguzu Saba* (described above). Warfield–Coppock (1992) surveyed 20 Rites–of–Passage programs throughout the country. All of the respondents emphasized the importance of these programs for "at-risk" African American youth. Boyd–Franklin et al. (2001) described a number of these programs and emphasized their significance in the effort to "take children back from the streets." It is extremely important that therapists who work with African American families familiarize themselves with such programs in their area.

Boyd-Franklin et al. (2001) describe the work of Dr. Asa Hilliard and the Onis Program, developed by Dr. Vernon Allwood in Atlanta, Georgia. Onis is a Rites-of-Passage program in a Black church, that utilizes older African American men to provide role models and "manhood training" for male adolescents. African and African American history, achievements. and cultural traditions are emphasized, along with the importance of academic achievement for these young men. The goal is to "help them to achieve a clearer understanding of positive African American manhood, [and] to strengthen their minds, bodies and souls through activities designed to build self-esteem, positive black racial identity, and strong bonds with other men in the community" (Boyd-Franklin et al., 2001, p. 215).

Jawanza Kunjufu (1985) developed SIMBA, a Rites-of-Passage program in Chicago, to counter negative street influences such as drugs, alcohol, gangs, and violence. SIMBA (which means "young lions" in Swahili) was a manhood training program designed to build a sense of solidarity and positive racial identity.

Another such program, which incorporates the seven principles of the *Nguzo Saba* (Harvey & Hill, in press) as well as Rites-of-Passage and mental health interventions for African American youth and their families, is the MAAT Adolescent and Family Rites-of-Passage Program in Washington, DC (Harvey, 2001; Harvey & Hill, in press). This program includes three interventions: (1) an after-school component; (2) family enhancement and empowerment activities; and (3) individual and family counseling (Harvey & Rauch, 1997). Its goal is to reduce the incidence of substance abuse and antisocial attitudes and behavior in 12- to 14-year-old African American males.

The after-school component consists of an 8-week program followed by a 3-day weekend retreat, at the end of which a Rites-of-Passage ceremony is held in which each youth is given an African name. Unlike many other Rites-of-Passage programs, which focus exclusively on youth, this program also incorporates a family component. Monthly 2-hour family group sessions emphasizing parenting skills, family involvement, bonding, and the development of a strong racial and cultural identity are scheduled, as is a parents' retreat. Later, the parent retreat evolved into a parent–youth retreat with the goal of enhancing family unity in which Afrocentric principles are taught and the family is included in the naming ceremony.

The final component involves individual counseling sessions with the youth and family sessions in the home that include the young male, his parents or guardians, siblings, and extended family members. Again an Afrocentric philosophy is combined with mental health principles to produce a therapeutic intervention, which is empowering to the youth and their families.

The staff members of the MAAT Center, as is the case with all

Afrocentric-based programs, are African American, live in the community, and identify with the youth and their families. The opportunity to work with Black staff as role models is an extremely important part of the program.

These programs provide an emphasis on racial and cultural identity, which is often lacking in conventional treatment approaches. Clinicians of all backgrounds should become familiar with Rites-of-Passage and other Afrocentric programs in their community so that they may refer the youth and their families to them. Also, as more African American families incorporate Afrocentric values and Rites-of-Passage programs into their lifestyles, it is important that clinicians from all backgrounds educate themselves on these beliefs. There is a growing literature on these approaches (see Boyd-Franklin et al., 2001; Harvey, 2001; Harvey & Hill, in press; Harvey & Rauch, 1997; Hill, 1992; Kunjufu, 1985; Warfield-Coppock, 1992).

The following case example illustrates the importance of this knowledge and intervention.

Karenga, a 14-year-old African American adolescent male living in Harlem, New York, was brought for treatment by Ms. Washington, his 34-year-old mother. They were referred by his school for treatment to an outpatient clinic at a large city hospital because of Karenga's aggressive behavior, truancy, and membership in an increasingly delinquent peer group. They were seen by John, an African American male clinician.

Ms. Washington appeared for the session in African dress. She explained to the therapist that she did not believe in therapy and was bringing her son only because the school was forcing her to. John explored her beliefs about what would be helpful for her son. She explained that she had tried very hard to expose him to Afrocentric values, to teach him about his African cultural heritage, and to help him to develop a strong Black identity. Her efforts, she felt, were undermined by the school, where she felt that her son had been wrongly labeled as a "troublemaker." She also felt that she was losing her son to his friends, who were both drug- and gang-involved, and she was very worried that he would be pulled into that lifestyle. Academic achievement of any kind was dismissed by his peers as "acting White." In despair, she reported feeling that there was nothing she could do to help her son and that therapy was "useless."

Karenga was a bright adolescent, who also felt that the therapy was useless. He repeatedly asked when the session would be over. At the end of the first session, the mother stated that she did not see "what once-per-week therapy was going to do for him." John told her that he agreed with her that therapy by itself was not going to be enough. He told her that he as therapist, her as mother, and Karenga himself were going to have to work together to "take him back from the streets." Ms. Washington and Karenga were both puzzled by this comment. The therapist explained that because Karenga was being strongly influenced by his friends, they needed to search for an intervention that would involve him in positive after-school activities and expose him to positive role models. Neither the mother nor Karenga knew of any such opportunity, but the therapist was aware of a Rites-of-Passage program at a community church, which he had learned about through another client. He empowered the mother to obtain information about this program before their next meeting.

By the next session, the mother had spoken to the director of the program. The therapist praised her and encouraged her to tell her son what she had discovered. Within the next 2 weeks, Karenga enrolled. Although he was initially resistant to going to an after-school program, he quickly became interested because he was very drawn to the Black male role models and mentors the program provided. As he became more involved with the program, he spent less time "on the streets" with his friends.

The therapist used Karenga's commitment to the program as an opportunity to praise his mother for taking the initiative and to praise Karenga for giving it a chance. The therapist encouraged the mother to share her concerns for her son with Karenga's mentors. They worked to reinforce appropriate school behavior and had a number of group activities on the *Nguso Saba,* which reinforced cooperative effort and violence prevention. Within 3 months, Karenga, his mother, and his school reported positive behaviorial change.

This case illustrates how a therapist with knowledge of Afrocentric beliefs and principles was able to help this family find a culturally compatible program that complemented his treatment interventions. He gained credibility with both the mother and the son by recommending a program that proved helpful to them. He empowered the mother to follow through and investigate this program on her own. His praise of the mother's and Karenga's efforts also reinforced his work with them and embraced the positive influence of the Rites-of-Passage program. It is important that therapists of all backgrounds be familiar with such Afrocentric programs in the communities in which they work.

DIVERSITY WITHIN BLACK COMMUNITIES

Caribbean Families

This book has primarily addressed the racial and cultural issues affecting African American families (i.e., those whose ancestors were brought to the United States from Africa during the era of slavery). But there are many Black families in this country who came to the United States from countries in the Caribbean or from the countries in the West Indies that were originally settled by the British. These countries include Jamaica, Trinidad and Tobago, the Grenadines, St. Vincent, St. Lucia, St. Kitts, Nevis, Montserrat, Grenada, Dominica, the Cayman Islands, the British Virgin Islands, Barbados, the Bahamas, part of Aruba, part of the Netherland Antilles, Barbuda, Antigua, and Anguilla. In addition, there are countries such as Bermuda, an island off the coast of South Carolina, and Haiti, a Caribbean island settled originally by the French. In most of these islands, the enslavement of Africans was practiced by the colonial powers until the mid-19th century (Brice-Baker, 1996; Gopaul-McNicol, 1993). Many famous African Americans come from families with Caribbean roots, including Harry Belafonte, Sidney Poitier, Colin Powell, and Minister Louis Farrakhan of the Nation of Islam.

New York, Boston, Washington, D.C., and Miami have large West Indian populations, but the high rate of mobility within the United States, particularly due to employment opportunity, signifies that therapists in other parts of the country may encounter such families. Although first-generation Caribbean immigrants can often be identified by their accent, therapists often make the mistake of assuming an African American cultural background for those of West Indian descent born in the United States. It is often helpful, once the therapist has joined with the family, to ask where the family is from. Therapists should be aware that Caribbean individuals identify strongly with their country of origin; when they are asked about their ethnicity or cultural background, they will often say "Jamaican," or "Trinidadian" rather than Caribbean, West Indian, or African American.

There are many similarities between families of African American background and those of Caribbean origin, including close extended family ties, close relationships with nonblood family members (often called "Auntie" or "Uncle"), a strong religious and spiritual values, strong educational orientation, and a very strong work orientation.

There are also many differences. For example, one major difference is that first-generation families from the Caribbean face similar hurdles to those faced by other immigrants coming to a new country—for example, a harsh winter climate, lack of contact with family and extended family members at home, and loss of prior skilled or professional employment status. Brice-Baker (1996) indicated that a pattern of immigration usually exists for this group. One family member comes to this country and gets a job. This person then obtains job referrals here for other adult family members, who then come to this country and live with the first person who immigrated. Children are often left behind with relatives; due to U.S. immigration laws, a parent may be separated from his or her children for many years (see the case example below). By the time they are reunited, they may be virtual strangers to each other.

It can take as long as 6 years or more for an individual to obtain a "green card" (the permit that allows an immigrant to work legally in this country) and to have enough money saved to bring his or her children into the country. U.S. immigration laws forbid those applying for green card status to leave the country, so that individuals cannot return home in emergency situations, such as the serious illness of a family member or to attend a funeral.

Another major difference is the divergent stereotypes of African American and Caribbean individuals in the United States. Brice-Baker (1996) stated that Caribbean families "have frequently been placed on pedestals by White society as examples of the 'good and industrious Black,' whereas African Americans have been stereotyped as lazy, criminal and willing to live on public assistance" (p. 87). These racist stereotypes have often created conflict between

African American families and those of Caribbean descent. Unlike African American families, who have a long history of experiencing the racism in the United States, Caribbean families are new to this country and are often more trusting of Whites and hopeful about their ability to achieve the "American Dream" (Brice-Baker, 1996; Gopaul-McNicol, 1993).

Sex roles in the Caribbean can be very traditional but there are often gender paradoxes (Brice-Baker, 1996; Smith, 1988). This is particularly true in the United States, where women are frequently the first to immigrate because of the availability of low-skilled employment. Similar to Latino families, women can have enhanced and powerful positions in the family here because of their wage-earning status, which may cause difficulties in their relationships with more traditional West Indian men. A practice often tolerated in the islands, that of men having extramarital affairs and even having more than one family with children, can create major conflicts in this country (Brice-Baker, 1996; Gopaul-McNicol, 1993).

Similar to children in African American families, children in Caribbean families are expected to respect their elders and other authority figures. Spanking as a form of punishment is customary. When working with families from both cultures, it is helpful if therapists avoid value judgments and instead indicate that they are aware of the fact that spanking is the expected form of discipline in their cultures. Therapists can indicate, however, that they care about the family and that they do not want to see them lose their children because of child abuse laws in this country. They can join with them to find new means of disciplining their children. As with many other issues discussed in this book, timing is critical, and these issues should not be raised until trust is established. There are cases, however, when child abuse is actually occurring and the children should be removed for their own protection. In cases of child abuse, therapists have an obligation to report these to child protective services. Therapists should confer with colleagues who share the family's cultural background to help in making this determination.

The following case example illustrates many of the issues described above, particularly the challenges of immigration and the separation issues that can occur between parents and children.

Lloyd was a 12-year-old boy who had recently arrived in New York from Jamaica. He was overwhelmed in his classroom and was often teased by the other children because of his accent. As a result, he was disruptive in class, which caused him to be referred for family therapy by his school counselor. The counselor had met with the mother and reported that she seemed unaware of her son's problems in school. The counselor was also very judgmental of this mother for having left her son for so many years.

Lloyd and his mother, Mrs. MacPherson (age 32), arrived at the clinic for their initial family therapy session. She appeared overwhelmed, uncomfortable, tense, and rigid in the session and obviously angry with Lloyd. She repeatedly corrected his behavior and posture, insisting that he sit still and listen. In this first session, the therapist learned that Mrs. MacPherson had immigrated to the United States 7 years earlier, leaving Lloyd in the care of her mother. Lloyd's father, her husband, joined her 2 years later. In the intervening years, Mrs. MacPherson and her husband had had two more children, Margaret (age 3) and Beth (age 1).

Mrs. MacPherson seemed very defensive about her decision to leave her son in Jamaica. She reported that it took her a year to find an employer who would sponsor her for her green card. She and her husband had saved all of these years to bring Lloyd to this country, but they could not do so until she obtained her own green card, which took over 6 years. In the last year, there had been a number of disruptions "back home" in Jamaica. Her mother, Lloyd's grandmother, had been very ill until her recent death from a heart attack. Lloyd had stayed with a cousin until Mrs. MacPherson could arrange to bring him to New York.

The therapist pointed out that it sounded like they both had been through a lot of loss and change in the last year. When she asked Lloyd about his grandmother, he burst into tears. He had referred to her as his "Nana," and it was clear that his primary attachment had been to her. As Lloyd was crying, his mother began to cry softly also. The therapist encouraged them to hug and comfort each other. Although both seemed awkward initially, they were able to hold each other for a few minutes.

The therapist asked what had changed for Lloyd since coming to this country. Again, he became tearful and his mother attempted to answer for him. The therapist, wanting to encourage some interaction between them, asked the mother to talk with Lloyd about what life had been like for him in Jamaica. The therapist was able to support her in giving him time to answer. Slowly, the story emerged. His grandmother had been the closest person in the world to him, caring for him even before his mother left while she was at work. He had been devastated by her death.

He remembered the time when his parents and he lived together in Jamaica, but his fondest memories of them were the Christmas and birthday gifts they sent. Because his grandmother did not have a telephone, he did not even have this limited method of contact with his parents while they were in the United States. When the therapist asked his mother how she felt after hearing Lloyd's words, she responded, "He doesn't even know me." She began to cry. Although both were rather stiff and distant at first, the therapist encouraged them once again to hold each other. She sat silently as they cried together. At the end of the session, the therapist asked that Mr. MacPherson and the two other children attend the next session.

Only Lloyd and Mrs. MacPherson appeared at this session to focus on Lloyd's school behavior because Mr. MacPherson could not take time off from work. The therapist encouraged the mother to talk to her son directly. Lloyd indicated that the schoolwork was not hard for him although math was taught differently in Jamaica. Mrs. MacPherson proudly told the therapist that she felt that the schools in Jamaica were more advanced. The most difficult issue for him in school was fitting in with his Black, Latino, and White peers at his middle school in Brooklyn. This was especially hard since he had started school in January, when everybody else had already made friends.

The only positive experiences he had with his classmates was making them laugh, but this was disruptive and made his teacher angry. The therapist empathized with Lloyd about the difficulty of starting a new school in a new country. She asked his mother if she could understand what he was going through and the mother shared some of her own difficulties fitting in and making friends when she first moved to this country.

In the next session, the therapist talked with the mother about discipline. She admitted that she had spanked him when the teacher called her. She told her son that he was lucky because "back home the teacher would have spanked you in school first and sent you home for another spanking." The therapist acknowledged that back home this was definitely the way children were raised. She explained the child abuse laws in this country and told the mother that she liked her and her son and did not want to see them run into problems here. She asked the mother if she would be willing to learn some new parenting techniques. Although the mother was not convinced that anything else would work, she agreed to try. For the next few sessions, a number of parenting techniques were introduced in the sessions. The therapist asked Lloyd and his mother to role-play these techniques and practice them in the sessions. Lloyd's behavior began to improve at home and in school.

The therapist praised Mrs. MacPherson and Lloyd for their progress and again asked to have the father attend a session. Again, she was told that he was working long hours in two jobs. She asked if there was a time when she could call him. The mother indicated that he was usually home on Sunday evening after returning from church. The therapist called the father and explained that out of respect for him as the father in the home, she wanted to ask his opinion about the work that she had been doing with his wife and son. He seemed taken aback by the request but responded very positively. Although he was never able to come in for a session, he agreed to talk with the therapist on the phone twice a month. He was willing to support the interventions that had been made. Lloyd's progress continued. The treatment continued for another 2 months.

This case illustrates many of the issues for families from Jamaica and other Caribbean islands. Many counselors do not understand that separations created by the process of immigration can often create a vacuum in the parent–child relationship. Moreover, some clinicians are prone to be judgmental concerning the parents. It is important that therapists indicate their awareness of the immigration laws and to acknowledge that separations are not the parent's fault. The issues of discipline in this case example, and the necessity for additional outreach to the father, can be very similar in the treatment of African American families. Although a comprehensive discussion of the issues facing Caribbean families is beyond the scope of this book, there is a need for more research into the needs of these families.

Biracial Children and Families

The numbers of biracial and multiracial children and families are growing in this country (Root, 1992, 1996). From the 1960s through the present, there has been an increase in interracial relationships and marriages. Consequently, there are also larger numbers of biracial or multiracial children (Daniel, 1996), many of whom identify as "biracial or multiracial" (Root, 1996).

In the 2000 Census, for the first time in history, individuals were allowed to indicate more than one racial category. According to the U.S. Bureau of the Census (2001b) brief on the Black population, "36.4 million or 12.9 percent of the total population reported Black alone or in combination with one or more other races" (p. 2); "34.7 million people or 12.3 percent reported that they were only 'Black.' An additional 1.8 million reported Black and at least one other race" (p. 1). "Within this group, the most common combinations were 'Black and White' (45 percent), followed by 'Black and some other race' (24 percent), 'Black and White and American Indian or Alaska native' (6 percent)" (p. 2).

Just as there is a tremendous amount of diversity among African American families, there are many factors that may contribute to the diversity among biracial families, including the race and racial identity of the mother and the father, the skin color of the children (i.e., how visibly Black they appear), the neighborhood or community in which they are raised, the racial composition of that community, peer experiences, the school experiences of the children, the philosophy of each parent about the racial identity of his or her children, the messages conveyed to them about how they should identify, and the quality of their relationships with each parent and extended family members. Although a comprehensive exploration of all the different forms of biracial families and the complex issues facing them is beyond the scope of this book, some of the issues for biracial families with one Black and one White biological parent will be discussed. (Clinicians should remember that biracial and multiracial children can also include Black and Asian, Hispanic, Native American, or other ethnic and racial combinations). Readers are referred to the growing body of research and scholarly literature now available on this topic (Brown, 1990; Buxenbaum, 1996; Daniel, 1996; Field, 1996; Funderberg, 1994; Gibbs, 1987; Gibbs & Hines, 1992; Gillem et al., 2001; Poston, 1990; Root, 1992, 1996; Tizard & Phoenix, 1993; Wardle, 1987, 1991).

Parents of biracial children often struggle with how to help their children to develop a positive identity and sense of self-esteem. This process can be particularly difficult from about age 10 throughout the teenage years. Although the preteen and teenage years are challenging for children from all backgrounds, these years can often be particularly difficult for biracial children because it is during this stage of their lives that they begin to struggle with issues related to their own identity.

The topic of interracial couples and families is particularly complicated because of the history of slavery, miscegenation laws, racism, racial identity, and skin color issues. As indicated earlier in this book, many African Americans come in a variety of skin colors and may have a family history that includes African, European, and Native American ancestry, although they identify as African American or Black primarily because the racial mixing occurred generations prior to their birth (see Chapter 2). The situation is often quite different for biracial children and families on issues of identity. In order to understand this complexity, it is important to place interracial relationships in the historical context of slavery, miscegenation laws, "Jim Crow" laws, and the "one drop" rule.

The racist institution of slavery has shaped the response to interracial relationships and the experiences of biracial individuals. Biracial children have existed in this country since the 16th century when the first Africans were brought here as slaves. Biracial children in that era were usually the result of White slave owners raping African women. These children were favored by the slaveowner and it was not uncommon for slaveowners to free them. Because a significant freed population threatened to devastate the economy of slave states, proponents of slavery felt the need for additional methods to control the slave population and justify their enslavement. One of these methods was the rule of hypodescent, known as "the one drop rule."

The "One-Drop Rule," or the Rule of Hypodescent

A crucial component of, and justification for, slavery was the belief in the inferiority of the Black race. In order to ensure White domination, a definition was constructed as to what made a person "Black." This "one-drop" rule, or the rule of hypodescent, deemed that any individual with one drop of African blood was black. Racist "miscegenation" laws, which forbade interracial relationships and marriages (Buxenbaum, 1996; Daniel, 1996; Davis, 1991) so that the White race might remain "pure," were first introduced in 1662. Such laws persisted in some states in this country until 1967, when they were repealed by the Supreme Court.

After the Civil War, segregation was built into the fabric of the society of many states in this country through "Jim Crow" laws, based on the "one-drop" rule, which were used to keep Blacks and Whites "separate, hostile and unequal" (Daniel, 1996; Hacker, 1992). It was customary that anyone with "one drop of Black blood" was deemed Black by other Blacks as well. The "Jim Crow" laws institutionalized racism and made it mandatory for Blacks to live separately from Whites. They were given their own inferior facilities, which were finally abolished as a result of the civil rights movement in the 1950s and 1960s. While many, if not most, Black Americans are aware of the history of racism, most White Americans (including many therapists) are not (Daniel, 1996; Davis, 1991).

Identifying as African American and being proud of one's cultural and racial background became an extremely important value in the Black community. In addition, African Americans were taught that it was very important to socialize children of African descent (even those of biracial ancestry) to have pride in themselves, their African American culture, and their history. This has been important even in the 21st century in order to prepare Black children for encounters with racism, especially the more subtle forms that exist today, and protect their self-esteem (Boyd–Franklin et al., 2001).

Many African Americans are aware that although children might be biracial or multiracial, they are often perceived by society as Black and treated accordingly. Thus, many African Americans advise biracial families to educate their children about their African American heritage and let them know that the world will view them as Black (Carter, 1995; Gardere, 1999). Gillem et al. (2001) describe the case of a young biracial woman who struggled with her own identity but currently identifies as Black. She was given very different messages about her racial identity by her mother, who was White, and her stepfather, who was Black, with "her stepfather urging her to take on the identity that society will ascribe to her because of her looks [a Black identity] and her mother wanting her to have more White friends and to feel more affinity with Whites" (p. 186). These types of mixed messages can create identity conflicts for individuals, especially during their adolescence and young adult years.

Within the last 10 years, there has been a movement by many more biracial and multiracial individuals to resist categorization as "Black" or "White." The champion golfer Tiger Woods, whose father is African American and whose mother is Asian, is a well-known example of an individual who identifies as "biracial" or "multiracial."

Organizations for biracial and multiracial individuals such as Shades (Buxenbaum, 1996) now exist on many college campuses in the United States. Gillem et al. (2001) quote Maria Root, one of the leading researchers concerned with biracial/multiracial identity:

> Root (1990) postulated that when racial identity and self-concept are difficult for biracial people, it is because of the tension between the two racial components of the self (which reflects the tension in the greater society between those two "components"). She asserted that biracial people demonstrate internalized oppression if they reject either part of their heritage. (p. 183)

Recent research (Brown, 1990; Buxenbaum, 1996) has shown that some of these individuals embrace a "public" and a "private" racial identity. Many of the individuals in both of these studies identified as "Black" publicly, but as "biracial" privately. It is important for therapists to recognize that biracial and multiracial individuals may identify in different ways. They should also recognize that these families may present with complex identity issues that can contribute to family conflicts. White, Black, and other ethnic minority group therapists should be aware that they may have a range of strong countertransferential reactions to individuals and families who identify themselves as biracial or multiracial. These reactions can impact and sometimes interfere with the treatment process. There is clearly a need for more research and clinical case material on the identity issues of these children and families and their experiences in treatment.

OTHER IMPORTANT ISSUES
IN AFRICAN AMERICAN COMMUNITIES

Challenges Related to the Educational Achievement of African American Children

African Americans have always valued education and have had strong achievement orientation (Franklin, Boyd-Franklin, & Draper, 2002; Hill, 1999a; McAdoo, 2002; Stevenson & Davis, in press). Many view education as the way their children can have a better life. For poor parents, education is viewed as their children's chance for upward mobility (Billingsley, 1992; Hill, 1999a). In a sample of over 3,000 Black, White, and Hispanic children in Chicago, Stevenson and Davis (in press) discovered that Black and Hispanic mothers were more invested in the academic achievement of their children than White mothers (Hill, 1999a). Studies conducted by the National Center for Education Statistics (1995) have demonstrated that high achievement orientation was also evident among poor Black parents (Hill, 1999a).

Many African American parents find that it is very difficult for their children to perform consistent with the parent's aspirations and goals for them (Hill, 1999a; McAdoo, 2002) In fact, the largest number of referrals for therapy for African American children and adolescents are for school-related academic and behavioral problems. It is important for clinicians to understand the reasons for this discrepancy.

One contributor is the self-fulfilling prophecy of low expectations. Researchers have found that low teacher expectations can profoundly influence the decline in academic motivation among Black students, particularly in the upper grades (Hill, 1999a; Stevenson & Davis, in press).

Some African American parents, particularly those whose children attend poor, inner-city schools, become discouraged by the racism inherent in the self-fulfilling prophecies and withdraw from active involvement in their children's schools; others become so angry in meetings that they alienate teachers, counselors, and administrators; and still others do not know they have the right to intercede for their child with the school system.

One of the most important contributions therapists can make to African American parents is to empower them to become more proactively involved in their children's schools. If a family member has exhibited what school officials perceived as hostility in prior dealings, therapists can often help to reframe these perceptions during phone conversations or school visits. Sometimes it is enough for the therapist to express the parents' concern for their child(ren) to change the school's perception of a parent's role. A therapist might also accompany a parent to school meetings, especially when the child is in special education and the entire child study team (CST) will be present for an IEP (individualized educational plan) meeting. This group, including CST members, teachers, and school administrators, can overwhelm parents and inhibit their speaking out on their child's behalf.

Therapists might also want to consider making a school visit to observe a child's interaction in the classroom if the child has been labeled as "disruptive." Boyd–Franklin et al. (2001) have documented teacher practices, such as ignoring certain African American children and being inappropriately critical of their work, which can lead to low self-esteem and high school dropout rates, particularly in inner-city schools. If the students' problems are precipitated by negative teacher behavior, this may be changed through the clinician's input. The therapist's support when helping parents deal with their children's school issues is often greatly appreciated (Boyd–Franklin & Bry, 2000).

The Disproportionate Placement of African American Children in Special Education Classes

Historically, African American children, particularly males, have been overrepresented in special education classes (Franklin et al., 2002; Russo & Talbert-Johnson, 1997; Serwatka, Deering, & Grant, 1995), in sharp contrast to their underrepresentation in classes for the gifted and talented (Ford, 1995; Franklin et al., 2002; Patton, 1992).

Kunjufu (1985) has described "the fourth grade failure syndrome" in which African American boys are often labeled as behavior problems or school failures at young ages in his multivolume study, *Countering the Conspiracy to Destroy Black Boys.* This labeling may occur as early as kindergarten (Boyd–Franklin et al., 2001). Such labeling often leads to special education placement and a higher risk for becoming a school dropout.

Given this pattern, child study team evaluations and special education placement can engender healthy cultural suspicion on the part of parents (see Chapter 1). Clinicians, school counselors, and CST members should anticipate this response and take the time to meet with parents and carefully review the child's rights and options. Unfortunately, because of the excessive placement of Black males in these programs, a child who genuinely needs smaller classes and resource room services may not receive them. A greater percentage of African American students are referred to these programs for behavior problems, particularly for fighting.

Boyd–Franklin et al. (2001) offer a number of guidelines that clinicians can use to empower African American parents to challenge school decisions and determine the appropriate educational placements for their children. See Boyd–Franklin and Bry (2000), *Reaching Out in Family Therapy,* for a case example illustrating the ways in which a family therapist can help African American parents making this type of decision.

Attention-Deficit/Hyperactivity Disorder and the Ritalin Controversy

In recent years, the media has focused attention on the increased diagnosis of ADD (attention-deficit disorder) or ADHD (attention-deficit/hyperactivity disorder), conditions which include many of the following behaviors: distract-ibility, difficulty concentrating, inattention, the inability to sit still, hyperactiv-ity, and impulsivity (e.g., blurting out answers or interrupting when others are speaking) (Barkley, 2000; Boyd-Franklin et al., 2001).

This diagnosis and the prescription of Ritalin (the drug prescribed to treat it) can present an enormous dilemma for therapists. African American families are aware that African American males have been disproportionately labeled with this diagnosis. Ritalin is often seen as a "drug," as is common with all psychiatric medications, and many African American parents adamantly re-fuse to allow their children to be put on these medications. Ritalin is especially suspect as it has been viewed by many in the African American community as an attempt to control Black children through drugs (Boyd-Franklin et al., 2001).

Clinicians will have to work to establish trust and credibility with Black families before raising the issue of medication. It is important for therapists to identify culturally sensitive psychiatrists and neurologists, particularly African Americans, who can work with Black parents struggling to make a decision about whether to allow their child to use medication.

Therapists can be helpful to African American parents by providing them with information on this condition and, if the diagnosis is inaccurate, helping to advocate for them and empowering them to challenge the school system on behalf of their children. A number of books are available to educate therapists and African American parents about ADHD and the Ritalin controversy (Barkley, 2000; Boyd-Franklin et al., 2001). Franklin et al (2002) and Boyd-Franklin et al. (2001) have described resources, websites, and advocacy organi-zations that therapists can utilize to help educate parents about these issues as well as others effecting a child's ability to succeed in school, such as learning disabilities and dyslexia.

Attitudes toward Achievement in the Black Peer Group

Another controversial factor effecting the academic achievement of African American children, particularly adolescents, is the influence of their peer group. Peer group influence is often a major concern of African American parents. It is important for clinicians to avoid stereotypical assumptions and to carefully question African American youth and their families about peer group influences since this influence can vary depending upon such factors as the achievement level of the peers, the culture of the school regarding achieve-ment, the socioeconomic level of the peers, and their parents' level of educa-tion.

Some African American youth, particularly in junior high and high school, struggle with the message from their peers that being smart in school is the equivalent of "acting White" (Boyd-Franklin et al., 2001; Kunjufu, 1988). African American parents may be surprised to discover that this pressure is prevalent at all socioeconomic levels and can be present in suburban neighborhoods as well as in inner-city schools (Boyd–Franklin et al., 2001). Because most adolescents desperately want to be accepted by their peer group, African Americans who want to do well in school adopt several coping strategies that Kunjufu (1988) has identified as clowning in the classroom, refusing to study in public, becoming a loner, fighting, and "tutoring bullies." In addition, Boyd–Franklin et al. (2001) have indicated that outstanding athletes may be immune from disparagement for academic achievement by the peer group because of their popularity.

Therapists should also be aware of the process by which some African American youth appear to "become raceless" (Fordham & Ogbu, 1986; Kunjufu, 1988). Kunjufu (1988) expresses the tragedy underlying this circumstance: "[They] have learned the value of appearing to be raceless—a clear example of internalizing oppression—in their efforts to make it. Many of these kids become very isolated and may struggle throughout their lives with a negative sense of their racial identity" (quoted in Boyd–Franklin et al., 2001, p. 96).

It is very important for clinicians to help African American adolescents and parents talk about the pressures they are experiencing. Black parents who are alarmed by this threat to their children's academic achievement may lecture their children. This can be counterproductive because adolescents in this position may "shut down." Boyd–Franklin et al. (2001) advise therapists and African American parents in this situation to work on developing active listening skills, which they describe in detail.

Therapists can also help African American parents to find enrichment programs that encourage bright African American adolescents to aspire toward college admission and meet other academically motivated adolescents, such as Upward Bound, or ABC (A Better Chance), (see Boyd–Franklin et al., 2001, for further information on relevant organizations). In addition, mentoring and tutoring programs are also available through local Boys and Girls Clubs, YMCAs, and many churches in African American communities. It is important for therapists to be aware of resources in their communities to which they can refer African American parents and children, including the Rites-of-Passage programs described above.

Substance Abuse and the Burden on the Older Generation

Like many families in the United States, some African American families have struggled with issues of drug and alcohol abuse. The burden of substance abuse has had a major impact on the older generation (e.g., grandmothers, grandfathers, aunts, uncles, and other concerned extended family members) when young men or women, who often became involved with drugs as teenagers, start to have children of their own (Burton, 1992). This may begin a devastating cycle in which their families are often placed in the double bind described below.

African American culture in its collectivistic roots has a strong legacy of not giving up on family members. As a consequence, the substance-abusing young person is still considered to be an integral part of the family system. Family members take in their children and raise them as part of the extended family. For older relatives, such as grandmothers and grandfathers, this may present a serious dilemma: they love their child and their grandchild but they are at an age when they hoped to retire, and now are faced with having to raise another generation of children. What makes this situation even more difficult is that the children may have severe health problems as a result of parental addiction. For example, children born to a drug-addicted or alcoholic mother are often born addicted and experience fetal drug or fetal alcohol syndrome, the symptoms of which include hyperactivity, cognitive deficits, and developmental delays in such things as gross and fine motor development. The following case poignantly illustrates one grandmother's predicament.

Mrs. Cellars was a 65-year-old African American grandmother. Her youngest daughter, Shakeera, was 25 and had been actively drug-involved since she was 15. Shakeera had given birth to two children, Kofi (age 4), and Malik (age 7). Throughout the boys' lives she had been only peripherally involved in raising them, spending most of the time living "on the streets" or in crack houses. Mrs. Cellars was the main parental figure for the boys. After Kofi's birth, Mrs. Cellars became the legal guardian of both boys. When Shakeera saw the boys, her visits were unscheduled and usually accompanied by requests for money. Money and other household items (the TV, VCR, or radio) often disappeared after Shakeera visited. All this time, Mrs. Cellars never lost hope that her daughter would go into a drug rehabilitation program and conquer her addiction.

The Cellars family was referred for treatment by Malik's school. He had been born with fetal drug syndrome and was showing signs of hyperactivity and disruptive behavior in school. His teacher also saw signs of developmental delays and was concerned about his language development. Mrs. Cellars appeared with the boys for the first session. She presented as exhausted from the demands of a full-time job, hypertension, and diabetes. She was overwhelmed by the care and responsibility for two very active children. That year would have marked her retirement, but she did not feel that she could afford to retire and still provide for the needs of her grandsons.

The therapist joined with Mrs. Cellars around her worry about the boys and also expressed her concern about Mrs. Cellars's medical condition. The therapist was the first person who showed any interest in Mrs. Cellars's needs. By the end of the session, Mrs. Cellars began to relax. They agreed to meet again to discuss the behavior of both boys at home and in school.

For the next four sessions, the therapist focused on parenting issues and strategies to help Mrs. Cellars address the boys' disruptive behavior at home. She also agreed to meet with her at the school with Malik's teacher and his guidance counselor. Malik had been classified as emotionally impaired and placed in a smaller, self-contained class the year before. The head of the CST joined the meeting to discuss an IEP for Malik. The teacher was very open to behavioral interventions and a time-out plan that she could use with Malik and other children in her class-room. Both she and Mrs. Cellars seemed relieved at having a concrete way to address his behavior. The teacher implemented a system of rewards in which the children earned "Pokemon" stickers for the completion of assignments and for positive behavior in the classroom. In subsequent sessions, Mrs. Cellars reported that he was doing much better.

About 4 four months after the start of treatment, Mrs. Cellars looked over-whelmed again and reported that she was "depressed." She stated that her daughter had become pregnant once more and Mrs. Cellars was agonizing over the prospect of having to raise another child. Although this was her "flesh and blood," she sim-ply could not take on any more responsibilities. The therapist explored the avail-ability of other family members who might help. A genogram was constructed. With the therapist's help, Mrs. Cellars was able to identify one of her older daugh-ters and a niece, who might be able to care for the child. A family therapy session was arranged to which Mrs. Cellars invited Shakeera, her older sister, Latisha, and Mrs. Cellars' niece, Bethany.

During the meeting, Mrs. Cellars cried and talked about her concerns for her unborn grandchild. She begged her daughter once again to go into a drug rehabil-itation program, which she refused. Shakeera's attention was caught, however, when her mother stated honestly that she could not take the responsibility for an-other child. She reported that she was "torn up" about the possibility of her grand-child going into the foster care system. Everyone agreed that this would be a very sad outcome. Shakeera knew from past experience that her child would be taken from her at birth due to her drug condition. Finally, Latisha (age 30) offered to raise the baby, provided that Shakeera agreed to have "her tubes tied" (a tubal liga-tion.) At first, Shakeera was very angry but finally she agreed when faced with the likelihood of this child being placed in foster care. With the therapist's help, Mrs. Cellars was able to express her ongoing need for support in raising the boys. Even though her dream of drug treatment for Shakeera never became a reality, she was able to create a stronger bond with Latisha and Bethany. In future sessions, the therapist worked with all of them to increase their family bonds and support net-work.

AIDS in the African American Community

While the tragic impact of the AIDS epidemic on persons of African descent and people of color worldwide (Rockeymore, 2002) is a major concern, a dis-cussion of the pandemic in Africa is beyond the scope of this book. This sec-tion will focus on the disproportionate incidence of HIV and AIDS in the Af-rican American community in the United States.

When AIDS first came to public attention over 20 years ago, reports in the media initially characterized the disease as one affecting gay men. In that early period, the organizations taking leadership roles as activists against AIDS were run almost exclusively by gay White men. This led to the mistaken belief by many African Americans that AIDS was a gay White man's disease and had no relevance to their own lives (Cohen, 1999; Rockeymore, 2002). Many chose to ignore the growing numbers of Black gay men, as well as heterosexual men and women, who were infected in the African American community. From the very beginning of the epidemic, however, the Centers for Disease Control reported that African Americans were "among the first cases of AIDS in America and that their rate of infection was disproportionate to their representation in the general population" (Rockeymore, 2002). In her chapter in *The State of Black America* 2002, Rockeymore (2002) reports the following:

> In 2000 alone, African Americans represented almost half (47%) of all reported AIDS cases even though they made up just 12 percent of the population. (p. 126)
>
> Indeed, 63 percent of all women and 65 percent of all children reported with AIDS in 2000 were African American. The rate of reported cases for African Americans was two times greater than the rate for Hispanics and more than eight times greater than the rate for whites. (p.125)

The numbers of African Americans infected presented a major challenge for traditional AIDS organizations:

> First, African Americans and Hispanics shared a history of oppression and exclusion that kept them outside of the social and economic mainstream of America. Unlike the high socio-economic status of gay white men, minority populations remained disproportionately represented among lower-income families. Their economic condition also dictated their relationship with the U.S. health care infrastructure. It is telling that African Americans, Hispanics and Asian/Pacific Islanders comprised 75% of all uninsured individuals in the United States—a disenfranchisement that exacerbated health disparities and created a climate conducive to the spread of the disease.
>
> Second, the primary mode of transmission among minorities proved to be different than that of gay white men. While men having sex with men would continue to influence transmission of HIV/AIDS among African Americans, substance abuse would prove to be the primary factor fueling its spread. Specifically, intravenous drug users and individuals engaging in sex with injection drug users were at risk because of their habit of sharing used needles and other contaminated drug paraphernalia. Again, poverty related issues often accompanied substance abusers and these factors would serve as a barrier for providing culturally competent care at traditional AIDS service organizations. (Rockeymore, 2002, pp. 129–130)

Clinicians should also be aware that because of the magnitude of the epidemic, many African American clients have experienced losses in their extended families and nonblood kinship networks. For some families, extended family members have stepped in to raise their grandchildren, nieces, and nephews when parents have died of AIDS.

AIDS is a multigenerational family disease when HIV/AIDS-infected mothers give birth to infected babies through perinatal transmission (Boyd-Franklin et al., 1995). Significant numbers of new cases of pediatric AIDS were prevented when it was discovered that zidovudine (formerly known as azidothymidine or AZT) and other AIDS medications taken during pregnancy were effective in reducing the rate of perinatal transmission. Women who receive no prenatal care, as is common with poor substance abusers, are at continued risk to transmit the HIV virus to their children. The multigenerational effects of unresolved mourning issues can manifest in mental health concerns such as depression, posttraumatic stress disorder (PTSD), and acting out in children and adolescents (Boyd-Franklin et al., 1995), as can be seen in the case example below.

Eric, an 11-year-old African American male, was referred for therapy for frequent disruptive behavior in school and persistent sadness. The referral came 4 months after the death of his mother, Charlene, from AIDS. Eric and his family were seen in therapy for 2 years; Eric also attended a weekly group therapy session for boys with behavior problems. During treatment Eric and his family moved from avoidance and silence regarding the illness and death of their mother to sadness and anger and eventually to open discussion of the matter. Although only about 10 sessions were spent dealing directly with these issues, the lifting of the veil surrounding Charlene's death eventually opened the door for intervention into other related issues plaguing family members.

Following his mother's death, Eric's maternal aunt, Donna, assumed caretaking of Eric, and his three siblings. (Eric's father died 6 months after Eric was born.) Donna, who was 36 years old and single, had no children of her own and was several years younger than Eric's mother. Donna was a very responsible individual who had been close to the children throughout their childhoods.

Eric's older sister, Delanya, was a 15-year-old "parentified child" who did well in school and assisted in the care of the younger children. She seemed to be in much private pain at the start of therapy, but refused to discuss her mother's death. Eric's younger half-brother, David, was a quiet, friendly, 9-year-old who usually presented as sad and with symptoms of attention deficit disorder. Eric's younger half-sister, Michelle, was an outgoing, cheerful, 3-year-old. She seroconverted and has tested negative for HIV since that time.

During the first 6 months of therapy, Eric was generally seen individually or with his aunt. Although neither AIDS nor the death of his mother was a central focus during this initial period, it became clear that these topics were not discussed in the family. It appeared that Eric was acting out the family's pain and silence. The whole family was invited to attend several sessions around the first anniversary of Charlene's death. All resisted discussing the topic. Eric, David, and Delanya insisted that they rarely thought about their mother anymore and that her death was not a relevant issue to therapy. At this point it was decided that family therapy would be best way to help Eric work through the loss of Charlene.

Secrecy was a central issue in the next few sessions. During this time, it was discovered that Donna was giving the children an implicit message that she did not want anyone to bring up Charlene's death. Before sessions or when the subject of Charlene's death came up at home, Donna would sometimes say to the children, "Now don't go talking all about your mother or you'll get me all upset." Indeed, at the beginning of treatment, Donna had said to the therapist, "I hope that you do not plan to spend much time having Eric and me discuss AIDS and Charlene's death. We have been over that enough already." In actuality the subject had received very little attention in the way of child–adult discussion.

In another session, Delanya and Eric expressed fear that people who learned that their mother had died of AIDS would view the family badly. Delanya was resentful at Donna and Eric for coming to therapy. Although Delanya soon became comfortable with the fact that the therapist would maintain confidentiality, she expressed fear that David and Eric would become comfortable discussing the topic in therapy and then be more likely to talk to one of their friends about their mother's having AIDS.

Eventually, as the topic became more readily available for discussion, issues of anger and guilt emerged. Eric in particular felt bad about discussing his mother in sessions. He felt that they were behaving disloyally by discussing family business with an outsider. Delanya eventually expressed anger about her mother's risky behavior, which had resulted in her leaving her children behind. Delanya also had a great deal of anger at her mother for not getting treatment early in her illness and for not continuing with regular treatment. Moreover, Eric and Delanya admitted guilt about their behavior when their mother had left for the hospital on the day of her death. Apparently she had awakened them early in the morning to do some favors for her and then to say goodbye. They related that they did not comply and got upset with her for waking them. They said that they did not realize the seriousness of her condition at that time and were shocked to learn of her death later that day. David then revealed for the first time his lack of response that morning, and cried about his insensitivity. In therapy, they worked on how they would like to have said goodbye to her.

Family myths surrounding AIDS and fears of abandonment also began to emerge during the 6 months following the first anniversary of Charlene's death. None of the children expressed a belief that they had caused their mother's death. However, Delanya expressed her conviction that if she had tried harder to convince her mother to get regular treatment, she would have survived much longer and perhaps even gotten rid of the virus. The children also believed that more compassionate behavior on their part on the day of their mother's death would have enabled her to live longer.

Eric indicated that many of his fights at school started because another student would make reference to his mother. In discussing the matter further, however, it became clear to Eric that none of his peers actually knew his mother or had any awareness of her illness. However, at the time of the insults he felt that everyone must be aware.

During one session, the family was very concerned because Michelle had a cold. They were fearful that her cold would make her vulnerable to recontracting HIV. Apparently, all family members were concerned about this possibility and had watched over Michelle carefully and fearfully during the past year.

Fifteen months after Charlene's death—shortly before Donna became engaged to her boyfriend, Alex—all three older children voiced their concern that Donna and Alex would one day marry, and that Donna would then move away and leave them behind. Alex began attending family sessions from that point on. Later, as they grew closer to Alex, Eric and Delanya became concerned that Donna and Alex might break up and they would lose him. On the second anniversary of Charlene's death, a few weeks before Donna and Alex were married, the children began to show apprehension about the upcoming wedding. David expressed concern that, during sex, Alex would give HIV to Donna, and she would die. (Alex and Donna both explained that they had both tested negative for HIV.)

Once the wedding passed the family wound down treatment over the next 2 months, although they occasionally returned for follow-up sessions. They emerged from therapy with the ability to communicate more effectively with one another about their issues and to better handle adversity. (Boyd-Franklin, Aleman, Steiner, Drelich, & Norford, 1995, p. 122–124)

Disparity in the Provision of Health Care for African Americans

Researchers (Chaisson, Keruly, & Moore, 1995) have concluded that higher AIDS death rates among African Americans can be attributed to disparities in medical treatment, including the unavailability of life-prolonging medication, health insurance, housing, and prevention services (Rockeymoore, 2002). As Rockeymoore states,

> Because of their exclusion from private health insurance and increased likelihood of living in poverty, African Americans with AIDS are more likely to rely on the Medicaid program for health care assistance. Indeed, Medicaid serves about 55 percent of all people living with AIDS and up to 90 percent of all children with AIDS in the U.S. Yet the assistance Medicaid provides is deeply problematic because it does not provide funding that would enable recipients to gain access to the lifesaving treatment and drugs that prevent full-blown AIDS until an individual can show financial need and prove that he or she has already developed full-blown AIDS. (p. 136)

She concludes with this chilling assessment: "When African Americans are finally eligible for Medicaid, they have little chance of surviving the disease for long" (p. 137).

Racial inequities also exist in other programs designed for AIDS patients. In her discussion of the AIDS Drug Assistance Program, which was established to help provide life-prolonging drugs to AIDS patients, Rockeymore (2002) indicates that "in 1999, 40 percent of individuals receiving assistance from this program were white, 31 percent were black and 24 percent were of Hispanic origin. . . . Because of the high costs of AIDS drugs, many states cap enrollment in the program creating waiting lists for drug assistance" (p. 137).

Similar racial disparity can be found in the Housing Opportunities for Persons with AIDS program (HOPWA), administered by the U.S. Department of Housing and Urban Development, which was established to prevent AIDS patients from becoming homeless due to their inability to work.

> Out of the total number assisted in 1999, 50 percent were white, 44 percent were African American, 12 percent were of Hispanic origin and 6 percent were American Indian/Alaskan native. The limited scope of HOPWA means that housing

slots are in limited supply and that many are left on waiting lists or shut out entirely. (Rockeymoore, 2002, p. 136)

In order to treat these clients, therapists must be familiar with programs for which their clients are eligible, funding available through the Ryan White Care Act, and case management issues. Their clients' survival and the welfare of their families may depend on the therapist's willingness to advocate for them and to empower them to obtain needed services. Many therapists have discovered that the systems and services described above are more responsive to poor Black clients who have advocates.

Given their experiences with biased practices in the medical, health insurance, housing, and social service systems, it is not surprising that many African American clients living with AIDS and their families approach the health and mental health system with a great deal of the "healthy cultural suspicion" described above and in Chapter 1. Attention to concrete survival needs initially is one way for a therapist to build credibility and facilitate the joining process in treatment.

Violence in the Black Community

African Americans are not strangers to violence, particularly in inner-city neighborhoods. White and Cones (1999) stated that "death and mortality from gunfire and violent assaults are frighteningly real and have invaded the psyche of today's youth." They report that homicide was the leading cause of death for young African American men between the ages of 15 and 34. Violence can take many forms, including racial profiling, police brutality, hate crimes and other incidents of racial bias, drive-by shootings, gang violence, Black-on-Black crime, drug-related violence, domestic violence, and child abuse.

Therapists are often called upon to help African American families deal with what White and Cones (1999) refer to an "epidemic" of violence on an individual, family, and, sometimes, community level. They referred to an article by Harris (1991) in the *Los Angeles Times*. Harris reported that

> students at predominantly Black Washington High School in South Central Los Angeles expressed concerns about being assaulted at parties, after school, while visiting friends, or just walking down the streets in their own neighborhoods. Every one of a hundred students expressed a fear of being shot. Almost all of the students knew of someone under eighteen who had been shot, stabbed, or assaulted. In three randomly selected classrooms, one-third of the students expressed a fear of being shot at or caught in gang gunfire. A seventeen-year- old boy was standing outside a school when a car drove by and started shooting. (White & Cones, 1999, p. 233)

These situations are all too common, as the next case example illustrates.

Jarron (age 17) was the only son of Vivian, his single-parent mother, and a good kid. One afternoon after school, Jarron was standing in front of a convenience store in his community talking to his friends. Suddenly, a car drove by and, to the horror of his friends, someone in the car shot Jarron. A friend called Vivian at work and she rushed to the hospital. As she stood at his bedside and looked down at her only son, her face crumbled in tears. The doctors had informed her that he had been mortally wounded in the stomach and that they did not expect him to survive the night. Weeks later in a therapy session, Vivian recalled that on hearing the doctors' words, she began to pray aloud for her son. Reverend Black, her minister, and some members of her church joined her and prayed with her. She asked God to take her son "home" to heaven. Shortly after, Jarron died in her arms. She cried in agony.

Much later, she went out to the waiting room and discovered a room full of Jarron's friends and other neighborhood youths. When she told them that Jarron had died, many sobbed and others were so angry that they threatened to reciprocate against the gang members who had mistaken Jarron (who was not gang-involved) for someone else. Vivian begged the youths not to "shame Jarron's memory by resorting to violence."

Vivian and her minister met with the youths for over 3 hours and then asked a Black family therapist in the community, Dr. Rockland, to join them. The minister and the psychologist talked with the youths about working together to stop the violence in their neighborhood.

In the next few days, Vivian, Dr. Rockland, and a minister in the community held a number of meetings with rival gang members. Dr. Rockland also did some violence prevention groups with neighborhood youths.

On the day of the funeral, Dr. Rockland accompanied the family to the church, to the cemetery, and back to the family home. During the funeral service, Reverend Black called for an end to the violence. He asked all of mourners, particularly the young people, to come forward, turn in their weapons, and pledge themselves to peace. This was a very powerful intervention. Many of these youth brought weapons forward, and stood at an "altar call" and prayed for peace. It was a moment that Vivian, her family, and the entire community will long remember because it began a process of community healing that has continued. Dr. Rockland continued to meet with Vivian, her daughter, Shayna (age 15), and her mother, Donna (age 55), for the next year to work through their grief and loss.

Jarron's death illustrates the tragedy of the loss of a young life, all too common in inner-city Black communities. It also demonstrates the unique roles that family therapists can be called upon to play. Dr. Rockland was called upon to do crisis intervention with Vivian, with her family, and ultimately with the youth in the community. Boyd-Franklin and Bry (2000) in their book *Reaching Out in Family Therapy: Home-Based, School, and Community Interventions* argue that family therapists, particularly those who work in minority communities, must be prepared to "reach out" beyond their offices and intervene in the community when it is appropriate and necessary. Dr. Rockland's proactive interventions, together with those of the minister, prevented further violence and gave support and therapeutic healing to Vivian, her family, and the community.

The Impact of Violence on Children

Recent research has shown that children living in violent urban neighborhoods can experience negative psychological consequences not only by witnessing violence but also by hearing about violent acts constantly (Fick, Osofsky, & Lewis, 1997; Lewis & Osofsky, 1997; Osofsky, 1997; Prothrow-Stith, 1993).

In many inner-city areas, very young children (as young as age 2) who have witnessed acts of violence have been diagnosed with posttraumatic stress disorder (PTSD) symptoms such as night terrors, repetitive play enactment of the experience, and flashbacks (Osofsky, 1997). Children often express their concerns about violence through repetitive play enactment and through the use of drawings (Lewis & Osofsky, 1997). These drawings can be used as a part of clinical interventions to help heal children and rebuild their sense of safety and trust (Osofsky, 1997), as the following case example illustrates.

Kyra, age 7, was brought for treatment by her mother, Mary Hubbard (age 27), after she witnessed the schoolyard killing of her cousin, Jakar, age 10, who had been targeted by a gang with a vendetta against his mother's boyfriend.

Jakar had been living with the family, which also included Martha Hubbard, Kyra's grandmother (age 50), and Kyra's baby sister, Imani (age 1), since his own mother's (Ms. Hubbard's younger sister) incarceration for drug dealing in the month prior to his shooting. Although her mother reported that Kyra was not particularly close to Jakar, she was very affected by witnessing his death and had frequent nightmares, was afraid to go to school, and often experienced flashbacks when she would begin crying or trembling uncontrollably.

Ms. Hubbard reported that Jakar's shooting was not the first experience Kyra had had with violence. About 2 months prior to Jakar's death, the whole family was awakened in the middle of the night by the sound of gunshots. Although no one was injured, the family discovered a bullet hole in the wall in the room that Kyra shared with her mother and her baby sister. Ms. Hubbard reported that Kyra was very "clingy" after this experience. Kyra had also heard many stories about violence in the neighborhood.

In the first session, as the therapist worked on building rapport with the mother and Kyra, Kyra appeared very anxious, clung to her mother, and often sucked her thumb. Whenever the therapist tried to ask Kyra a question directly, she would turn her back and cling to her mother. The therapist encouraged her mother to hold Kyra on her lap and to comfort her when she began crying in the session.

In the second session, the therapist provided crayons and paper. Initially, Kyra sat on her mother's lap and refused to touch the drawing supplies. As the session progressed, however, she picked up a crayon and doodled idly. The therapist encouraged the mother to comment on the drawings and ask her some questions about what they were. Kyra shrugged and would not talk at all.

This pattern continued in the next two sessions. By now the mother and the therapist were also drawing pictures during the session. In the fifth session, the therapist asked Kyra to draw a picture of her family. She drew stick figures of her mother, her grandmother, and two tiny girls. She identified one as her "baby sister" and the other as herself. Both were the same size in the picture. She continued to create doodles on another page and seemed to enjoy the process of drawing.

In the next session, Kyra came into the room, immediately left her mother's side, and sat down at the table and drew a small mound with a cross over it. When the therapist asked what it was, she reported that it was Jakar's grave. The therapist then asked her to talk about Jakar. She responded, "He was shot." Her mother asked if she could draw a picture of what happened. Kyra drew a tiny stick figure of Jakar and a very large gun pointed at him. She began to cry softly. The therapist encouraged her mother to comfort her and to ask her gentle questions about the incident. Haltingly, Kyra described how she was playing in the schoolyard with some friends. She heard a shot and turned around to see Jakar fall. She remembers screaming but was not sure what occurred after that. She spontaneously began a stick figure drawing of this event.

In subsequent sessions, Kyra would enter the session and begin drawing. She drew a number of pictures of guns, usually large, with no connection to a human being. In the 12th session, she drew a large gun, which was pointed at four small stick figures. The therapist asked her to tell her about the picture. Kyra reported that the gun was trying to kill her family. Her mother asked her if she was scared. She whispered "Yes." Her mother then shared with her that Jakar's killers had been caught and put in jail. Kyra spontaneously drew a picture of two men in jail. For the next few sessions, her drawings vacillated between pictures of shootings in the neighborhood and pictures of criminals in jail. In one session, the therapist commented that the jail seemed very far away from Kyra's neighborhood. The mother, the therapist, and Kyra played a game in which the picture of the jail was moved farther and farther away from the picture of her neighborhood. Gradually, the violent themes began to decrease.

Initially, Kyra had been afraid to go to school. Gradually, her mother had been encouraged to go with her and to remain for the first few minutes until Kyra became involved in schoolwork. Because Kyra was afraid to walk to school, a friend of the family dropped Kyra and her mother off at school on his way to work, and a school aide would drive them home in the afternoon.

The therapist discussed the ways that they could protect themselves in the neighborhood. The mother was encouraged to draw pictures of the family walking to school and of the criminals in jail. She also drew a number of pictures of the police protecting the neighborhood. Police cars began to appear in Kyra's drawings. Ms. Hubbard confirmed that there had been a more visible police presence in their neighborhood in recent months. Also, a group of parents had started a community patrol. She was able, with the therapist's encouragement, to talk to Kyra about this and to include these in their drawing sessions. Almost 6 months after the incident, Kyra no longer needed her mother to stay with her once school started.

Over the next 6 months, Kyra's drawings began to change. She drew a picture of a stick-figured boy surrounded by sun and clouds. When asked what it was, she reported that it was Jakar in heaven. The therapist asked how he was feeling and Kyra said "Happy." She also drew a number of drawings of herself walking to school with her mother. There were increasing signs of hope in her drawings. The figures were smiling, and the gun had disappeared. Apartment buildings and trees were depicted with more representations of the sun. At the time of completion of treatment, 1 year after the incident, Kyra no longer experienced nightmares, flashbacks, or periods of crying. She was able to walk to and from school with her mother or her grandmother.

This case illustrates the ways in which PTSD can be addressed in family treatment. Building upon the work of Eliana Gil (1994), who often uses play and drawings in family therapy, the therapist was able to utilize the symbolism of the drawings to help a traumatized little girl and her mother to communicate about her inner fears for herself and her family members after witnessing the violent death of her cousin.

Racial Profiling and Police Brutality: The Fears and Anger of African American Parents

Boyd-Franklin et al. (2001), in their book *Boys into Men: Raising Our African American Teenage Sons,* reported that many of the African American parents they interviewed expressed fear, worry, and anxiety about the safety of their children, particularly their sons. In addition to the fears about youth or gang-related violence and random incidents, many reported fears about issues such as racial profiling, DWB ("driving while Black," in which Black males are routinely stopped by the police while driving just because they are black), and police brutality.

Examples of racial profiling and police brutality are alarming to many African American families. The case of Amadou Diallo has become particularly notorious. Amadou Diallo was an African immigrant returning to his home when he was mistaken by police for a serial rapist who was attacking women in the neighborhood. Although Diallo was unarmed, the White police officers fired 41 shots at him, alleging that when he reached for his wallet to show his identification they thought he was reaching for a weapon (Boyd-Franklin et al., 2001). Incidents of racial profiling and police brutality are not confined to the inner city, as the case below demonstrates (see also Chapter 10, in the "Narrative Therapy" section, for the case example of Robert).

Kenyata was a 17-year-old African American senior in a predominately White suburban high school. He was walking through the school halls on his way to his next class when he observed a uniformed police officer choking a friend of his.

He approached the police officer, who had been stationed at the school since the Columbine school massacre, and yelled, "Stop it! What are you doing to him?"

He then called out to the school counselor, whose office was down the hall.

The police officer knocked Kenyata out of the way and continued choking his friend. Pinning him against the wall, he radioed for backup. When two other officers arrived, he yelled at them to "take both of these guys down to the station." One of the officers hit Kenyata over the head and shoved him into a wall before throwing him into a police car.

At the police station, Kenyata learned that his friend, Mark, had been choked because when told to "move on" in the hallway he had allegedly "talked back." Kenyata and Mark were both charged with resisting arrest, interfering with a police officer making an arrest, and aggravated assault.

Hours later, Kenyata was finally allowed to call his parents, who quickly arrived at the police station, accompanied by their lawyer. The police scheduled him for a court date the following week, and refused to release him into his parents' custody. At his parents' insistence, the police finally allowed Kenyata to seek medical attention at 10:00 P.M. He was escorted to the emergency room by an armed guard, and then placed in a juvenile detention facility to await trial. His parents, who were Black middle-class professionals, were appalled to see their son treated in this way.

They had moved to a suburban neighborhood in the hope of protecting their son and did not contemplate that their son would meet violence at the hands of the police. They met with their lawyer, the school counselor, and the students who had witnessed the incident. All corroborated Kenyata's account and agreed to testify in court.

The parents also reached out in the community for support. Other parents, their minister, fellow parishioners, and community representatives arranged to meet with the local police chief, the principal, and the superintendent of schools. In a very heated exchange, the police and school officials defended their actions. Kenyata, who was still in juvenile detention, was angry and dejected when told of this by his parents.

Kenyata's parents, their minister, and friends from the community arrived to support him at the court hearing. His lawyer introduced his excellent school record and sworn statements from the other witnesses, and asked that the charges against him be dismissed. The judge ordered that he be placed on probation and have weekly appointments with his probation officer. Another court date was set for 4 months later, at which time his probation records would be reviewed and a decision would be made about further prosecution.

At the suggestion of their lawyer, the family was referred for family therapy. The therapist, a young White woman, felt overwhelmed by the anger in the room during the first session. Kenyata was angry and withdrawn, and the parents were furious about the treatment their son had received by the police, the court, and the school system, which had suspended Kenyata indefinitely. As the session proceeded, she realized that this anger was not directed at her, but at the authorities who had mistreated Kenyata. She was then able to join with all family members and to allow each of them the chance to vent their anger.

At the end of the session, she asked if each was comfortable, given their recent experiences, working with a White therapist. They all agreed that a Black man, who could understand what Kenyata had experienced, would be preferable. The therapist empathized, but explained that there were no Black therapists in the clinic. She asked if they would be willing to contract to work with her for 4 weekly sessions. If they still felt they needed to work with a Black male therapist at that point, she would do her best to find them a referral in the area. The family members agreed.

The family used the early sessions to continue to express their anger about the racism their son had experienced. The therapist encouraged the parents to talk with their son about this. In one session, they heard for the first time about his frightening experiences in juvenile detention. It was clear that the family was solidly supporting Kenyata, and the therapist praised them for that support.

The family also used the sessions to talk through important, painful consequences of Kenyata's arrest. For example, despite a great deal of community pressure, the police chief and the principal refused to replace the officer who had beat Kenyata. This made Kenyata so uncomfortable that he did not want to return to his old school once his suspension was lifted, which surprised his parents because he had so many close friends there. The parents agreed to explore the possibility of a transfer to another school. In the meantime, the therapist encouraged them to insist on daily home instruction for him so that he would not fall too far behind.

By the fourth week of treatment, Kenyata was enrolled in a new school in a nearby town and was doing well. The therapist praised both Kenyata and his parents for what they had been able to accomplish. At the end of the session, the therapist reminded the family of their original contract and asked if they wished to continue treatment or to obtain a referral. The family agreed to continue in treatment with her.

The therapist used the remaining months of treatment to help focus the family on the future for Kenyata. She had a number of sessions in which she met with Kenyata individually to discuss his feelings and plans. He worried that it was too late in the year to apply to college. The therapist encouraged him to discuss this problem with his guidance counselor. Together, they found colleges that were still accepting applications.

In a family therapy session, the therapist helped Kenyata and his parents prepare a strategy for submitting his applications in the short time remaining. They worked together to help Kenyata accomplish this and visited several schools. Kenyata received a number of college acceptances before his court date.

On the day of the court proceedings, the therapist accompanied the family and was prepared to testify in the hearing if necessary. At his lawyer's request, she had already written a letter discussing his progress in treatment, his excellent school performance, and his college acceptances. The judge dismissed the charges, released Kenyata from his probation and, at his lawyer's request, removed all charges from his record.

The family completed treatment at this point. The following Christmas, the therapist received a Christmas card from the family telling her how well Kenyata was doing in college and thanking her for her help in this difficult situation.

Therapists are referred to Gardere (1999) and Boyd-Franklin et. al. (2001) for clear examples of the ways in which they can help African American families to talk to their children and adolescents, particularly their sons, about these kinds of incidents of racial profiling and prepare them to handle these experiences.

II

MAJOR TREATMENT THEORIES, ISSUES, AND INTERVENTIONS

9

The Therapist's Use of Self and Value Conflicts*

The previous chapters of this book focused on cultural and racial issues related to the treatment of African American families; subsequent chapters address the theoretical contributions of the major schools of family and systems therapy and present a model for a multisystems approach to the treatment of Black families. There is, however, a missing link between these two areas of discussion. If we are to successfully treat African American families, we must first explore ourselves as people, as men and women, and as therapists. In this context, this chapter provides an opportunity to explore the therapist's use of self and the values, perceptions, and cultural similarities and differences that have an impact on our personal frame of reference and on our work as therapists. Without this essential link I risk the possibility that the later theoretical chapters will be applied in a rote fashion, without careful attention to the human element—that is, the essential relationship between the therapist and the family.

Although this relationship is central to effective therapy with all clients and families, it is particularly crucial with African American families because of the many psychosocial factors specific to this ethnic group that can complicate this process and lead to premature termination (e.g., racism [Chapter 2], resistance, "healthy cultural suspicion" [Chapter 1], and mistrust of mental health services [Chapter 1]). Given these factors, the most important process in working with African American families is "joining," that is, initiating therapeutic intervention by building a relationship with the family. The first half of this chapter is intended to help therapists explore the general issues and as-

*I would like to express my appreciation to Dr. Cheryl Thompson and Dr. Sandra Lewis for their suggestions and contributions to this chapter.

177

sumptions they themselves bring to therapy and to be sensitive to those of the Black families they treat so that the therapy process can be facilitated. It will also point out some of the obvious pitfalls for African American, European American, Asian, Hispanic, and therapists from other ethnic and racial groups in working with African American families. The second half of this chapter deals more specifically with common value-related areas of conflict between the clinician's own biases, perceptions, and cultural orientation and those of certain Black families.

GENERAL ISSUES OF THERAPEUTIC INTERACTION WITH AFRICAN AMERICAN FAMILIES

The Concept of "Vibes"

Over 30 years ago, Scheflen (1973) and Birdwhistell (1970) first sensitized the social science and mental health fields to the ways in which social cues such as body language, tone of voice, and social distance influence social interactions. Scheflen (1973) had a major impact by raising the awareness of the mental health field to the differences in sensitivity to social variables among different ethnic groups. African Americans, because of the often extremely subtle ways in which racism manifests itself socially, are particularly attuned to very fine distinctions among such variables in all interactions—with other Blacks, with White people, with persons from other ethnic and racial groups, and with "White" institutions. Because of this, many African Americans have been socialized to pay attention to all of the nuances of behavior and not just to verbal messages. The term most often applied to this multilevel perception in African American culture is "vibes." A clinician (whether Black, White, Asian, Latino, Native American, or from another ethnic or racial group) needs to be acutely aware that every African American client and family member is "checking out" her or him in terms of appearance, race, skin color, clothing, perceived social class, language, and a range of more subtle clues such as warmth, genuineness, sincerity, respect for the client, willingness to hear the client's side, patronizing attitudes, condescension, judgments, and human connectedness. While for some cultural/ethnic groups (e.g., White Anglo-Saxon Protestants, Jews), the intellectual connection tends to be the more important for some of its members, in African American culture the vibes or the human connections are most often of greatest significance in establishing bonds with another person or group of people. These perceptions are not just based on what is seen or what is said but on a very basic "gut feeling" level.

Subsequent chapters stress the importance of making this gut-level joining connection with African American families before extensive historical or family background information is taken. Because of the history of racism and their own experiences with the welfare and other social systems, African American families are particularly sensitive to information gathering that is perceived as prying when conducted before the joining process has gotten underway and a bond of trust has been established. Well-meaning therapists can lose a family by doing this prematurely. Chapter 11 details specific suggestions for facilitating the joining process with African American families.

One very important vibe among African Americans is the sense of whether they are being treated with respect. Many African Americans are very sensitive to clinicians who convey the impression that they know a great deal about African American families. It is far more productive for the clinician to assume that each Black family is somewhat different and to make no other assumptions, allowing families to teach her or him about themselves and their own cultural backgrounds. Once again, I must stress the idea that there is no such thing as *the* African American family. Clinicians sometimes make the error of using their cultural knowledge to show families how well they are acquainted with African American culture. It is far more useful to treat cultural material of the type presented in this book as hypotheses to be explored with each family.

Therapists are often surprised to learn that they have to establish credibility with African American families. This is very different from their interactions with clients from other cultural groups. Some Latino or Hispanic families, for example, will give automatic respect to "the doctor," "the therapist," or any person who is perceived as holding a position of authority. With African American families, that credibility has to be earned. Some African American family members will be constantly assessing whether they can trust the therapist.

Thus, the person-to-person connection is the most important in work with African American families; without it, all of the therapist's carefully applied treatment techniques are useless. African American families will leave treatment very quickly in the initial stage if this connection is not made with *each* family member.

Another vibe to which some African Americans are particularly sensitive is that of "missionary racism." In this situation, the clinician (often without conscious awareness) conveys to the family that his or her goal is to "save them from their plight" or to "take care of these poor people." This is often a very subtle vibe, particularly notable as an attitude characteristic of the well-meaning clinician (Black, White, or those from another ethnic or racial group), who unwittingly conveys a patronizing stance to an African American family without intending to.

The Insidious Nature of Racism

In Chapter 2, I attempted to convey the insidious and pervasive nature of the racism that African Americans experience in this country. The issue of race is almost never a neutral issue for African Americans; it is always present on both a conscious and an unconscious level. It is important to reiterate at this juncture that because African Americans comprise the only ethnic group in this country that was brought here almost exclusively as slaves, the slave–master aspects of racism have persisted in the psyches of Black and White people alike (Grier & Cobbs, 1968). Since this psychological structure has persisted in both subtle and overt negative stereotypes and discrimination, race is a lens through which many African Americans view the world and by extension the therapist, be she or he Black, White, or from another ethnic or racial group. Race is equally a lens through which many therapists (often unconsciously) view Black families.

Racial Countertransference and Racial Stereotypes

The term *countertransference* has not been a popular one in the family therapy literature. It is, however, particularly relevant here when it is applied to the conscious and unconscious racial stereotypes that we all hold and that inevitably influence the treatment process (Sanchez-Hucles, 2000). It is extremely important that all therapists explore their own stereotypes (positive and negative) about African American families (Sanchez-Hucles, 2000). Part of the development of any clinician who wishes to work effectively with Black clients and families must include the process of "soul searching." This chapter is intended to help therapists explore and struggle with their own subtly manifested, ingrained beliefs. For example, many clinicians, African American, White, and those from other ethnic and racial groups, harbor a subtle fear of Black men. Unless they are made consciously aware of this fear, they will convey it on a number of levels to their clients.

Other clinicians have struggled with a belief that African Americans are to blame for their problems. This may be articulated conceptually as, "They are poor because they want to be" or "They should pull themselves up by their bootstraps" or "All other ethnic groups made it; why can't they?" This process is called "blaming the victim." It is very important that therapists, who discover these beliefs within themselves, create an opportunity to work on these issues either with their supervisors, in their own treatment, or through experiential groups or courses on diversity topics.

In Chapter 1, I explored a very common assumption, the "class not race" view. In this view, the clinician totally ignores racial and cultural differences and sees the problems of African American families as arising primarily from a culture of poverty (Hill, 1999a). Still other therapists make the reverse error, seeing only the strengths of African American families, which makes it difficult for them to identify the true pathology in the Black families they treat. They deny problems or collude with families to avoid opening up "secrets" because they have been told that African American families are sensitive to prying. This book is intended to assist therapists with the struggle to strike a balance in the handling of such sensitive areas in their treatment of African American families.

The next sections of this chapter explore particular issues for White, Black, and therapists from other ethnic and racial groups in developing cultural sensitivity when working with African American families. They also explore some common errors that therapists make. If therapists can be sensitized to their own issues, they will be consciously aware of them and thus can devote their attention to the family that they are treating. They will also be less likely to reject African American families who are difficult to engage initially. The therapist's use of self is his or her most powerful intervention tool in the treatment of Black families. It can be refined and sharpened by this exploration.

The Importance of Exploring One's Own Culture

One of the important contributions of the Bowenian school of family therapy has been the emphasis on the therapist exploring his or her own family of origin (Bowen, 1978; Nichols & Schwartz, 1998). In addition, it is very important that each therapist explore his or her own cultural identity (or lack of it), family values, beliefs, and prejudices (Sanchez-Hucles, 2000). Chapter 16 will address in detail the ways in which this can be incorporated into training programs. However, for many clinicians in the field, this process may need to be done on a more personal level. It is important for therapists who work with African American families to find an informal support group of other clinicians so that they can share and get feedback on their observations. Many national conferences of mental health associations now have workshops on race, ethnicity, and the treatment of African American families. In working with any ethnic group, the ability of the clinician to effect change is greatly increased by the exploration of the aspects of his or her own culture, ethnic group, and family of origin she or he likes or dislikes. The clinician should be asking her- or himself, "Which parts of my 'family culture' have I accepted and rejected?" (Pinderhughes, 1989).

It is also important for clinicians to explore the question, "Why do I want to work with African American families?" Such a question can be very helpful in forcing all of us as therapists to acknowledge any missionary tendencies before they are transmitted to the families we treat. The next three sections will discuss the particular issues for White therapists, Black clinicians, and those therapists from other ethnic minority groups working with Black families.

Issues for White Therapists and Those from Other Ethnic and Racial Groups in Working with African American Families

Although this section addresses many of the common issues that White therapists and those from other ethnic and racial groups often experience in the process of learning to work with African American families, it is important to recognize that the discussion is not meant to be exhaustive or representative of all therapists. It is intended to point to some problem areas and encourage therapists to search within themselves for their own particular areas of concern. Many White therapists and those from other ethnic groups come to their work with Black families with little or no firsthand experience of African Americans. Some may have known Black individuals in their school or work settings but have never been to an African American's home. Many are very aware of the differences between their backgrounds and those of the African American families they treat. In their eagerness to practice therapy effectively, they often unwittingly make some serious errors.

For example, some beginning White, Asian, Latino, and Native American therapists are so afraid of making a mistake with African American families that they may adopt a very tentative, subservient, or humble role. This is neither necessary nor helpful, since it conveys to the Black family a lack of confidence on the part of therapist. A variation on this pattern is a situation in which a White trainee is overly impressed with a very street-wise African American client or family member and his or her ability to "hustle" the system. Some African American clients, particularly adolescents, will resent the fact that their therapist is taken in by this "street-wise" attitude. In many of these situations, family members may interpret the therapist's admiration as phony, which in turn may lead to the family leaving therapy feeling very resentful. It is not unusual in these situations particularly for the beginning therapist to mistakenly believe that he or she has "connected with" and understood this family even though the opposite has happened. Sometimes therapists will inappropriately attempt to use slang that they believe is representative of Black dialect in a mistaken attempt to join with the family. Such use of dialect, even though made with the best intentions, is often viewed by African American families as condescending (Hunt, 1987).

There are a number of useful strategies that White, Asian, and Latino clinicians who become aware of this kind of behavior in their sessions can employ. It is often not helpful to a new therapist for his or her supervisor or colleagues to simply point out that these attempts are counterproductive. They need to suggest concrete changes that the new therapist can make to further his or her efforts to connect with Black clients. It is important to help clinicians understand when this behavior is occurring. Videotapes of family sessions that can be stopped and replayed are very useful for this purpose. Ultimately, the goal is for clinicians to be able to recognize their inappropriate behavior and correct themselves during the session. It is also useful for therapists in this position to carefully examine their own racial issues that may interfere with treatment. African American families are often new to therapy, and they need to be clearly joined with, prepared, and brought into the process. Counterproductive behaviors will interfere with that joining.

There is a belief among some clinicians that African American families are not appropriate for therapy. This is a variation of the "blaming the victim" response. Such clinicians often report that "these families can't be helped" or that "you can't do *real* therapy with these families." Therapists must explore their own expectations in this regard, or these negative feelings will be transmitted to their clients, where they could promote feelings of inferiority (Hunt, 1987). Therapists who find themselves caught in this process may need to enlist the help of their supervisors and/or their colleagues to explore these issues. Moreover, they need to seek out training experiences that will equip them with the skills to be effective in cross-cultural and cross-racial situations.

Another type of problem commonly encountered by White therapists and those from other racial and ethnic groups who are new to work with Black families is a tendency to expect to do excellent work immediately with these families, and to judge themselves harshly when they cannot be "super-therapists" (Hunt, 1987). Often trainees who were high achievers in school feel totally inadequate when they find that many of the techniques they have learned are either ineffective with Blacks or have never been "translated" for use with this population. They often become sensitive, self-deprecating, and anxious about their perceived inadequacies. Sometimes these clinicians cope with their anxiety by making desperate attempts to acquire knowledge about African American culture in the hope that this will help them in working with families. Therapists experiencing this issue can change their behavior with Black families by confronting the ways in which their own self-doubts and feelings of inadequacy interfere with establishing a therapeutic alliance. It is also helpful for them to realize that establishing this alliance with African American families often takes time and persistence. Expectations of an immediate joining are often unrealistic (Hunt, 1987). It is my hope that this book will provide an anchor in terms of this knowledge and give the therapists permission to relax, to be themselves with African American families, and to temper their expectations of perfection. Working with families leads to the development of a certain sense of humility in all of us that can be balanced with a feeling of our own competence as clinicians.

The opposite problem can also occur. Sometimes therapists believe that they are effecting change but audiotapes or videotapes of sessions or interviews with a supervisor behind the one-way mirror reveal no progress. For apparent change to become actual change, therapists must work with their supervisor's help to (1) allow African American families to express feelings of anger and/or rejection, (2) appreciate their right to reject therapy, and (3) recognize that issues that have nothing to do with the therapist, such as the "healthy cultural suspicion" (Chapter 1) that many African American families feel, may interfere with the initial joining process. Once again, I must reiterate the central theme of this chapter: in order for clinicians to develop this therapeutic alliance with African American families, they must be willing to extend themselves and establish a human bond or connection. Hunt (1987) reinforces this point. Although her writing focuses on work with individual African American clients, it is very relevant to family therapy as well. She states that it is not "what you know but who you are and how you use information about a person's cultural characteristics that eventually allows the client to trust [you]" (p. 116). This ability to convey who one is and to be "real" is essential in establishing a true therapeutic bond with African American families.

Raising the Issue of Race in Cross-Racial Therapy

Another dilemma faced by many White therapists and those from other ethnic and racial groups in working with Black families relates to the question of when and if the issue of race or racial difference should be raised. Many therapists received their initial training in the psychoanalytic school of thought and have been taught that "transferential" issues should not be raised until they are broached by the patient. Such therapists are therefore very hesitant to raise the sensitive issue of race in cross-racial therapy. Unfortunately, this omission can have serious consequences for the development of an open trusting relationship with an African American family. As stated earlier in this chapter, it is important for the White, Latino, or Asian therapist (and therapist from other ethnic and racial groups) to recognize that although they may not feel that differences in race or ethnicity are an issue for them, they often are for Black families. Although this does not always interfere with the treatment process, at least on the overt level, the willingness of a clinician to raise the issue of race with an African American family often gives the message that "anything can be discussed here," clearing the air and removing a possible obstacle to the development of trust. Although there is considerable debate in the field, in my experience it is far better to raise the issue with African American families than to run the risk of it obstructing the therapeutic process.

As stated above, many African Americans are very aware of the race of any individual they encounter. They can usually tell on the telephone if the therapist is Black, White, or from another ethnic or racial group. They are also taught from an early age to distinguish light-skinned Blacks from Whites. This sensitivity is ever present and often operates on a level at which White therapists and those from other ethnic and racial groups have no awareness.

Sometimes inexperienced therapists collude with African American families to deny the issue of race. It may not be discussed or it becomes an "unspeakable" topic. If a therapist asks a family directly, "How do you feel about working with a White [or a Latino or Asian] therapist?," the issue is then available for discussion. Therapists need to be prepared for the possibility that this question may elicit feelings of anger. Some family members may even verbalize their reluctance to work with a White therapist or one from another ethnic or racial group. The more able the therapist is to remain nondefensive and nonapologetic while discussing this issue with the family, the greater the likelihood of enhancing the therapeutic connection. It is very important that the therapist from a different background avoid personalizing the client or family's response. These responses are usually a direct reaction to the client's past expe-

riences with racism and not necessarily directly related to their current therapeutic relationship. A word of caution: Timing is very important. It is best if
this issue is raised after the clinician has had at least one session (or more) to
join with the family and establish a therapeutic alliance. It is not necessary to
belabor this issue with African American families. A young White therapist
whom I supervised was so anxious about the implications of cross-racial therapy that she unwittingly raised it repeatedly in a number of sessions with a
Black family, thereby conveying her ongoing anxiety to the family.

It is not helpful for the White therapist or one from another ethnic or racial group to try to convince a Black client or family that he or she "under-
stands" their problems and that his or her experiences are similar to theirs.
Many African Americans experience this assurance as condescending or patronizing. It is far more useful to avoid thinking of the family members in stereotypical ways but to invite them to share their experiences. This can often
open up areas of discussion that will be beneficial to the family and to the
therapist's understanding of them. Often African American families have never
really discussed or shared the expectations they have of each other that were
formed by their childhood experiences, the area of the country in which they
were raised, their family structure (e.g., single-parent, intact, or extended family), their religious views, and what they have learned from peers about male–
female relationships. The therapist can learn a great deal about the couple's
cultural backgrounds and the family's own culture and use it very effectively to
reframe their experiences as different from each other rather than as "good" or
"bad."

Special Issues for Therapists
from Other Ethnic Minority Groups

The first edition of this book focused primarily on issues for Black and White
clinicians. The last 15 years witnessed a growing trend in the clinical field of
increased numbers of therapists from other ethnic minority groups. This has
been a very important development given the ever-rising numbers of clients
from these cultures. There is a need, however, to begin to explore the challenges faced by these therapists in their work with African American families.

One challenge for some of these clinicians has been to begin to identify
the areas of similarity and difference of Blacks in relation to people from their
own cultures. Although a careful exploration of these comparisons is beyond
the scope of this book, McGoldrick, Giordano, and Pearce (1996), McGoldrick
(1998), and Sue and Sue (1999) have begun this process. There is definitely a
need for further exploration of this type of cross-cultural work in the research
and clinical literature.

The particular history of slavery, racism, and discrimination faced by generations of African Americans have shaped their response to therapy as well as
their reactions to those from other groups. Many Latino, Asian, and Native

American therapists, as well as therapists from other ethnic groups, are initially surprised to discover that the "healthy cultural suspicion" of some Black clients (discussed in Chapter 1) may also be applied to them.

An error that can sometimes be made by very well-meaning therapists from other ethnic minority groups has been to assume a kinship or connection with an African American family, based on their minority status, that the family may not experience. It is very important that therapists in this position try to avoid taking this response personally and recognize that some African American families may well have experienced racism and discrimination from members of other ethnic minority groups. They should be aware of the importance of cross-racial or cross-cultural joining. The use of self is crucial in this process. It may be helpful in some cases for these therapists to inquire as to how an African American client or family might feel in working with someone from their background. Once again, as discussed above, timing is a crucial part of this process and the therapist should take care to join and connect with all family members before raising this issue.

Issues for African American Therapists Working with Black Families

As African Americans learn more about treatment, they are becoming more sophisticated assessors of what the field has to offer. Whether they seek out a private practice or a community clinic, they will often come in asking for a Black therapist. When an African American therapist is available, the factor of shared race often eases the transition into treatment for a family. Sometimes African American clients are less suspicious and guarded when they are working with a Black therapist. African American families frequently expect something different from a Black therapist on a personal level. They are searching not just for an expert but also for someone whom they feel they can trust.

Often African American families are more relaxed initially with a Black therapist because they have made assumptions about a certain level of understanding. They more closely identify with the Black therapist, who is therefore drawn closer into the family circle. This often results in a more assertive use of the therapeutic process by the family. In such cases, an easy familiarity is more likely to develop between the family and the therapist, which can be utilized in treatment when appropriate.

Many African American therapists have found that sharing their own experiences can be extremely useful with Black families, as can identifying common experiences such as normalizing the reluctance of African Americans to enter treatment. Use of Black dialect, when appropriate, can be helpful if it is comfortable for the therapist and is syntonic with the family. It is most important, however, that the therapist be true to him- or herself. Since the Black therapist runs the risk of overidentification with the family, and of losing therapeutic objectivity, he or she must be aware of this danger in order to guard against it. Use of self-disclosure is best done in a careful, thoughtful, and very selective way.

Male–female issues are often important in the treatment of African American families and couples. Any couple therapist is well aware of the seductiveness, alliances, and competitiveness that can develop with one or more members of the couple. (See also Chapter 5 for issues specific to African American couples.) This can be enacted in a variety of ways in the interaction between the Black therapist and the Black family. African American male therapists who were interviewed for this book stressed that they were very aware of potentially competitive postures between them and male family members. A number of these therapists were conscious of attempting to neutralize this competition.

Because of the socialization around "macho" beliefs, for example, some African American men may find it difficult at first to undergo the process of "opening up" in front of another Black man (i.e., the therapist). The husband/ father frequently enters treatment afraid that his problems with his spouse and/ or children will be interpreted as weakness by the therapist. The African American male therapist may be perceived as a professional, less streetwise, and so on. There may even be suspicions about the therapist's masculinity because he does not assume a more traditional Black male role. An important aspect of the credibility that the African American male therapist must establish in these situations is that of establishing himself as a peer. Nonverbal cues, for example, when the therapist seats himself behind a desk and thus distances himself from the couple or family, often inhibit the development of trust, increasing the possibility of these types of suspicion arising.

For the African American female therapist working with Black couples and families, the issues can be slightly different. She can be seen by the woman as a competitor by virtue of her education, appearance, age, socioeconomic level, and so on. Unless she carefully prepares the family and/or couple for treatment, openly discussing the purposes of her actions, her attempts to join with the African American man can be misinterpreted by the women in the family as seductiveness. Given how loaded the issue of fidelity is with many African American couples, this can interfere prohibitively with the treatment process. Some African American men, on the other hand, feel more comfortable initially seeing a Black female therapist because they feel less threatened. It is sometimes easier to acknowledge weaknesses or problems with a Black woman than with a Black man, a situation particularly true if sexual problems are involved.

It often comes as a very painful surprise to young African American clinicians when they discover that Black families are also "checking them out." The "healthy cultural suspicion" described in Chapter 1 extends to most "White" institutions, including mental health centers and hospitals. It can, in some cases, also extend to the African American clinicians who work in them. Jackson (1980) has discussed the fact that some Black clients and families may initially view the Black therapist as a member of "the White establishment" and even as a threat to their existence. These African American families will often question whether the Black therapist is an "Uncle Tom" (someone who meekly serves the White man), an "oreo" (Black outside, but White inside), or a "token" (a Black person who is placed in a position merely to meet affirmative action guidelines). In a smaller number of African American families, the Black therapist may even encounter a projection of the family member's feelings of self-hatred, wherein she or he secretly feels that a Black therapist is second-rate and not as good as a White therapist. Some of these Black clients may be very White-identified and be at the preencounter stage of racial identity (Cross, 1991; Helms & Cook, 1999; see Chapter 2). Occasionally a Black family such as this may even refuse to work with an African American therapist.

These responses from Black people are particularly painful, especially for beginning African American clinicians. It is very important that they be discussed openly in the supervisory relationship so that they can be understood. African American therapists who have struggled with their own self- and racial identity will be in a better position to join with such families and to recognize that these reactions are a product of the racism in U.S. society and not a personal affront. It is therefore very important for African American therapists to understand that even though the joining process may be at least superficially more comfortably undertaken, they must never neglect it and must not assume that because they are Black, all Black families will immediately give them their trust. This trust must be earned by the therapist, irrespective of race.

African American therapists are often very surprised to discover that they may have their own unique issues to resolve if they are to treat Black families effectively. There is a direct relationship between the degree to which Black therapists are comfortable with themselves, their own families, their own racial identity, and their ability to work with African American families. Since Black people vary considerably on the degree to which they view their racial identity as important to consider, it is not surprising to learn that Black therapists vary considerably also. To the degree that a Black therapist denies or rejects his or her own racial identity, he or she may be cut off from African American families and may have difficulty establishing therapeutic bonds (Helms & Cook, 1999; Hunt, 1987). Conversely, if African American therapists overidentify with Black families, they may miss important issues, losing their objectivity and their ability to act as therapeutic agents of change.

In their work in the mental health fields, African American therapists often experience a double bind. It is not unusual for an African American therapist to be the only Black on staff and thus to find her- or himself particularly concerned about the treatment strategies that are applied to Black families. She or he may come to feel like "the voice in the wilderness," the sole person repeatedly stating these concerns. Black therapists, like most Black people who work in predominantly White fields, must struggle with maintaining their racial identity while interacting with Whites (Helms & Cook, 1999; Hunt, 1987). Some African American therapists also struggle with considerable guilt over having "made it," thus having left other Black people "behind."

Class and socioeconomic differences are difficult issues for all middle-class therapists, but they present even more of a dilemma for the African American middle-class therapist who is working with poor Black families. Many Black therapists can recall experiencing the anger of African American families around this issue, a form of rejection by Black clients that often heightens their feeling of not quite belonging anywhere. These are very important issues that must be addressed by every Black therapist at some point in his or her development. Some African American therapists are fortunate enough to have had therapy of their own with an African American colleague. Many find themselves in a dilemma, however, because some White supervisors are not aware of or equipped to address these issues with the Black therapist. When supervisors approach this in an insensitive or clumsy way, it can often be experienced as judgmental or accusatory by the African American therapist.

African American therapists attempt to deal with these dilemmas in many different ways. Some are very productive. They look for other African American mentors and role models outside of their agencies and programs or join Black professional organizations such as the Associations of Black Psychologists, the National Association of Black Social Workers, and the Association of Black Psychiatrists. These individuals and groups can be used as support networks for African American therapists to explore their beliefs about Black families, therapy, and the development of their own self-identity.

Some of the ways in which some well-meaning African American therapists attempt to cope with this dilemma are counterproductive and in fact undermine effective service delivery to Black families. One role sometimes assumed by African American therapists in training has been referred to as "the saboteur" (Hunt, 1987). Because many African American therapists experience the rage common to Black people in response to racism, they often respond with what Hunt (1987) characterizes as "indirect hostility and anger in their communications with White and Black professional peers" (p. 116). Because of their concerns that some "White theories" often do not work for African American families, these therapists can sometimes resort to stereotypical comments about African Americans: "Presenting themselves as experts on the Black race allows their assumptions to go unchallenged by many peers" (Hunt, 1987, p. 116).

Many of these African American therapists are expressing their anger at a system that they perceive as not accepting or valuing them or their clients. However, rather than working toward developing ethnically appropriate treatment strategies, they sometimes overprotect their clients and avoid addressing important therapeutic issues. They sometimes engage African American clients and families in an "us against the system" type of discussion, which may confuse the families they treat. African American families often come into therapy in crisis, needing help on a number of problems, and thus are suspicious of Black therapists who have the need to present themselves as "protectors of the race" (Hunt, 1987). To further complicate these issues, supervisors are frequently reluctant to raise these issues with African American therapists, which means that they may never be addressed.

Another role that can be counterproductive occurs when the African American becomes the "moralizer" who is going to "raise the consciousness of Black people" (Hunt, 1987). Instead of using therapy to empower African American families, these therapists sometimes adopt a "preacher/teacher" model in which they "deliver impromptu lecturettes to their unsuspecting Black clients" (Hunt, 1987, p. 117). The key to recognizing this pattern when reviewing videotapes or audiotapes is noticing whether the therapist "preaches" or talks more than the family. In such situations the therapist, instead of addressing the problems that the family brings to the session, discusses political or racial problems in society and ignores or minimizes the family's concerns. It is important for supervisors to help these therapists learn to distinguish between lecturing and doing therapy with African American families.

Due to the increased empathy that African American therapists often feel for Black families, there may be a tendency to set themselves up as their "rescuers," becoming overinvolved in the family's issues and treating family members with pity for their life experiences. Therapists who make this error often "wallow in their client's emotional content as a release of their own personal guilt for having made it into the mainstream of society" (Hunt, 1987, p. 118). It is important to note that although Hunt describes this as a pattern in some Black therapists, it is also quite common among White therapists as well. Sometimes therapists engaged in this pattern overextend themselves for the African American families they treat, so that they "[are] available at all times, make little or no demands on the clients and inappropriately do favors for them, thus creating new dependency" (p. 118). This pattern is not only counterproductive for African American families but it quickly "burns out" the therapist. An African American therapist whom I supervised some years ago paraphrased a line from the play *River Niger* in describing this feeling: "Everybody wants a piece of my toe." Eager young Black therapists who want to do therapy with African American families need to be helped to guard against this pattern and set limits with the families they treat. They need to address the guilt discussed above and the conflict about having "made it."

In conclusion, although the patterns described above clearly do not apply to all therapists, whether Black, White, or from another ethnic or racial group, they do illustrate some of the common pitfalls and dilemmas. A number of the examples that are described as more common to Black, White, or other ethnic minority therapists can clearly occur in all of these groups. It is important, however, for therapists to be aware of their own particular issues and to seek out someone in their own lives whom they can trust and with whom they can address these problems: a therapist, supervisor, mentor, colleague, coworkers, other trainees or therapists, or sensitive friends.

VALUE-RELATED ISSUES IN THE TREATMENT OF AFRICAN AMERICAN FAMILIES

The pervasive impact of values on the therapeutic alliance and process has been discussed throughout this book within a variety of contexts. This section will present some of the conflicts in this area that may not have been explored or examined in sufficient detail.

In this section, it is very important to reiterate a theme that has been stated throughout this book: there is no such thing as *the* African American family. By the same token, there is no one set of values that is common to *all* African American families. The most important lesson to be learned by therapists is that all therapy is a process of negotiation of values and beliefs. It is crucial for therapists to clarify their own values for themselves and to explore with the family their particular beliefs. It is the ultimate sign of disrespect to any person or family to assume a knowledge of her, his, or their beliefs or values without asking for clarification. Similarly, it is the greatest acknowledgment of the dignity of a person or family to ask him, her, or them to tell or teach one about himself, herself, or themselves and the things that are important to him, her, or them.

Values Clarification for Therapists

Values clarification is an ongoing, lifelong activity. It is not a task done once in training and then completed, but a process of continuously exploring one's own reactions, countertransferences, and beliefs as one works with families. Because family therapy and other systems approaches are such active forms of therapy, the therapist's own values and perceptions are constantly "on the line."

It is important, therefore, for the family therapist, particularly during the training years, to use supervision and peer support to explore his or her countertransference reactions to the families he or she treats. For example, a family therapist who is hesitant or even afraid to confront issues with an authoritarian parent may have some unresolved issues with his or her own parent. If these patterns recur frequently and interfere with the therapeutic interaction, therapy for the therapist may be indicated.

Values and Therapy

Aponte (1994) makes the following statement about the role of values in the therapeutic process:

> Values frame the entire process of therapy. Values are the social standards by which therapists define reality, identify problems, formalize evaluations, select interventions, and determine therapeutic goals. All transactions between therapists and clients involve negotiations about the respective value systems that each party brings into the therapeutic process. (p. 170)

Given these issues, there are a number of areas in which well-meaning therapists can encounter serious value differences and/or conflicts with African American families. The following are among the most significant: (1) "casual" versus "formal" styles, (2) different political views, (3) religious beliefs or values, (4) the importance of race and discrimination, (5) teenage pregnancy and abortion, and (6) parenting and discipline.

All of these issues have been or will be discussed in detail in other chapters. This section will therefore focus exclusively on the areas of difference or conflict within therapy.

Casual versus Formal Styles

Most therapists spend many years in school, where attitudes and interaction tend to follow along more "casual" lines than they do in many families. Students call professors by their first names and refer to each other informally. When they begin to join with families and engage them in family therapy, their natural tendency is to view an informal, "first-name basis" style as putting people at their ease. With African American families, and particularly with older, more traditional family members, this may be a serious error. This may be especially true if the therapist appears to be very young from the client's viewpoint.

The most important lesson here is for the therapist to take his or her cues from the family. Although many younger African American families allow children to call adults by their first names, many older or more traditional Black families are offended by this practice, seeing it as a sign of disrespect. In my own family of origin, for example, all of my parents' adult friends were referred to as "Aunt" or "Uncle" in order to indicate their closeness to the family but also their status as elders to be respected. It would have been unthinkable for us to call them by their first names alone.

"Old school" Black families often object to children referring to therapists, teachers, or other adults on a first-name basis. Similarly, they may object to a therapist, particularly a young one or one whom they do not know well, referring to them by first names. It is usually helpful to start with a more formal introduction and allow the family to indicate their preference.

During my internship at the Philadelphia Child Guidance Clinic, a family taught me this lesson very graphically, as the following case example illustrates.

The Jefferson family appeared for a family session. In the waiting room, there were many members of the extended family. Mrs. Martha Jefferson (age 36) had originally brought her son Jeffrey (age 12) for treatment. When it became clear that they were part of a large extended family household, the other members were asked to come in.

I was very young and very new to the process of family therapy at the time. As the family sat down, I asked them to go around and introduce themselves. Martha Jefferson began and gave only her first name. Her brothers and sisters (Jeffrey's aunts and uncles) did the same. When we came to Martha's mother, she looked at me directly and said, "I am *Mrs. Jefferson.*" Her message was clear. She was making an emphatic statement about her role and power in this family and about the respect she demanded as the grandmother and a member of the older generation.

Naming can also be used to elevate someone's status within the family structure. For example, in a three-generation family in which a grandmother, a young unwed mother, and a child live in a household, the entire family including the child may refer to the mother by her first name as if she were a sibling. The therapist can begin to help draw the generational boundary by referring to her as "Ms." or "your mother" in the presence of her child and other family members.

Working with African American Families with Different Political Views from the Therapist

The issue of political views and values can often be a very difficult and painful one for Black and White clinicians as well as those from other ethnic and racial backgrounds, who hold strong political beliefs that they may find are not shared by the Black families with whom they work. It is easier to see this difference and acknowledge it openly if the therapist is a blatant racist or is largely condemning of poor Black families, Black families on welfare, or Black single-parent families. It is much more difficult to see and acknowledge in more subtle situations. Political views are important parts of our value system and must be addressed and brought to our conscious awareness so that we do not unwittingly impose them on others or reject those who do not share our views or priorities.

The two examples that can best describe this dilemma are the struggles of a young White woman therapist with a strong feminist orientation and a young Black male therapist who adopted a "Blacker than thou" posture with the families he treated. The struggle in both of these situations involved a well-meaning therapist who wanted to help but who encounters a Black family or family member with radically different views. It is important to underscore here that both of these therapists hold very deeply felt and sincere political views, which contribute positively to their own lives. The important point here is that even the most positive view can become oppressive if it is imposed on someone else.

Gloria, a 28-year-old White woman, was a social worker with a strong feminist orientation. She was a member of the National Organization of Women (NOW) and had a great deal of concern about the ways in which women have been victimized by men. She was working for the first time at an inner-city community mental health center and had a number of single-parent Black families in which mothers were involved with boyfriends whom she felt "demeaned them as women." She routinely denigrated the treatment these women received by men, encouraged them to leave their relationships, preached to them about the role of women in society, and had never included any of these Black men in the treatment process. Black families typically stayed with her through the first few sessions and then dropped out of treatment.

This scenario illustrates the mismatch that can occur when a therapist is so invested in her or his political views that they dominate her or his view of the world. In this case, her strong feminist values did not allow Gloria to truly join with the African American families with whom she worked. It was clear that no matter which issue they brought to treatment, the mistreatment of these women by men became the primary focus. In many of her cases, Gloria had in fact correctly assessed very problematic couple relationships, but she always moved immediately to "politicize" these women rather than to address the presenting problems that they brought to therapy. In addition, Gloria was so angry at men in general that she was unable to reach out to the African American men in these families and involve them in the treatment process. The sad motif in this situation was that Gloria was never consciously aware of these discrepancies. She thought she was helping and raising the family's "political consciousness" without recognizing and accepting the family's presentation of their needs.

In an earlier paper (Boyd-Franklin, 1983), I addressed the fact that many African American women prioritize their feminist values differently from many White women. Thus some African American women will respond first to being Black and then to being a woman. Women of different races who presume a bond based on gender can sometimes find that some African American women experience this assumption as patronizing. This is particularly unfortunate when the well-meaning therapist is totally unaware of this perception and proceeds as if a bond has been formed. It is helpful to ask people their views in an atmosphere of respect rather than in one of conversion.

An example of a similar dilemma for an African American therapist can be seen in the case of Kwame.

Kwame was a 26-year-old psychologist with a strong sense of his African-American identity. He had adopted an African name, wore an Afro hairstyle, and often wore African clothing as well. He strongly and genuinely believed in the necessity for Black people to accept their "blackness," and he had worked hard to nurture a strong Black identity in his own life.

In 1990, Kwame was working in a community mental health center and was assigned a Black family in which a young Black woman was referred because she was on academic probation from her college and was profoundly depressed. In the first session, Kwame met with the young woman and her parents. The young woman had an Afro hairdo and wore a red, black, and green pin in the shape of the continent of Africa. She stated clearly that her parents could not accept her Black identity and were very rejecting of her. Her parents were a middle-aged, middle-class Black couple who were very angry at their daughter for trying to act "too Black" and getting involved in Black student political activities rather than focusing on her studies.

Kwame identified immediately with the young woman (whose situation replicated his struggle with his own parents). In his mind he labeled her parents as "bourgie" and proceeded to lecture them on how they were making their daughter depressed by not accepting her need to express her own African American heritage. While this was one possible treatment dynamic, it became Kwame's total treatment focus. The parents refused to return for family treatment. Kwame then saw the young woman individually and allied with her against her parents. He told her that they were "Uncle Toms" who could not understand her. The young woman stayed for two sessions and did not return to treatment.

Kwame's approach has become known as the "Blacker than thou" syndrome. He was genuinely committed to his own African American identity but had conflicts about it. This young Black woman and her family replicated his own unresolved issues with his family of origin. Kwame believed strongly in his political convictions about his blackness but he was not able to put his values aside and join with these parents to help them discuss their conflicts with their daughter. His politics caused him to become judgmental of the family and to unwittingly lose his therapeutic neutrality. He formed a generational alliance with the young woman and became so overidentified with her that he was unable to conduct treatment on an individual or a family level.

These two cases admittedly are extreme examples of a problem that may manifest itself in many subtle ways. They are presented here, however, as a word of caution for well-meaning therapists of all races who are not in touch with the powerful influence that their political views may carry and the ways in which they may have difficulty in working with family members who hold different orientations, regardless of the color of either the therapist or the client family.

Religious Beliefs

The training of many therapists has tended to disregard religion or spirituality as an issue in treatment or to pathologize it (see Chapter 7). The difficulties that can arise from the presence of different religious or spiritual orientations can immobilize the therapist and bring therapy to a virtual halt. Therapists may be unable to help family members resolve differences in religious perspectives and renegotiate rules because of their inability to clarify their own religious values. The following case example illustrates this dilemma.

The Williams family consisted of Mrs. Williams (age 32), Mr. Williams (age 33), and their two boys, Robert (age 9) and Ronald (age 10). Ronald was displaying acting-out and aggressive behavior in school. He "talked back" to his teacher and often fought with other children. At home he was described by his mother as being a "bad child." Mr. and Mrs. Williams were active as Jehovah's Witnesses. They were involved in their Kingdom Hall and spent many evenings in Bible study and weekends "pioneering," that is, doing door-to-door missionary work. The boys often went with them to the Kingdom Hall, and Robert was described as the good child who never gave trouble. Ronald was clearly scapegoated by the family. In the course of exploration about behavior and rules at home, it became clear to the therapist that there were many restrictions on the boys. Mrs. Williams stated angrily that Ronald was a "terrible sneak" who had brought small toys resembling the television characters "Voltron" and "Transformers" into the house. She was very angry because these were considered "demonic" by her religion. The children were not allowed to play with other children in the neighborhood or at school. The therapist was appalled. She felt strongly that this family was stifling the children's social development. Her first reaction was to side with the children and encourage them to stand up to their parents.

Her supervisor helped her to see that she was becoming caught in the family's structure and was actually forming a cross-generational alliance with the children against the parents.

The therapist was encouraged to join with the parents by asking them to teach her about their religious beliefs and their concerns for the children. In the course of this process, it became clear that these beliefs were primarily Mrs. Williams's and that Mr. Williams had been going along with her program. She was clearly the strength and power in the family. It also became very clear that Mr. Williams secretly encouraged Ronald's rebellion against his mother. The therapist was then able to help these parents discuss their differences, particularly in terms of childrearing. They were able to agree on the beliefs that they felt were most important for the children to understand. The therapist then encouraged Mr. Williams to discuss these issues with Ronald, who was able to tell his parents how he was often ridiculed by his classmates because of the things that he was not allowed to do. Mr. Williams empathized with his son and asked his son how his parents might help him with this. He was also able to be clear with Ronald about the rules that he had to follow and the reasons for them. Mrs. Williams was able for the first time to stand back and support this process without intruding.

The therapist in this situation was able to recognize her own value differences with the family, discuss them with her supervisor, and avoid a collision with the family that would have exacerbated rather than resolved the family conflict.

Racism and Discrimination Issues

While issues concerning racism and discrimination could be included under the discussion of political views, it is important to note that racial considerations are often pervasive enough in character to extend beyond the political outlook. Often, the most difficult African American families for many therapists to treat are those who "deny" their blackness or minimize its importance. This is also an issue for many politically active White therapists and those from other ethnic and racial groups. There are some Black people, particularly those who live and work in all-White settings and who may have gone to schools or professional training in an all-White atmosphere, who see a real value in being "color-blind." This is particularly difficult for African American therapists who feel strongly about issues of Black pride and racial identity. The question is often compounded because these families tend to come into treatment when they are confronted by the realities of racism and their worldview is threatened. The question that frequently arises in supervision is, how does one join with or convey respect to a person or family whose beliefs are radically different from one's own? This is a very basic struggle, one for which there are no easy answers. In these situations, the therapist must assess his or her own values and clarify his or her own beliefs. The following case example illustrates these issues.

Alice Downing was a 15-year-old African American adolescent who had grown up in an all-White suburb for most of her life. She and her family were referred for treatment after she made a "suicidal" gesture in which she took 10 aspirin tablets. Her family consisted of her parents, Mr. Carl Downing (age 45) and Mrs. Anne Downing (age 42), and her sister Mary (age 11). In the first session with the family, the therapist was struck by the fact that Alice looked quite different from the other members of her family. She was in fact the only family member with "Black features." She was light brown in complexion. Her mother, father, and sister were very light-skinned and "White" in facial features, and her mother and sister had light hazel eyes. In the course of the first few family sessions, the therapist discovered that Alice was scapegoated by the family and had been for most of her life. Her mother and father both stated that she had "always been in trouble." In an individual session with Alice, the therapist learned that the precipitant for the suicidal incident had been a rejection by her boyfriend, who was White. His family had objected to his seeing a Black girl. She had never shared this information with her family.

In a family session, with the therapist's help, she was finally able to do so. Both her mother and her father became very angry with her and told her that she had created this problem herself by raising the issue of race at all. Ms. Downing proudly stated that race was never an issue for her and then she claimed that she had many relatives who "passed" for White and were married to White spouses. Mr. Downing described his rise in a White corporation and told his daughter how he had always tried "not to stand out or be different."

The therapist, who was Black, had an extreme reaction of tremendous anger toward these parents. She recognized that this family had very different values from her own. In a discussion with her supervisory consultant, she carefully analyzed her own anger at this family. With the consultant's help, she was able to clarify her reaction and separate out her own countertransference. Once this was accomplished, she was able to challenge the family's avoidance of the color issue in their home and help them see that their daughter had always felt "different." She helped the daughter to talk directly to her mother about this pain for the first time in her life, and helped the mother to talk to Alice about this and to try to understand her daughter's need to develop her own cultural identity. Mr. Downing strongly objected and stated that he felt that if she focused on her "difference" she would never "fit in." The therapist asked Mr. and Mrs. Downing to discuss what they had been told about racial identity by their own families and to share the times when it had caused them conflicts in their lives. For the first time, they were able to discuss in front of their children their own struggles with racial identity and the reasons why they had made their choice to live a "color-blind" lifestyle.

In another session, the therapist asked the parents to discuss the possibility that they had made their choice but that their daughter might feel trapped and unable to make a choice for herself. She asked if they loved their daughter enough to allow her the right to make her own choice and struggle with her own decision on racial identity.

Although the parents' views on racial identity changed very little in the course of therapy, they were able finally to support their daughter's need to struggle with her own racial identity and her own appearance as a Black woman. The issue of color difference had long been a taboo issue in this family but it was now opened sufficiently to promote some possible differentiation for the children.

The struggle of this therapist was a very difficult one: her own values conflicted with the family's values; her own cultural identification and sense of African American identity contrasted sharply with those of the family; and she overidentified with the daughter. She used her supervisory consultant to work through her own countertransference and value issues so that she could intervene appropriately in the family. Had she simply expressed her anger at the parents, she would have been drawn into the family dynamics and would have repeated the family's pattern of nonacceptance and blame. There is a very valuable lesson to be learned from this example: it is crucial for family therapists to be willing to seek out a consultation with a trusted supervisor or colleague when these reactions occur. This is an essential part of the process of value clarification and the differentiation of one's own beliefs from those of the family that is in treatment.

Teenage Pregnancy Versus Abortion

One potentially explosive issue for therapists and African American families relates to the question of teenage pregnancy versus abortion. Clearly, this is a value-laden issue that taps a very powerful response in many individuals in this country. There are strong feelings and opinions on the part of both "pro-choice" groups and "right-to-life" groups. Therapists are clearly not neutral or immune to opinions on this question.

There are many different views within African American communities on this issue also. Some very religious African American families are very opposed to abortion. Other Black families, because of moral, cultural, and/or Afrocentric beliefs, feel very strongly that children have a right to be born. This often taps multigenerational beliefs and decisions to choose to carry a pregnancy to term that have been made by other members of the family, such as a mother and/or a grandmother. Stack (1974) in her description of a discussion between a 15-year-old girl who is pregnant and her mother captures the cultural beliefs of many Black people on this issue:

Lottie talked with her mother during her second month of pregnancy. She said, "Herman told my mama I was pregnant. She was in the kitchen cooking. I told him not to tell nobody. I wanted to keep it a secret but he told me time will tell. My mama said to me 'I had you and you should have your child. I didn't get rid of you. I loved you and I took care of you until you got to the age to have this one. Have your baby no matter what, there's nothing wrong with having a baby. Be proud of it like I was proud of you.' My mama didn't tear me down; she was about the best mother a person ever had." (p. 47)

This view is by no means universally held by African Americans. There are many Black leaders, such as Jesse Jackson, who have argued that "babies having babies" must stop. There are those who feel very strongly that teenage pregnancy seriously compromises both the teenager's and her child's future. Planned Parenthood has extensive educational programs for teenagers in African American communities.

Within one African American family or extended family, many different views may be represented and this issue may be a very loaded, volatile one within the family. In addition, therapists may find themselves in a serious values conflict with a family regarding these issues. This can sometimes result in a premature termination of treatment by the family, as the following case illustrates.

Janice Valentine (a 14-year-old Black adolescent) was referred for treatment by her physician, who had discovered that she was 4 weeks pregnant. Her mother, Connie Valentine, age 31, appeared for the intake session with her. Both Janice and her mother expressed concern and ambivalence about her pregnancy. Connie Valentine had been pregnant with Janice at age 15 and was very concerned that Janice was now pregnant at the same time in her life. When the therapist asked them to discuss the issue, it became clear that the grandmother, Connie Valentine's mother, had taken a strong stand that "nobody was gonna kill my great-grandchild." The therapist, supported by Janice's physician, pushed strongly for an abortion, arguing that having a baby at 15 would seriously alter Janice's life. They became very concerned with the number of weeks the family had in which to make a decision as to whether or not to have the child.

In one session, the therapist, becoming more concerned as the decision point for a therapeutic abortion was approaching, pushed the mother to help her daughter make a decision. The family dropped out of treatment. Many months later, the therapist learned from the physician that Janice had had her baby.

This case illustrates a number of points. First, it is a classic example of a value conflict between the "helping persons" and the family. The therapist and the physician, because of their own beliefs, became so invested in the outcome, that is, the "decision," that they lost touch with the structural issues in this family. They in fact re-created the family structure by becoming rigid parental figures who accepted both Janice and her mother's definition of helplessness. First, the family system had presented as two ambivalent, uncertain adolescents, a structure that was never challenged. The mother was never helped or supported to assume a parental stance with her daughter. Second, the therapist disregarded information concerning a very important value conflict between herself and the grandmother in this family. She did not correctly read the grandmother's level of power in the family structure. Since the grandmother was never engaged, the therapist unwittingly became locked in a value struggle with the grandmother over the outcome of the decision. Third, the family structure was not changed because Janice Valentine was once again left "in the middle" and was given conflicting messages.

The decision of the family to have the child might have been the same whatever the therapist had done, but the family structure could have been altered significantly if the therapist had engaged the grandmother in the therapeutic process and helped her and her daughter to openly discuss their concerns about Janice's pregnancy. This opportunity was lost because the therapist became equally enmeshed in the family dynamics and tried to convince Janice and her mother of her point of view.

Parenting and Discipline

Another area in which therapists often clash with African American families is that of parenting or disciplinary issues. Many African American families take pride in being of the "old school," firmly upholding such beliefs as those expressed by the maxim "spare the rod, spoil the child." McGoldrick (1982) points out that there are often good reasons for this response by African American parents. She discusses the concept of African American parents providing strict discipline for their children in the hope of protecting them from the severe societal consequences of acting-out behavior, particularly in adolescence.

Peters (1981), in her discussion of approaches to discipline among Black people, makes the following observations:

> Discipline techniques of Black parents have often been noted by observers of Black parent–child interaction. Although definitive studies of discipline in Black families have yet to be done, many researchers have described the Black parents' more direct physical form of discipline that differs from the psychologically oriented approach preferred by mainstream families, such as withdrawal of love or making approval or affection contingent on the child's behavior or accomplishment. The strict, no-nonsense discipline of Black parents—often characterized as "harsh" or "rigid" or "egocentrically motivated" by mainstream-oriented observers (Chilman, 1966)—has been shown to be functional, appropriate discipline of caring parents. (p. 216)

There have been a number of studies of childrearing practices. Lewis and Looney (1983), although their study of working-class Black families did not focus specifically on childrearing practices, note that they "were impressed with the firm but supportive and understanding push of children toward responsible autonomy. The concern about keeping children busy in meaningful activities was particularly apparent in the most competent families" (pp. 134–135).

In their work, they cite a number of authors who have studied child-rearing practices in African American families. For example:

> They note that in this very poor neighborhood child play is commonly characterized by fighting, and discipline by frequent "whippings." Mothers are authoritarian in their approach to their children, pushing them toward early autonomy but then punishing them corporally for transgression. The children express strong loyalty and affection for their mothers, suggesting that she is the center of the family. "She assigns chores, sees homework, metes out punishment, and warns against hazards" (p. 205). (Lewis & Looney, 1983, p. 133)

Lewis and Looney (1983) also point out that "the most competent adolescents in our sample saw the fact that their parents were strict as a source of family strength" (p. 134). This is extremely important because in many African American families this "strictness" or strength is seen as a protection against the influences of "the street" (i.e., drugs, delinquency, crime, lack of interest in education, etc.).

Peters (1981) reports on her own work with working-class Black families.

> Mothers became more dynamic in their disciplining as their young children began to understand the appropriate behavior parents expected. Most parents emphasized obedience. However, obedience was not viewed negatively; it was an important issue, often of special significance to a parent. Parents said that they believed obedience "will make life easier for my child," "means respect," "is equated with my love," or "is necessary if my child is to achieve in school." (pp. 216–217)

In my own work with African American families, I have found it helpful to join first with these families and to build trust with them before challenging the issue of discipline. It is very important that the therapist avoid an attacking or judgmental posture with the family. The therapist may try to understand the protective posture, referred to above, in which some African Americans firmly believe that physical punishment will change their children's behavior and protect them from the often harsh censure of society. (Remember that understanding does not necessarily mean agreement.) This issue is complicated by the fact that some child welfare agencies in the past have overreacted to the word "spanking" and have prematurely removed children from African American families for child abuse, without exploring this issue further. On the other hand, it is very important that therapists not collude with families to deny child abuse and put children at risk. Therapists in all states are now required to report families in which child abuse has occurred or is suspected. This is sometimes a painful but necessary process. Given these realities, it is often helpful for new clinicians, particularly those from other ethnic and racial groups, to confer with an African American supervisor, clinician, or another knowledgeable member of the African American community before making the decision to report.

In my own work with these African American families, I have often found that, once trust has developed, I can say to the family: "I care about your family and I understand that spanking was the way that you were raised, but I am deeply concerned that, given the laws in this country, you could lose your children if you continue to spank them. I don't want to see that happen because I know how much you love them. Are you willing to work with me to try to come up with some new ways of disciplining her [him]?" Therapists should not expect immediate agreement but should be willing to be honest about the constraints of the law and have an open discussion with their clients about this issue.

Negotiation of Values in Therapy with African American Families

Upon recognition of the value issues in family therapy, the therapist is faced with a dilemma. Many African American families enter therapy with very unclear notions as to the process of therapy or very different expectations from those of the therapist as to what the process will provide. It is very useful to ask family members directly what they expect from the process. This, however, can lead to another level of difficulty for the therapist. There are many situations in which the family may want one thing (i.e., "fix the child") and the therapist may view the problem differently (e.g., "this is a family problem"). This impasse is extremely common in therapy in general and is particularly relevant to the struggles between therapists and Black families.

In order for this dilemma to be resolved, a negotiation process must occur between the therapist and the family. Aponte (1976, 1994) was one of the first family therapists to discuss the negotiation of values and/or perception of the problem between the family and the therapist. Ultimately the inevitable points of difference, particularly in cross-racial therapy, must be addressed by this negotiation process.

When I present workshops on this topic, I am often asked "Can White therapists or those from other ethnic and racial groups treat Black families?" Clearly there is no one answer to this question. Although many Black families express a wish to work with a Black therapist, the reality is that it is more likely that they will be involved in a cross-cultural treatment process. This is due to the shortage of African American therapists in many agencies and in training programs. It is imperative that this issue be addressed and efforts be made to recruit African American therapists for all training programs throughout the mental health field.

At the same time, given this reality, therapists of all races must learn to work with African American families. In my experience the cross-cultural and cross-racial differences are most successfully negotiated if the therapist (of any race or ethnic background) views family therapy as a negotiation process (Aponte, 1994) in which the family is asked for its expectations of treatment, these values are clarified, and the therapist is clear on his or her own goals, values, and beliefs. The process can then be negotiated from a position that conveys respect for the family's belief system.

10

Major Family Therapy Approaches and Their Relevance to Treating African Americans*

With most ethnic groups, but particularly with African American families, the family therapist must be willing and able to be flexible and to draw from the work of many different schools of family therapy. Given the centrality of the joining process to therapy with Black families, the most effective approach incorporates both the use of self and the theoretical approach best suited to the family at hand. This chapter summarizes some of the major family system approaches and views them in terms of their relevance to the treatment of African American families.

The first section of the chapter explores the structural family therapy model, paying particular attention to the work of Minuchin, Montalvo, Guerney, Rosman, and Schumer (1967), Aponte (1976), Aponte and Van Deusen (1981), Haley (1976), Minuchin (1974), and Nichols and Schwartz (1998). In section two the Bowen model is examined, as well as the contributions of those influenced by his theory (Bowen, 1976, 1978). As an outgrowth of the Bowenian school, some therapists now incorporate a "family therapy with one person approach" (Carter & McGoldrick-Orfanidis, 1994), discussed in the third section. The fourth section considers the applications of the paradoxical, strategic, or systemic approach. In the fifth section the narrative and postmodern approaches are explored in terms of their utility in the treatment of African American clients and families (Epston & White, 1992; Nichols &

---

*Sections from an earlier version of this chapter, with some editorial changes, are adapted from Boyd-Franklin (1987).

Schwartz, 1998; White & Epston, 1990). The concluding section examines integrating all these different approaches.

STRUCTURAL FAMILY THERAPY AND THE TREATMENT OF AFRICAN AMERICAN FAMILIES

Structural family therapy provides a comprehensive model for the treatment of Black families that can be effectively employed in combination with other approaches. Minuchin (1974), Minuchin et al. (1967), and Minuchin and Fishman (1981) developed this approach. It provides a method for assessing the structure of a family, identifying its areas of difficulty, and restructuring the family system in order to produce change. Developed initially for work with minority families, it contains many of the strategies that are most effective at engaging and changing their familial structure.

The structural approach is primarily a problem-solving one (Haley, 1976). This aspect of the structural school makes it particularly useful in working with African American families. It is focused, clear, concrete, and directive. For many African American families, the idea of going for treatment is a very new one. As mentioned in Chapter 1, historical approaches that appear to pry into "family business" before trust can be established are often rejected. The problem-solving focus of the structural approach is therefore an important way to engage Black families initially. This is particularly helpful for "multiproblem families" who are overwhelmed with life's demands. This approach can help a family to clarify and prioritize its problems. With its focus on change, it directs the energy of the family toward the future and improvement rather than toward the past and blame. For African American families who may feel powerless to change their lives, this approach provides a sense of empowerment and accomplishment as each problem is resolved and the family is restructured.

The use of family prescriptions and tasks serves an educative function and often provides strategies for change. The emphasis on clear treatment contracts at the end of the initial session (Haley, 1976) is also important when one considers that the treatment process is so new for many Black families. This model quickly engages the family in an interaction process with each other and with the therapist. It is also particularly effective in engaging the peripheral members of extended families in the treatment, and it helps to dismantle the "resistance" of many Black families. An additional therapeutic benefit is that it gives family members a hands-on experience with change.

Minuchin (1974) and Minuchin et al. (1967) were among the first family therapists to discuss the utilization of African American and Hispanic extended families in the treatment process. They focused on two aspects of extended family organization that are very common in Black families: the role of the grandmother or the three-generational family, and the role of the parental child. Both of these are discussed in detail in Chapter 4.

Boundaries

Aponte and Van Deusen (1981) state that "the structural dimensions of transactions most often identified in structural family therapy are boundary, alignment and power" (p. 312). These three areas are an important part of the early assessment process.

Minuchin (1974) defines "the boundaries of a subsystem" as "the rules defining who participates and how" (p. 53). Aponte and Van Deusen (1981) clarify this point:

> These rules dictate who is in and who is out of an operation, and define the roles those who are in will have vis-à-vis each other and the world outside in carrying out that activity. The unit directly engaged in the operation may be one member of a family with all the others excluded, or any combination of family members plus persons outside the family. (p. 312)

As Part I of this book has established, these boundary issues may be very complex in African American families. For example, a child, his mother, his grandmother, his babysitter, and his child welfare worker may all be involved in an issue concerning his behavior. The concepts *enmeshment* and *disengagement* are related to boundary issues (Minuchin, 1974; Nichols & Schwartz, 1998). Aponte and Van Deusen (1981) elaborate on these concepts:

> At the enmeshment end of the continuum, the boundaries among some or all of the family members are relatively undifferentiated, permeable and fluid. . . . At the disengaged end, the family members behave as if they have little to do with one another because within their families their boundaries are so firmly delineated, impermeable, and rigid that the family members tend to go their own ways with little overt dependence on one another. (p. 314)

Minuchin (1974) proposes a continuum stretching from extreme enmeshment to extreme disengagement:

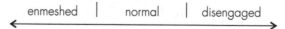

enmeshed | normal | disengaged

The vast majority of U.S. families typically fall within the normal range, but many Black families tend to fall more within the enmeshed range. Normal, functional African American families often have very close relationships, with a great deal of interaction and reciprocity (Billingsley, 1968, 1992; Hill, 1972, 1977, 1993, 1999a; Stack, 1974). However, this is a very vulnerable area in Black extended families because this closeness often results in roles and boundaries becoming very blurred (see Chapter 4). This can be true cross-generationally as well.

At the other end of the spectrum, some African American families are more disengaged. For example, a child may be raised in a large extended family, but he or she may be essentially ignored. Children in some of these families seem to grow up by themselves. They are often sent to school and so on by themselves. No one seems to notice them until there is a crisis.

Alignment

The concept of alignment (Aponte & Van Deusen, 1981) within families encompasses two concepts: alliance and coalition. *Alliance* refers primarily to the patterns of family members working together on something of shared interest (Aponte & Van Deusen, 1981). Haley (1976) defines *coalition* as "a process of joint action against a third person" (p. 109). In complex African American extended families, the alliances and coalitions are often cross-generational and may include key individuals who are outside the family but who are very involved and often consulted on key issues, such as close friends, godparents, babysitters, ministers, church members, and so forth.

Power

Aponte (1976) equates "power" with "force" and defines it as "the relative influence of each family member on the outcome of an activity" (p. 434). This issue is often a very complicated one in African American extended families. As shown in Chapter 3, which describes these complex extended patterns, often another relative or nonblood relative has considerable decision-making power in a family. This person might be a grandmother, grandfather, aunt, uncle, mother, father, minister, boyfriend, or girlfriend. From a therapeutic perspective, this creates a complex situation because these individuals often do not appear early in the treatment process and are frequently not even mentioned by those who do attend sessions. Therapists may proceed to have many family therapy sessions with a mother and her children and may even begin to see initial changes. These changes can often be sabotaged later by a very powerful family member who has never been involved in the process. These powerful family members can also have a great deal of influence over the family's continuation in treatment. Therefore, the therapist must begin to explore early in family sessions who the true decision makers are. The following questions may be important:

1. To whom did you speak before you made that decision?
2. Did anyone disagree with you on that issue?
3. Who has the final word on that issue in your family?
4. To whom do you listen when you need advice?

These issues need to be clarified before the introduction of any interventions. Questions regarding such issues should be asked in terms of extended family and people outside the family who may be involved in the therapy.

THE BOWENIAN MODEL AND THE TREATMENT OF AFRICAN AMERICAN FAMILIES

The work of Murray Bowen (1976, 1978) and subsequent work of Bowenian therapists is very relevant to the treatment of African American and other minority families. However, it must be modified for use with different cultures and its obvious contributions must be explored and clarified. The Bowenian approach has two major strengths that can be particularly useful to therapists working with African American families: (1) it provides strategies for exploring extended family dynamics (particularly in the midphase of family therapy), and (2) it provides a theoretical framework that can be useful in generating hypotheses about family dynamics. There are important reasons why the Bowenian approach is more useful in the midphase of family therapy than during the initial stage. Given the resistance and suspicion with which many African American families approach treatment, the fact that the Bowenian approach is more historically focused may raise anxiety and cause the family to flee before trust can be developed. The structural approach quickly establishes a problem to work on and introduces a specific contract between the therapist and the family to solve that problem together. Once an initial problem has been addressed, the therapist has some credibility with the family. The process of establishing trust has begun. In the midphase of treatment with Black families, once trust has been established, the therapist often learns for the first time the "real" family structure of a Black family. It is during this phase that the therapist finally becomes aware of the presence of a man in the home or of a sibling who has been raised by family members "down South."

Bowen's theory relies on the use of the family tree (later called "genograms" by Guerin and Pendagast, 1994, and McGoldrick and Gerson, 1985) to help the family map its family organization and membership with the therapist. This process should never be conducted in an initial session with an African American family; it should always be delayed until trust is clearly established. Any attempts to gain this information prematurely will often prove futile, may be incomplete, and may cause the family to leave treatment. Guerin and Pendagast (1994), Bowenians by training, describe the wealth of family dynamic information that can be gained from this process. Elsewhere, I have given examples of the use of the genogram in family therapy with African American families (Hines & Boyd-Franklin, 1996). A number of points are highlighted. For example, Black families are often complex in organization and frequently have permeable boundaries. Therefore family members may live together or apart at different points in their lives. Because of the process of "informal adoption" (Hill, 1977, 1999a), extended family members will often raise other parents' children during times of crisis. The family therapist must be careful to include both biological and nonblood relatives, many of whom may be very significant in the family's life, in a genogram. For example, a neighbor, church member, minister, boarder, babysitter, boyfriend, or girlfriend may play a very significant role in the family structure. This is often not apparent until a broader genogram is constructed after careful questions are asked.

The conceptual framework of Bowenian theory also has a great deal to offer family therapists who are working with African American families. The following concepts will be discussed: differentiation, the family projection process, the multigenerational transmission process, family emotional cutoff, and extended family issues. (See Chapter 11 for a genogram example.)

Differentiation

In the complex extended family in which many African American children are raised, it is not unusual for an enmeshment, or blurring of boundaries (Minuchin, 1974), to occur (see Chapter 4). In the extreme, this can be seen as a fusion or lack of self-differentiation (Bowen, 1976; Nichols & Schwartz, 1998). In the more enmeshed African American family, this lack of differentiation of self can be exaggerated. The therapeutic task is to help family members differentiate and still remain connected to the core family and the extended family. This differentiation issue is particularly toxic for many African American young adults who are going beyond their families in terms of education, profession, and social class. The level of differentiation necessary for this mobility is often frightening to many young Black adults and their families, which can result in the development of symptoms in family members.

The therapist's task in these situations is to help open the channels of discussion in a family where differentiation may be viewed as desertion. In such cases an "emotional cutoff" (Bowen, 1976) can occur. Many African American families who come to clinics are in fact cut off from their support systems. In these families, when the therapist initially asks about family or extended family, he or she will be told that there is "no one." When trust is gained, however, and the genogram is constructed (usually during the midphase of therapy), one often discovers a fairly extensive extended family—which may even live close by—that has been cut off. This has often occurred because the family system could not tolerate the differentiation of an individual. Since the extended family has been historically so important for African American families, this is a very significant loss and can lead to the emergence of symptoms in individuals in all of the generations involved. The family therapist who is aware of this process can often help a parent who may be re-creating that emotional cutoff with his or her own child to reconnect with his or her own parents while maintaining his or her own differentiation of self. The Bowenian technique of "coaching" can be very useful in helping an individual to resolve issues with the family of origin.

The Family Projection Process

Bowen (1976) defines the *family projection process* as the process by which parental undifferentiation impairs one or more children. There are many ways in which a child becomes the focus of this projection process. Sometimes this is related to what the parent may feel toward the child prenatally and at the time of birth. In many African American families, the birth of a child is met with factors that can significantly increase parental anxiety (e.g., financial burdens, unwanted pregnancy). All of these may contribute to the way in which the arrival of a child is viewed by a particular African American family. Secrets often form around the facts of a birth, and these secrets can create a charge of anxiety around a certain child that is never resolved. That child can then become the focus of parental and extended family anxiety and can develop symptoms.

Knowledge of this family projection process can be an aid to therapists when exploring questions of parenthood, paternity, skin color differences, and roots, as well as in the exploration of the genogram. It can also help clarify the reasons why a particular child has been singled out in an African American family to become the object of this projection process.

The Multigenerational Family Transmission Process

Bowen (1976) has clarified the ways in which the family projection process is transmitted through many generations. In ethnic groups that have strong connections to extended family networks, it is particularly important to be aware of this process. The concept of family repetitions is very useful in understanding certain phenomena in African American families. The case of Anna illustrates a fairly common example.

Anna was a 14-year-old African American girl who was brought to a community mental health center by her mother. She was referred by the school because her academic performance had deteriorated in the last year and her behavior toward teachers was increasingly oppositional. Her mother reported that she also "talked back" to her a great deal at home. In the course of her treatment process with this family, the therapist discovered that Anna had not manifested these symptoms until shortly after her own 14th birthday. Further exploration revealed that the mother had become pregnant with Anna shortly after her 14th birthday and had been terrified that Anna would repeat her "mistake." She therefore had "cracked down" on Anna at this point and became extremely restrictive, refusing to allow her to leave the house except to go to school. Once this was clear, it could be pointed out to her mother. She was then helped to discuss her own history of rebellion from her mother and her agonizing experience of her pregnancy with Anna. Anna's maternal grandmother was invited to join a session with Anna and her mother in order to discuss this. Anna was able to understand her mother's seemingly disproportionate fears for her, and they were able to renegotiate the rules for Anna. The therapist was then able to help put Anna's mother in charge of enforcing these rules in a more realistic way.

This example demonstrates the ways in which a multigenerational transmission process can operate in an unconscious way in a family. In many Black families these family repetitions are all too common. The involvement of the maternal grandmother paved the way for some resolution of the mother's unresolved issues with her own mother. This example also demonstrates the value of combining the Bowenian and structural approaches. Once the multigenerational issues were clarified, the generational boundaries were restructured, placing the mother in charge.

FAMILY THERAPY WITH ONE PERSON

Ongoing relationships with members of the family, extended family, and significant others are frequently major presenting issues for African Americans. While African Americans often raise their children to be "independent," in many families there is also a concurrent assumption of "interdependence," where the needs of the family are often placed above those of the individual. It is often difficult for mental health practitioners, especially those from more "individualistic" cultures, who have been trained to value separation/individuation and differentiation, to understand "collectivistic" cultures, such as that of African Americans and others (e.g., Hispanic, Asian, Italian, etc.).

One extension of the Bowenian model that is particularly useful in individual treatment with African American clients for whom the conflict between individual and family is a complex and even paradoxical dilemma is "family therapy with one person" (Carter & McGoldrick-Orfanidis, 1994). Based on the work of Murray Bowen (1976, 1978), it incorporates the systems concept that "if one person changes, all others in emotional contact with him will have to make compensatory changes" (p. 193).

The therapist uses the process of coaching to work with an individual on family-of-origin issues. After the therapist joins with, or engages the client in the treatment process, the next step involves the therapist's attempt to understand the historical context underlying the client's current issues or problems. To help the therapist understand the nature of large and often complex extended family relationships, it is often very useful (once trust has been established) to do a genogram (see Chapter 11) with the client. To facilitate this process, the therapist might suggest that the client bring in pictures of extended family members. The genogram can play a major role in helping the client to identify multigenerational family transmission processes (Bowen, 1976) and to clarify the roles that the client had assumed in childhood and adolescence and the way in which they manifest in his or her adult life. For example, many individuals who assumed the role of "parental child" in their family of origin continue to play that role with their own siblings and parents throughout life.

Another very useful technique, recommended by Carter and McGoldrick-

Orfanidis (1994), is the development of a family chronology, or a time line. The activity of depicting critical family events and stresses in chronological order can reveal the "motion of family patterns over time" (p. 205). This technique can bring clarity to families who have experienced multiple stressors over time when the relationship between major events has been obscured due to anxiety.

Once the foundation of the family history is established, the therapist may introduce the client to basic systemic concepts such as triangles, the family projection process, the scapegoat, the parental child, or multigenerational transmission. Clients, who are immersed in guilt, blame, or anger may welcome the opportunity to see their problem from a different perspective. This is a very crucial juncture in treatment. Initially, many clients feel very trapped by their family circumstances. They are so used to doing things in a certain way that they cannot imagine changing, but once they have a more clear understanding of the role that they play in their family, they are in a position to begin to consider how they want that role to change.

Many African American women, for example, enter treatment because they feel overwhelmed by the demands of their own family and extended family members. Some have tried to engage their family members or partners in therapy, but have been unsuccessful. Family therapy with one person (Carter & McGoldrick-Orfanidis, 1994) can be a very effective approach for these clients. The following case example illustrates the use of this approach in treating a young African American woman who assumed overwhelming family responsibilities consistent with the cultural expectations of informal adoption.

JoAnn, a 29-year-old single parent, was referred for therapy by her physician. Her blood pressure had risen dramatically in the last year due to excessive stress.

She was the mother of two young children, ages 2 and 3, and had been divorced from her husband for 2 years. Within the last 6 months, her younger sister, Pat, had died suddenly of breast cancer, leaving three orphaned children. Her sister had never been married and the children's fathers were not involved in their lives. Having been very close to her sister, JoAnn took the children, ages 4, 5, and 9 months, into her own home. They shared a small two-bedroom apartment with JoAnn and her two children.

During the first week after her sister's death, JoAnn's extended family, consisting of her mother, two aunts, their husbands and children, and her brother and his wife, had been supportive and had helped out Then they all returned to their homes in North Carolina. Within 6 months, the tremendous stressors of caring for five children under age 6 were beginning to overwhelm JoAnn.

In the first two sessions, the therapist joined with JoAnn and learned that she came from a large, enmeshed extended family, from which she was emotionally cut off (Bowen, 1976). She and her sister had both been sexually abused by their stepfather, their mother's second husband. After a long period of abuse during which JoAnn had been subject to many threats from her stepfather, she finally told her mother. JoAnn was devastated when her mother sided with her husband instead of with her. When JoAnn was 20 and Pat was 18, they had "run away" together to

New York City. They had both gotten secretarial jobs. JoAnn went to school at night at a local college. One year prior to her sister's death, she had become the first person in her family to graduate from college. Her degree in computer sciences had helped her to get a high-paying job in a major company.

JoAnn had two young children, Ronnie, age 2, and Ressie, age 3, who were in daycare while she worked. Her ex-husband had remarried and did not see their children or contribute to their support. JoAnn now had the expense of five children in daycare.

The first few months of treatment focused on JoAnn's feelings of grief at the loss of her sister. They had been exceptionally close. They had lived nearby and helped each other with childcare. JoAnn found herself crying "all the time," and feeling very alone. She reported that she and her sister had been each other's support and that she had no other support system. The therapist listened empathically and helped to normalize her grief. The sense of being overwhelmed that she felt in caring for all of the children was exacerbated by her feelings of depression. She "was not herself," and did not feel that she could comfort her sister's "babies" when they cried for their mother. In those early sessions, the therapist helped her to express all these complex feelings. Gradually, she began to connect a bit more with the children and to resume some of her normal activities.

Her feelings of loss and abandonment were stirring up many old memories of times when her family had not "been there" for her. In the fourth month of treatment, the therapist introduced the process of doing a genogram. JoAnn was willing, although somewhat skeptical of its usefulness. One of the first patterns that emerged was that her mother had had a very similar experience. Her mother's mother and father had been killed in a car crash when she was 18 and her sisters were 9 and 10. Her mother had essentially raised her own sisters (JoAnn's aunts) alone, with some help from friends in their church and community. Because the circumstances of the deaths were so different, JoAnn had not noticed the similarities. The therapist was able to talk with her about the Bowenian concept of the multigerational family transmission process (Bowen, 1976). The therapist asked JoAnn if her mother might have experienced some of the sense of grief, loss, overwhelm, and obligation that JoAnn herself felt.

The therapist also learned that JoAnn had felt very close to her aunts when she was growing up. They had lived with her mother in her early childhood until each married and moved into her own home in the same community. When the therapist explored her current relationship with them, JoAnn revealed that although they had been cut off from her for many years, they both had called JoAnn often since her sister's death and had been very supportive of her. The therapist asked if she had discussed her circumstances with them. She replied that she had not because they had their own problems and she had always been very independent.

As the therapist began to explore this independence, it became clear that JoAnn had functioned as a parental child (Minuchin, 1974) during her childhood and adolescence and had cared for her sister, Pat, and her brother, Larry, while her mother worked. She had often served as her mother's confidante and support until her mother married her stepfather, Harry, when JoAnn was 15. She felt displaced by the marriage. The sexual abuse began when JoAnn was 16 and continued until she and her sister left home 4 years later. Her mother and Harry separated a year after the girls left and divorced 5 years later. Harry died of a heart attack shortly after the divorce.

JoAnn decided to tell her mother about Harry's abuse at age 19 when she learned from her sister that her stepfather had also abused her. When, after a very emotional exchange, JoAnn's mother "sided with him," JoAnn was devastated and began to emotionally distance herself from her mother. She began working long hours after school to save enough money to leave home. She did not tell anyone else about the abuse and continued to take care of herself and her siblings until she and her sister left their hometown on a bus on JoAnn's 20th birthday.

In order to clarify this complicated history, the therapist also completed a family time line with JoAnn. This was helpful, when coupled with the genogram, because it enabled the therapist and JoAnn to look at the sequence of her history and to understand major family events.

Once the family genogram was complete, the therapist worked with JoAnn on her own feelings about sexual abuse. She reported that such abuse did not occur often because her mother was usually at home. But when her mother visited her relatives in another city, JoAnn's stepfather came into her room at night and threatened to harm her sister if she resisted or told anyone. When the therapist explored her feelings toward her stepfather, she reported feeling rage at the time that had still not abated. She also reported that she was angry that he had died before she could confront him. The next 10 sessions focused on her feelings of anger at and betrayal by her stepfather and her mother. As a part of this process the therapist asked her to write a number of letters to Harry and to her mother, which she would not mail. She poured out her hurt, anger, rage, and feelings of betrayal. The therapist also used the "empty chair" technique and asked JoAnn to imagine that first her mother and then (many sessions later) her stepfather was in the chair. Initially, she felt too unsafe to contemplate her stepfather sitting in the chair. The therapist asked her to imagine a protective, unbreakable, see-through shield surrounding her. She was then able to state her feelings toward him. She found these exercises very cathartic and helpful.

Utilizing the genogram again, the therapist began exploring the family members to whom JoAnn felt closest. She named both her aunts. The therapist encouraged JoAnn to welcome their phone calls and to initiate an e-mail correspondence. E-mail was successful. They wrote about their families and traded photographs. At one point, her Aunt Cora came to visit her and the children. The therapist and JoAnn discussed the possibility of her sharing with her aunt her history of abuse. Cora was not surprised at the revelation because she had recently been informed by her younger sister, May, that Harry had sexually abused her—a secret May had kept for many years. They cried together about their hurt, sorrow, and anger, and the fact that they had all had to suffer alone and be so isolated in their pain. Cora also shared with JoAnn that her mother had been sexually abused as a child by another neighborhood child, whose family was friends with her own. Cora encouraged JoAnn to talk with her mother about her feelings and to write to May, although JoAnn was so overwhelmed by these disclosures that she felt that she could not act on them right away.

In their next therapy session, JoAnn and her therapist processed her feelings of anger and outrage at her stepfather for his abuse of her aunt. They also discussed the multigenerational nature of the sexual abuse in her family. She was able to feel some sympathy for her mother, but this did not allay her anger at her for not responding to her cries for help.

Although she was not yet ready to discuss these issues with her mother, with the therapist's help, she wrote to her Aunt May to tell her about her own experiences and her sadness following Cora's disclosure of May's abuse. May called her upon receiving the letter and they cried together on the phone. After this call, she, Cora, and May began planning for a visit by JoAnn and the children to North Carolina.

As the relationships became closer, the therapist encouraged JoAnn to share with them the intense sadness she felt at the loss of her sister and some of the burden that she felt in raising the children alone. This was still very difficult for her, as she felt that the disclosure threatened her hard-won independence. A month later, an unexpected event intervened: JoAnn was laid off from her job. She was left with nothing but a small severance package from her company and unemployment insurance. Upon learning of her burdens, her mother called and asked JoAnn to move back to North Carolina to live with her. JoAnn felt very conflicted. While a move to North Carolina seemed appealing, given her history, JoAnn felt that she could not consider moving back unless she worked through her intense anger at her mother and her extended family for not helping or protecting she and her sister during the period when they were sexually abused. While she was growing closer to her Aunts Cora and May, who were encouraging her to move back, their relationship was still new.

Although she and Pat had remained in contact with their extended family over the years, JoAnn had not seen any of her family until Pat's funeral and Cora's recent visit. JoAnn and Pat had formed their own "extended" family unit and had raised their children together in New York.

The therapist helped coach JoAnn to speak honestly with her aunts and to tell them of her dilemma. They role-played these discussions in therapy. When she called her aunts to share her concerns, they were both very supportive, and encouraged her to at least visit with the children. Although both offered to help with the children if JoAnn moved back to North Carolina, JoAnn explained that she could not imagine living with her mother. Cora offered to have her stay with her and her family until they could find a more permanent solution.

In her next therapy session, JoAnn expressed very conflicted feelings. Although she had grown close to her aunts, she had had only occasional casual chats with her mother, primarily about the children, since her sister's death. She had not raised the sexual abuse issue that had prompted her and Pat to leave. The therapist asked whether JoAnn felt that she could write a letter to her mother explaining that she was coming home for a visit and that she would be staying with her aunt. She also encouraged her to tell her mother what she and Pat had experienced and her feelings toward her.

JoAnn wrote several versions of this letter over the next few weeks. As is often the case in this type of coaching, the first letters were very angry. JoAnn poured out her feelings of abandonment and betrayal. But in her final version, she was able to clearly tell her mother how she felt and to make clear "I statements." She also thanked her mother for her offer of a place to stay but explained that she was not ready for that at this time.

To her surprise, her mother wrote back immediately and confessed her sorrow at the hurt that she had caused her and her sister. As soon as JoAnn and her sister left, she regretted the loss of her daughters, which she attributed, correctly, to her decision to support her husband. Shortly thereafter she and Harry had a big fight and she "threw him out." She shared that she herself had been abused as a child and had felt particularly guilty because she had been unable to protect JoAnn and her sister. Her weakness had made her afraid to confront Harry with the truth and leave her marriage. She stated that she had never stopped loving JoAnn and her sister, even though they had had very little contact for a number of years. Pat's death had also been very difficult for her—she was filled with regret that she had missed so many years with her daughter.

In her next therapy session, JoAnn discussed her reactions to her mother's letter. She stated that her mother's admission of her own victimization by sexual abuse made JoAnn feel some sympathy for her, but did not end her anger. After this session, she wrote a letter acknowledging her mother's letter and told her that she and the children would be visiting and that they would stay at Cora's house.

The next week, her mother called. JoAnn and her mother had a long emotional phone conversation about their feelings for each other and her mother's regret at not being able to protect her and her sister. Her mother told JoAnn that she was looking forward to her visit and hoped that she and the children would relocate to North Carolina.

Prior to her trip, JoAnn and her therapist had a session exploring the question of her own "space" and where she would feel safest during the trip. She felt comfortable staying in Cora's home with the children, but was not sure how much time she wanted to spend with her mother or her brother, with whom she had had very little contact. The therapist supported JoAnn's idea of structuring short interactions with her mother and brother initially, and encouraged her to talk with Cora and May about her concerns.

JoAnn had a very successful trip. She and the children enjoyed the visit and she acknowledged the help and support not only of her aunts, but of her mother and her brother and his wife as well.

She and Cora and May grew even closer and had many discussions about their experiences and about JoAnn's feelings about returning home. During her time at home, she had a number of visits with her mother in which they talked about some of their feelings. As she and her therapist had discussed, she kept these meeting brief, and left whenever she became overwhelmed. She later described to her therapist very "mixed-up" feelings toward her mother, including sadness, love, hurt, and anger.

At her aunts' urging, she explored employment opportunities during her visit. She was offered an excellent position with a company that had an on-site daycare center for their employees' children. She found an apartment near her aunts' homes and, after leaving her children in their care, she returned to New York to pack and arrange to give up her apartment.

During her last few weeks, she had a number of sessions with her therapist in which she processed her experiences during the visit. Although she felt much closer to her aunts, she was still ambivalent about her mother. The therapist helped to arrange a referral for her in North Carolina, and they discussed the need for her to continue in therapy. The possibility that she and her mother and other family members would have family sessions together in the future was discussed.

This case illustrates many important aspects of "family therapy with one person" and the role of "coaching." As Carter and McGoldrick-Orfanidis (1994) have discussed, it was important for JoAnn to process her own feelings toward her family gradually, over time. She first had to deal with her intense grief at the loss of her sister and her feelings of being overwhelmed by caring for five children. Once she and her therapist constructed the genogram, they were able to explore her emotional cutoff from her family related to sexual abuse by her stepfather. Contact first with her aunts, with whom she had once had a positive relationship, allowed her to gradually reenter her family. Writing letters was used in many instances, as Carter and McGoldrick-Orfanidis (1994) have advised, "to open difficult emotional issues without having to deal immediately with the reactivity of the system" (p. 203). Keeping family contact time-limited also gave JoAnn a sense of control and allowed her to relate to family members individually initially and gradually.

PARADOXICAL/STRATEGIC/SYSTEMIC APPROACHES WITH AFRICAN AMERICAN FAMILIES

Papp (1981) states that "paradox is primarily a clinical tool for dealing with resistance and circumventing a power struggle between the family and the therapist" (p. 244). In this respect, it can be particularly useful with African American families who are often very resistant to the treatment process. Papp (1981) stresses, however, that "paradox is neither always necessary nor always desirable" (p. 245). Careful consideration of when or how this type of strategy should be introduced into the process is very important in the clinical application of these approaches.

There is a need for caution in the use of the paradoxical approaches with African American families. These techniques are particularly problematic in the beginning of the family therapy process because of the suspicion with which many Black families approach therapy. Once the family has been introduced to the treatment process and their trust in the therapist has been established, the paradoxical/strategic/systemic approach can play a very important part in a treatment plan with an African American family. It is easily incorporated into an overall structural approach.

Papp (1981) divides paradoxical approaches into three types: (1) redefining the symptom, (2) prescribing, and (3) restraining. The first of these, the process of redefining the symptom, can be particularly useful in the process of reframing a negative interaction in a positive way. For example, in many African American families living in inner-city environments, there is a constant recognition of the dangers of the street. Parents, particularly single mothers who are raising children alone, are often terrified of the street influences of drugs, crime, and death that threaten their children. A frequent outcome of this process is the tendency of many of these families to restrict children to the house. Many parents will frankly acknowledge that they become more over-protective and restrictive as their children approach adolescence.

Aponte, in a masterful videotape interview with an African American single-parent mother and her three teenage daughters, reframed her overprotectiveness as "loving too much" and was able to help her negotiate with her children a balance between legitimate concern and protection and age-appropriate independence. This type of reframing is extremely useful in Black families, who often feel overwhelmed, beaten down, and unsuccessful in their parenting function. By the process of reframing, one can often tap a well-spring of love and concern.

Selvini-Palazzoli, Boscolo, Cecchin, and Prata (1978) have developed systemic approaches for treating very disturbed families. Their approach includes the use of paradoxical letters that contain a prescription for the family. This approach can prove useful in the treatment of Black families in which key members of the family or the extended family are resistant to coming in for treatment. Often this resistant person or persons may hold the real "power" in the family. In Black families typically men in general and older female family members such as grandmothers in particular are the most difficult to engage. Paradoxical letters can be particularly useful after initial structural change has occurred among the family members present and it is clear that another key person must be involved in order for the change to be a lasting one.

Madanes (1981) has developed techniques of strategic family therapy based on the theories of Milton Erickson described by Haley (1973). These techniques are also very "goal oriented and directed toward alleviation of specific dysfunctional aspects of the family" (Minuchin & Fishman, 1981). According to this approach, the identified patient is viewed as having the symptom to protect the family.

In many single-parent African American families, it is not uncommon for a mother who is raising children alone to become overwhelmed with the pressures and demands of her role. In these situations, because of the absence of a male partner to share the burdens, the oldest child—particularly the male child—can be very vulnerable to a process involving the reversal of generational boundaries. Often this child assumes spousal or parental responsibilities for the parent. The child may become his or her mother's confidant at a very young age. These responsibilities eventually become too much for the child, and he or she develops symptoms. In such a situation the strategic use of a "pretend" paradigm can be very helpful (Madanes, 1981). The following case illustrates this point.

A young African American mother, age 27, brought her 10-year-old son to our clinic. She complained that he had once been very helpful to her and had taken care of her three younger children (ages 6, 4, and 2). In the last year he had begun to have angry outbursts at home, where he would throw things and become enraged over seemingly small requests. His mother felt that she had no control over him. The therapist asked the child to demonstrate an angry outburst. He did so and his mother threw up her hands in a gesture of helplessness. In the next session, he was directed to pretend to have an angry outburst, and the mother was instructed to pretend to calm him down. She was then instructed to pretend to have an angry outburst herself in which she complained about the burdens of her life. Her son was to pretend to calm her down. They were instructed to perform both of these pretend sequences in the evening each day after the younger children were in bed (thereby giving them a special time for themselves). The angry outbursts stopped within 2 weeks.

This approach is particularly useful in Black single-parent families with young children, where protection of an overwhelmed parent is clearly a dynamic.

A variation of this protection theme is a "sacrificial paradigm," which can be used very successfully in African American families with adolescents involved in serious and potentially dangerous acting-out behaviors such as drug use. Once again, the child's symptom is seen as protecting the family from dealing with other problems. In this case, the behavior is so potentially dangerous that the danger is exaggerated and reframed as a "sacrifice" on behalf of his family. The symptom is prescribed and the family is told that this sacrifice will have to continue until they are ready to deal with the real issues in the family. The case of Jimmy illustrates this process.

Jimmy was a 17-year-old Black male who was brought by his family for treatment because of his poor school performance, truancy from school, and extensive marijuana use. The family consisted of his mother, father, three older sisters, a brother, and his maternal grandmother. The older siblings had left home, and Jimmy was beginning his senior year of high school. The parents were a very child-focused older Black couple who had no relationship beyond their parental tasks. Jimmy's mother had a very close relationship with her own mother, who was dying of cancer.

It became very clear that Jimmy's acting out was serving a very major function in this family by protecting his parents from dealing with their concerns about their pending empty nest. After numerous attempts to restructure the family and put the parents in charge, the therapist learned that the parents exercised considerable denial regarding the extent of Jimmy's problems. He would often sneak back into their home when he was truant from school and smoke marijuana in the basement. Both parents consistently ignored these "signs."

Finally, a meeting of the entire family was held in which the therapist told Jimmy and his family that Jimmy was sacrificing himself to protect them from dealing with their concerns about having an empty nest. It was obvious that he loved them so much that he would continue sacrificing himself until he flunked out of school and became hooked on more serious drugs. He would then become so dysfunctional that he would have to stay with them forever. The family was told that Jimmy was to continue to sacrifice himself for them until they were able to demonstrate their love by stopping him.

The parents at first were stunned by this reframing. The prescription was repeated in two subsequent sessions. The parents began to discuss ways in which they could work together to set clear limits for Jimmy. Within 3 weeks, Jimmy had returned to school and the parents had become more adept at confronting his marijuana use. Subsequent sessions were held with the mother and father alone to talk about the issues of loss for them, particularly for the mother as all of her children grew up. She was able to ask her husband's support in helping her through her mother's illness and her need to establish a new role now that her job as "mother" was coming to an end.

NARRATIVE AND POSTMODERN APPROACHES WITH AFRICAN AMERICAN FAMILIES

In the 1980s, leading theories in the field of family therapy were challenged radically by postmodern approaches. Nichols and Schwartz (1998) describe this postmodern period as one of skepticism in which

> accepted practices and knowledge were "deconstructed." That is, they were shown to be social conventions developed by people with their own biased perspectives and motivations. . . . Postmodern psychologies concern themselves with how people make meaning in their lives, how they construct their realities. (p. 318)

In the same time period, Kenneth Gergen, a social psychologist, introduced a postmodern psychology known as "social constructionism" (Gergen, 1985, 1991a, 1991b), which emphasized the power of "social interactions in generating meaning for people" (Nichols & Schwartz, 1998, p. 323). Ironically, this work opened the door for the exploration of the ways in which people from different backgrounds and social experiences might construct their beliefs and values quite differently.

It was in this postmodern atmosphere, following the political activism of the 1960s, that family therapy along with the fields of psychology, social work, and mental health began to explore race, culture, and ethnicity as having a major impact on the beliefs and values of the individual or family and their response to therapy (Boyd-Franklin, 1989; Hardy, 1989; McGoldrick et al., 1996; Nichols & Schwartz, 1998). Hardy (1989) began to challenge the "theoretical myth of sameness" in the entire mental health field.

Within the context of this exciting new era, another postmodern approach, known as "narrative therapy" began to develop. Based on the work of Michael White (1989) and David Epston (Epston & White, 1992; White & Epston, 1990), narrative therapy has particular relevance to the treatment of African American families. Unlike many of the earlier family therapists discussed in this chapter, who were interested in "the family's impact on the problem, narrative therapists are interested in the problem's impact on the family" (Nichols & Schwartz, 1998, p. 402).

White's work was influenced, at least in part, by the writing of the French philosopher Michel Foucault (1965, 1975, 1980, 1984), who looked at the ways in which institutions can oppress and dehumanize people and the ways in which those in power can often dominate and marginalize other social groups (Nichols & Schwartz, 1998). In the 1980s and 1990s, these ideas influenced some politically conscious family therapists to integrate feminism, racism, sexual orientation, multiculturalism, and the impact of social class into their work. As Nichols and Schwartz (1998) have shown, the narrative therapy movement gave family therapists a clear method for incorporating cultural narratives into the therapy process and understanding problems in their cultural context (Freedman, 1996).

White (1989) was concerned about the tendency of some earlier forms of family therapy to be perceived as "family blaming," and challenged the belief of many family therapists that symptoms serve functions in families. He posited that people in families are often oppressed or dominated by their problems. Nichols and Schwartz (1998) summarized the following ways in which narrative therapists work to change this:

> (1) take a collaborative, listening position with strong interest in the client's story; (2) search for times in a client's history when he or she was strong or resourceful, (3) use questions to take a nonimposing, respectful approach to any new story put forth; (4) never label people and instead treat them as human beings with unique personal histories; (5) help people separate from the dominant cultural narratives they have internalized so as to open space for alternative life stories (White, 1995; Freedman & Combs, 1996). (Nichols & Schwartz, 1998, p. 402)

Rather than see the problem as in the individual or even in the family, narrative therapists often "externalize the problem." The client and the family are encouraged to unite to find ways of becoming victorious together over the problem that is dominating and oppressing everyone. This is a very empowering message that can be applied very effectively to the lives of African Americans and other groups who have experienced racism and oppression. Afrocentric family therapists such as Makungu Akinyela (in press) have incorporated narrative therapy principles in their work with African American families.

The next example illustrates the case of an African American family whose son was a victim of racial profiling.

Robert (age 18) and his family were referred for family therapy by a friend of the family. Mr. and Mrs. Brent, his parents, and his older brother, Joe (age 20), accompanied him to the first session. The Brents were a middle-class African American family, living in a predominantly White suburban community. Robert was in his last semester of high school, looking forward to graduation and attending college the following fall.

As he was driving home from his job at a video store one night at about 11 P.M., he was pulled over by a police car with two White officers inside. He was driving his mother's car at the time.

One officer roughly pulled him from the car, yelling "Get out." He was thrown up against the car and searched. When he resisted, he was brutally beaten and then taken to the police station. He was detained for a number of hours before he was allowed to place a call to his parents. When his frantic parents arrived at the station, they were told that he was a suspect in a series of local robberies. They called their lawyer immediately. The perpetrator of the crime was later apprehended and charged by the police. Brent described the incident angrily as a case of racial profiling and police brutality. Joe added that "they saw a young black man in a nice car in a White neighborhood after dark and decided that he was a criminal."

The therapist, an African American woman, had a very strong countertransference reaction of anger at the police. With the help of her supervisor, she was able to separate herself enough from these emotions so that she could appropriately validate the family's anger at the racist acts that had occurred. She also felt deeply concerned for Robert, who had been afraid to leave the house alone since the attack and was suffering from a number of posttraumatic stress disorder (PTSD) reactions, including nightmares, daytime flashbacks of the event, and severe anxiety and depression.

The therapist agreed to meet with the family and to see Robert individually once a week. In his individual sessions, Robert talked about the incident in great detail. In the first discussion, his hands were shaking so much that he could barely control the tremors.

He described his dreams, his flashbacks, and his fears of going outside his home alone. He was mortified that he had been treated in such an aggressive and demeaning way. To the therapist's surprise, he was actually blaming himself for taking a job that required him to drive home so late.

With Robert's permission, the therapist helped him to share these concerns with his family in the next session. Mr. Brent again became angry and said, "This is not your fault—it's racism." The therapist observed Robert's trembling response and said to the father, "You are saying something extremely important, but I think that Robert is reacting to the anger in your tone. Can you help him understand that you are not angry at him but at these racist acts?" The father and mother both looked at the therapist in surprise. The father explained this to Robert and asked if he understood.

The therapist then asked the father to talk with his son about the incident and help him understand how racism was operating. Again, the father was surprised. The therapist asked why he was surprised. He said, "Doesn't he know about racial profiling?" The therapist encouraged the father to ask his son. Again, the father was surprised at Robert's lack of knowledge. The father eloquently explained to his son how police sometimes target Black men by pulling them over, searching their vehicles for no reason other than the color of their skin. Joe spoke and reminded Robert that he had been stopped while driving home from college about 2 years previously. As they spoke, the therapist helped to underscore the message that this incident had not been Robert's fault but had been the result of racism. In the next three sessions, this theme continued, with the therapist using the narrative technique of externalizing the problem of racism (White, 1989).

All of the members of the family had been taking turns driving Robert to school for almost 3 months. With his family's support and his ongoing individual therapy, his PTSD symptoms had begun to lessen. But he was still afraid to drive alone. The therapist worked with the family to gradually have Robert drive with one of them in the car. When he was able to do this a number of times, the therapist asked the entire family to take Robert driving at night. For the first few trips, another family member drove. These trips were discussed carefully in the session. Gradually, Robert began to drive, first, with the whole family in the car, then with one family member at a time. He still refused to drive alone. The therapist focused only on the positive and reframed each positive gain as Robert and his family's personal "victory over racism"—they were not allowing racism or the racist behavior of those police officers to defeat Robert or the family.

The therapist shared with Robert and his family that she felt he was still fearful about another incident occurring and was not sure how he would handle it. She took out a pad of paper and asked Robert to write down any memories he and his family had of times in which he was strong in the face of racism. Joe reminded Robert that he "stood up for" another Black child in school who was being attacked and called racial epithets. His mother added that Robert had always been a strong young man, who was not afraid to do things or take on challenges. As Robert wrote down his family's ideas, his demeanor and body posture began to change. He actually appeared stronger and less anxious.

In the next session, the therapist asked for suggestions that Robert's family might have about how he might handle the situation if another racist incident occurred. His mother spoke first and said, "Whatever you do, don't resist them." His brother said, "Don't stoop to their level; keep your dignity as a Black man." His father said: "Say I'm not armed."

The therapist added, "Don't back-talk them."

The therapist then asked the family what they thought they could do to help him with this. The mother suggested buying him a cell phone so that he could reach someone quickly in an emergency. Robert liked this suggestion and said to both of his parents, "Yeah, you better carry your cell phones too and keep them on." The family agreed to do this as soon as possible. Over the next few weeks, the therapist asked the family to role-play various scenarios with Robert. At first, the therapist provided the scenarios. Gradually, the family members began to suggest new ones. Finally, Robert began to suggest his own. As the weeks went by, Robert began driving a few blocks alone. Within the next few months, he was able to venture further. Once again, each of his gains was framed as his victory over racism and his ability to not allow racism to defeat him. At the time of this writing, their lawsuit against the police is still pending. The officers involved were given a warning but were not suspended or removed from the force.

This case illustrates the deep psychological damage that racist acts of racial profiling and police brutality can cause. This African American therapist was able to deal with her own countertransference in order to help the family members to process their anger and fear. The Brents, like many other African American middle-class families, believed that they did not have to prepare their sons for incidents of racial profiling and police brutality. As Boyd-Franklin et al. (2001) have indicated, they thought that "their zip code would protect their children" from racism. They learned that they must prepare their children for racism, not to make them bitter, but to help prepare them for the realities that they may face. (See Boyd-Franklin et al., 2001, for a more complete discussion of how to prepare young Black adolescents for these situations. Many of these suggestions can be used with African American families and incorporated into family therapy sessions.)

This case also illustrates a successful incorporation of the narrative therapy approach (Epston & White, 1992; Freedman & Combs, 1996; White, 1989, 1995; White & Epston, 1990; see also Chapter 7). Robert's narrative was that he was a victim of racism (in the form of racial profiling and police brutality). He was traumatized by the incident and afraid to resume his usual lifestyle. With his family's help, the therapist was able to "externalize the problem" by labeling it as "racism" and mobilizing Robert and his family to fight against it and not allow it to win.

CONCLUSION: THE INTEGRATION OF THESE DIFFERENT APPROACHES

Many family therapists now incorporate a more integrated approach to family treatment (Mikesell, Lusterman, & McDaniel, 2000). The approaches presented in this chapter can be combined very effectively in an overall process of family therapy with African American families. In my experience, the multisystems model presented in Chapter 11 provides the best overall framework for the treatment of African American families. It is particularly useful in the early "joining" and "problem" stages of treatment (Haley, 1976). The other treatment approaches described in this chapter can be easily incorporated. For example, in the early stages of treatment the structural approach, with its emphasis on engagement and problem-solving techniques, provides the family initially with concrete solutions to pressing problems and establishes the restructuring of the family system. It takes into account the varying constellations of extended family structure in many African American families and provides a structural "road map" for therapists who are treating these families.

Once trust has been established and the therapist has gained credibility through this restructuring, the Bowenian approach can be very useful in the midphase of family therapy. By using genograms, the therapist can further clarify the "real" extended family network. A choice can then be made to include specific extended family members in sessions or to "coach" family members to handle their issues directly with their family of origin. Often lasting structural change cannot occur until these significant sources of "power" in the family can be included. The conceptual framework provided by the Bowenian model can be very useful to the therapist in clarifying the family projection processes and the multigenerational transmission process evident in African American families. Similarly, the family therapy with one person approach can be extremely useful in situations where African American clients present individually, but have many issues with their family members, or where key family members refuse to come in for treatment.

The paradoxical/strategic/systemic approaches should be used with caution in the initial stages of treatment with African American families. Because of the suspicion with which many Black families approach treatment, they are best incorporated into an overall multisystems approach. They can then be utilized when necessary with resistant African American families in which the symptom is a metaphor for a particularly toxic family issue.

Finally, the narrative and other postmodern approaches emphasize the importance of obtaining the family's own story or narrative of their experiences. This is an important perspective in treatment in that it helps therapists to avoid stereotyping and to recognize each family's view of its own history. Externalizing the problem, particularly when racism is clearly a factor, can track the cultural and racial narrative of many African American families and can be a very powerful intervention. As demonstrated in the case example above, it aligns the family members together against racism.

Many of the approaches described above were designed to work with nuclear and, in some cases, parts of the extended family. There is another level of family involvement that must be explored if effective work is to be done, particularly with poor African American families: the involvement of outside systems or agencies that have an impact on the life of the family. All of these levels of involvement are considered in relation to each family and to the structure of therapy in the chapter that follows.

11

The Multisystems Model

In my experience as a teacher of family therapy, a thoughtful self-examination and use of self by the therapist (discussed in Chapter 9), combined with the multisystems model, defined by Boyd-Franklin and Bry (2000) as "a problem-solving approach that helps families with multiple problems to focus and prioritize their issues and that allows clinicians to maximize the effectiveness of their interventions" (p. 4), can help facilitate the crucial processes of joining with and engaging African American families. It can allow therapists to build credibility more quickly by providing a model that is immediately useful in resolving the problems presented by the family. Henggeler and Borduin (1990) and Henggeler, Schoenwald, Borduin, Rowland, and Cunningham (1998) have empirically demonstrated the effectiveness of multisystemic approaches, particularly with at-risk populations such as conduct-disordered youth.

Many therapists were originally trained with very rigid boundaries in terms of therapeutic function. Work with extended families, churches, outside agencies, and so on, was seen as the job of the social worker in an agency. Unfortunately, clinicians from other mental health disciplines were not trained to see these interventions as a part of their job description. So traditional dichotomies and professional boundaries in the mental health field often inhibit clinicians from providing effective treatment for African American families. It is very difficult to divide functions between service providers without further complicating the "system" confusion that many families endure. It also deprives clinicians of one of the most important ways in which they can establish rapport and build credibility with many African American families—joining first around "real-life" problems, such as housing, food, clothing, financial help, and medical care—that a therapist's interventions may empower the family to obtain. This is particularly true in the treatment of poor Black families (see Chapter 13).

As the previous chapter has indicated, effective therapy with African American families requires the therapist to be flexible enough to draw theories from different family systems approaches and incorporate them into the treatment plan. It also requires the therapist to be willing and able to intervene at a variety of system levels, such as individual, family, extended family, church, community, and social services. This complexity often overwhelms clinicians because most have never been given a model within which they can organize their levels of intervention. This chapter offers that theoretical framework as well as an alternative to a long-accepted dichotomy between modalities of treatment (e.g., between individual and family therapy) and may be particularly useful to therapists beginning to develop their own model of treatment.

The multisystems approach presented herein was developed from my own clinical experience. It is not intended to provide rigid constraints for the therapist or to be the "absolute" model of treatment for African American families. It is offered as a flexible set of guidelines that can be adapted to the needs and problems of different families and that can be adjusted to the therapist's own personality and style. It should also be noted that this model has broad-based applicability in the family therapy and mental health fields and has relevance to the treatment of all ethnic groups.

In order to treat African American families effectively in therapy, a therapist must be able both to conceptualize and to intervene at multiple levels and in multiple systems. These systems might include the individual, a subsystem (Minuchin, 1974) of a few family members, a nuclear family unit, an extended family, significant others and nonblood family members, church and community resources, and, particularly in the case of poor African American families, the social service system (Boyd-Franklin & Bry, 2000). The approach discussed here is built upon the structural family systems model (Minuchin, 1974), the ecostructural approach (Aponte, 1976, 1994), ecological approaches (Bronfenbrenner, 1977; Falicov, 1988; Hartman & Laird, 1983; Holman, 1985), and multisystemic models (Boyd-Franklin, 1989; Boyd-Franklin & Bry, 2000; Henggeler & Borduin, 1990; Henggeler et al., 1998).

This chapter addresses three main aspects of the multisystems model: (1) Axis I: The Treatment Process, (2) Axis II: The Multisystem Levels, and (3) Home-Based Family Therapy with African American Families. Unlike most treatment approaches, which are based on linear models, the multisystems approach is composed of two main axes based on the concept of circularity. The first axis includes the basic components of the therapeutic process: joining, engaging, assessing, problem solving, and interventions designed to restructure and change family systems. Each of these components does not occur only once, as it might in a linear model; they can and do recur repeatedly throughout the treatment process at all systems levels. In order to work effectively with African American families, the therapist must be flexible and willing to intervene at different levels. The second axis explores the multisystems levels including the individual, family subsystems, the family household, the extended family, nonblood kin, friends, church and community resources, social service agencies, and other outside systems. The third aspect, home-based family therapy, allows the clinician the opportunity to reach out to important family members who may not come in for treatment.

AXIS I: THE TREATMENT PROCESS

Haley (1976) delineated five stages to the first interview in a problem-solving structural approach: social stage, problem stage, interaction stage, contracting stage, and closing stage. Within the multisystems approach, this framework is useful as a model for one session, a series of interviews, and an overall treatment plan at each system level. With this in mind, the flow of treatment should be as follows (see Figure 11.1):

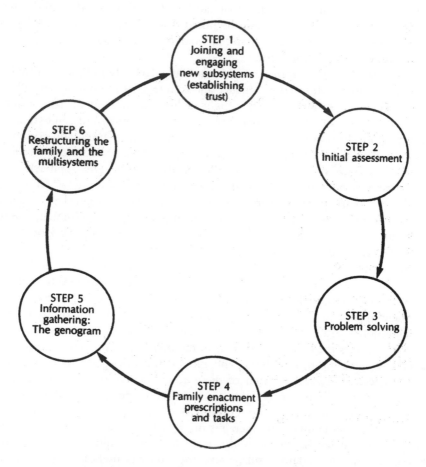

FIGURE 11.1. Axis I: The therapeutic process.

Step 1. Joining and engaging new subsystems
Step 2. Initial assessment
Step 3. Problem solving (establishing credibility)
Step 4. Use of family enactment, prescriptions, and tasks
Step 5. Information gathering: The genogram
Step 6. Restructuring the family and the multisystems

Joining and Engaging African American Families

Joining has many different aspects. It is important to convey to each family member who attends a family session that his or her input is valued and important. Conveying respect is important—African American families are very sensitive to a sense of being condescended to. For example, many therapists address family members by their first names (as described in Chapter 8). This is a mistake, particularly with older family members. It is best to refer to people as "Ms.," "Mrs.," or "Mr." until the family member indicates otherwise or the therapist asks for and receives permission to use first names. It is also helpful to ask family members what they would like to be called.

According to Hunt (1987), because of the reluctance with which many African American families come to treatment, "the most difficult aspect of therapy with African American clients is establishing the relationship" (p. 118). Joining frequently involves outreach in working with African American families. Key family or extended family members may be unwilling or unable to come in for treatment sessions. Therefore, it is often important for the therapist to reach out by means of letters, phone calls, and even home visits in order to engage such crucial family members. It is important for the therapist to contact family members directly rather than conveying messages through other family members.

The engagement of men in all cultures has long been an issue in the family therapy field. This is even more exaggerated in relationships with African American men because of the issues discussed in Chapter 5. It is critically important to reach out directly to them. For example, the therapist might tell a mother that it is agency practice to contact all of the key family members and ask her advice as to the best time to call a father (or father figure). She should be given some degree of choice but should not be asked for "permission" to call him. It is important to underscore here that a man may have a number of relationships to the child and to the child's mother. He may be the child's natural father, who may or may not live in the home. He may be the mother's live-in boyfriend or the child's stepfather, and he may be the mother's brother or an "uncle" or family friend who exerts a great deal of influence over this child. In joining with this person, it is important for the therapist to convey the message that his help is needed and that he has a special relationship with this child. Often that statement or reframing will open the door to his involvement.

Many poor African American families have no phone in the home. In other cases, the therapist leaves phone messages, but his or her calls are not re-turned. In these circumstances a letter may "break the ice" between the thera-pist and this key family member. The following is an example of such a letter:

Dear Mr. _____

Your son Johnny has told me a great deal about you. I am his therapist and I have been working with your family at our clinic now for 3 months. We have been trying to deal with his school problem. I've reached a point where I need your help if we are to go further.

You are one of the most important people in your son's life and there are things he will listen to from you that he won't hear from anyone else.

Please give me a call as soon as possible at [phone number] so that we can figure out some ways to help him together. I know you are working most days, but I'd be happy to call you in the evening or to stay later at the clinic to see you.

Many African American fathers will return a call if it is framed in this way. The therapist may also adopt a strategy in which she or he corresponds with a resistant father to keep him informed of his son's progress and to ask his help when necessary.

As stated above, there are often key extended family members who may object to and sabotage certain aspects of the treatment. Contact with these members is essential, as can be seen in the following case example.

James was a 14-year-old African American adolescent who was being treated in a day hospital program. His family consisted of his mother, his stepfather, and his two younger siblings. He had come to us following hospitalization. He had been hallu-cinating, had paranoid ideation, and had threatened to harm his mother during a fight with her. His father, although he had never lived with him, saw him regularly and was a very important figure in his life.

Family sessions had revealed that there was a great deal of friction between James's mother and his natural father, who was very critical of the way in which she was raising James. An issue arose in our treatment program when James refused to take his medication and began hallucinating again and had a major aggressive outburst with a staff member. In a subsequent session, James's mother reported that James's father was a recovering drug addict and opposed to any form of drug use. The therapist therefore contacted James's natural father and asked him to come in alone to see her. When the father arrived, he appeared very angry and stated that he didn't want his son to be on drugs. He reported that he was now a counselor in a drug program and did not believe in them.

Resisting the urge to try to convince him otherwise, the therapist joined with him by asking in what ways he was concerned about James. His father accurately described his observations of James during the period prior to his hospitalization. He was obviously very worried about his son. As he relaxed, he began to share some of his own history of drug abuse. He had begun experimenting with drugs at about James's age and felt very guilty because he had been an addict for many years and had only recently reentered his son's life.

It became clear that his anti-drug stance was partly a strong belief system but also his way of having some influence in his son's life.

The therapist joined him in his concern for his son and shared her own fears for his safety "on the streets" if he became inappropriately aggressive. The father hung his head and asked her if she had children. She replied that she did. He asked, "What would you do if you were in my shoes?" She replied, "I would agonize just like you are but I'd be afraid to leave him with no help. I'd give him the medication but I'd hound the doctors, and get involved so I could monitor what was going on." After much thought the father decided to agree to a trial of medication and also agreed to "talk to his son" with the therapist and come in regularly for sessions with his son.

The above example clarifies the importance of joining or connecting with African American men in face-to-face contact. Joining must be accomplished before the therapeutic agenda is pursued. This issue of joining with men or fathers has been carefully discussed by Haley (1976). In his discussion of the initial interview he clarifies some strategies that are useful in this process. He points out that even when the mother is designated as the spokesperson for the family, it is very important to also seek out the father's opinion.

This example is particularly important when one considers that men, especially African American men, often do not appear for the first session of therapy. It therefore may be important for the therapist, who may have already seen the rest of the family, to "balance the scales" by meeting with the father alone initially or by giving him "his say" in his initial family sessions.

This is also true of other extended family members who may be asked to enter the treatment process at different points. It is crucial that the therapist take the time to join with each of these members before moving on to the agenda or "problem stage" (Haley, 1976) of the session.

An important aspect of joining is the willingness to include those who come in. I have repeatedly seen therapists walk into a clinic waiting room and invite in the "family" for a session and leave the friend or neighbor they brought along sitting outside. With all families, but particularly with African Americans, it is necessary to find out who these people are and to assess their contribution to the presenting problems.

One aspect of joining and engaging, outreach—leaving our "ivory tower" to meet with a family in their home or community—goes counter to the training of some mental health professionals. Home visits, however, may be the only way to connect or join with significant family members unwilling to enter treatment.

Initial Assessment

The initial assessment phase in a multisystems approach is an observational one wherein the therapist observes the family and begins forming initial hypotheses about the family structure and the areas that will need to be restructured or changed. This process might be aided by considering the following questions:

1. How do family members seat themselves?
2. Who is the family's spokesperson?
3. Do family members allow each other to speak or are they constantly interrupting?
4. Is this the whole family or are key family members missing from the session?
5. What are the boundaries in this family? Are they clear?
6. Who has the power in this family? Is that person present in the room?

These are not questions that will be asked directly of families, but they will help therapists to form their own hypotheses about the family structure and the areas that will need to be restructured or changed.

For therapists working with African American families, a number of other important questions should be considered:

1. How is the family responding to the therapist? Is the joining complete? Are key family members beginning to trust the therapist?
2. Should the issue of race (or class) be raised at this point?
3. Who referred the family? (This is important since many African American families are not self-referred.) Has the therapist made a clear distinction between her- or himself and the referral agency?
4. How does the family feel about being "in therapy"? How do other key family members (not represented at the meeting) feel? This is important because, as I have stressed, many African American people feel that therapy is only for "crazy people."
5. Why does the family believe they are coming to therapy and what do they want from the process (as distinct from the goals of the referral sources or the therapist)?

Assessment is a process of hypothesis generation and then the gradual testing of those hypotheses in subsequent sessions. The testing of these hypotheses is begun immediately in the initial session. The other clear advantage of this multisystems model is that intervention begins early and is combined with problem solving and assessment. Assessment is cyclical and ongoing.

Problem Solving

Problem solving, from a systems perspective, does not occur one time but instead is a cyclical process throughout treatment. The value of the problem-solving focus of the structural family therapy approach (Haley, 1976; Minuchin, 1974) to the treatment of African American families was discussed earlier, in Chapter 11. It serves many functions with African American families. First, it is educative in that it quickly initiates families who are new to the treatment process. Second, many of our families are "multiproblem families" who feel overwhelmed by a vast number of problems and often flit from problem to problem and never focus on any one issue long enough to reach resolution. Still others feel so powerless to effect change that they become immobilized. Clear attention early on to identifying and rating the priorities of the problems that the family feels are most pressing will help to mobilize or empower the family by identifying specific problems that can be solved.

The third positive aspect of the problem-solving process at the early stage of treatment is that the therapist begins to gain credibility and to benefit from a sense of trust with the family as problems are addressed and solved. Depending on the family, this initial process may take one session or many; trust too is an evolutionary concept with many African American families.

Families with Multiple Problems

African American families referred for treatment often present with many problems. These problems can overwhelm even the most experienced therapists (Boyd-Franklin & Bry, 2000; Berg, 1994; Henggeler & Borduin, 1990; Henggeler et al., 1998; Kagan & Schlossberg, 1989). Berg (1994) has given the following suggestions for therapists who are working with these families:

1. Do Not Panic! . . . be calm.
2. Ask the client what is the most urgent problem that he wants to solve first. Follow his direction, not yours. Be sure the goal is small, realistically achievable and simple.
3. Ask yourself who is most bothered by the problem. Make sure it is not you; you do not want to be the "customer" for your own services.
4. Get a good picture of how the client's life would change when that one goal is achieved. . . .
5. Stay focused on solving that one problem first. Do not let the fact that the client is overwhelmed affect you. . . .
6. Find out in detail how the client made things better in the past. . . .
7. Be sure to compliment the client on even the smallest progress and achievements. Always give the client the credit for successes.
8. When one problem is solved, review with the client how he solved it. What did he do that worked? (p. 199)

Use of Family Enactment, Prescriptions, and Tasks

Minuchin (1974) and Haley (1976) have stressed the importance of encouraging families to interact with each other or to enact their family drama in our offices. This is particularly useful with African American families because it quickly involves family members in the therapeutic process. If individuals feel peripheral to the therapeutic process, they often will not return.

Some African American families enter treatment thinking of therapy as a "quick fix." These families often don't see the connections between talking about their problems and actually solving those problems. The use of family prescriptions and tasks can be effective in such situations because they continue the therapeutic impact beyond the session. When a family therapist assigns tasks or prescriptions, the family therapy process is moved out of the office and into the home. This causes other family members who may never come into the office to become curious about and often indirectly engaged in the process of therapy.

For example, in a family where a powerful grandmother has refused to come in, asking a mother to discuss the issues from the session with her mother in private without the children present and to come back and share the grandmother's ideas establishes dialogues between the mother and the grandmother and between the therapist and this absent family member. The therapist might then follow up with a letter or a phone call.

Tasks and prescriptions are important whether or not they are carried out as requested. For example, if the grandmother refuses to share information with the mother, the therapist needs to determine if this resistance represents a long-standing lack of communication between the mother and grandmother on important issues.

A major task of this stage is the process of enactment whereby therapists should encourage family members to "act out" what they do at home. They might "stage an argument" or enact a typical family pattern. The therapist can then ask other family members how close this enactment was to the actual interactions at home. This kind of role play can provide very valuable information for the therapist as well as for the family.

Enactment is very central for many African American families. Often, by the time a family comes in for treatment, the lines of communication have completely broken down. A family from an ethnic group with a strong belief in therapy may be more likely to understand that therapy can help to reopen communication channels. Because many African American families are new to the concept of therapy, enactment or role play that forces two or more family members to communicate with each other in the session gives a very powerful message to the family that the facilitating of communication is a central purpose of family systems therapy.

Enactment and the assignment of tasks in and out of sessions also comprise a very important component of the empowerment of African American families in the treatment process for those who feel powerless to change the "system." As they accomplish assigned tasks, they begin to feel that they have the power and ability to rein in their children and achieve a functional family. If the therapist does not actively involve family members—particularly parental figures or adult extended family members—in the process of change, then the therapist will place him- or herself in the parental or executive role in the family. Throughout this book I have stressed the difference between "helping" and "empowering" African American families to change. When a process is initiated whereby the family does the work in the session and members speak directly to each other rather than through the therapist, the likelihood of generalization outside of the actual sessions is far greater.

Information Gathering: The Genogram

Contrary to the training of many mental health professionals, who are taught to gain a great deal of background information early in the process, clinicians working with African American families often find that they have to postpone information gathering until after trust has been established. This often means that extensive joining, initial attention to assessment, and problem solving occur before the collection of extensive historical data, such as the construction of a genogram, can take place. This is consistent with the structural approach, which stresses the importance of joining and a problem-solving focus in the first session.

The genogram is essentially a family tree. It is a tool, borrowed from the field of anthropology, that can be very useful to clinicians. A number of family therapists trained by Murray Bowen have used the genogram to illustrate his system concepts (Guerin & Pendagast, 1994; McGoldrick & Gerson, 1985). Hines and Boyd-Franklin (1996) found this work to be particularly valuable when working with African American families because genograms provide a way to organize complex extended families. A word of caution is important here. Because of the resistance and suspicion that many African American families bring to the treatment process, the therapist must develop an alliance of trust with the family before this process can be completed in a meaningful way. I have often seen therapists attempt to apply this instrument prematurely with African American families, with the consequence that the family feels as though the therapist is "prying into their business." The information given under such circumstances is often merely the bare outline of a complex family tree. Crucial individuals and key information are often left out until the family feels trust.

As this chapter emphasizes, an important step in building this trust is joining with the family around the problems that they feel are most pressing. If this is done in the first session, the therapist can begin exploring the household composition and extended family supports soon thereafter. I emphasize this here because this is the reverse of what constitutes the intake procedure in many clinics, that is, collecting extensive histories in the first interview.

Once trust has been established, the information for the genogram can be collected in a variety of ways. With some families, it may be helpful to sit with the whole family and draw out the family tree. With others, it is useful for the therapist to simply record the information as it emerges and then to construct the genogram at another time. Often as trust grows, other family relationships are clarified. Indeed, therapists often discover that their concept of family organization expands over time.

Figure 11.2 illustrates the family tree of the Bell family. Mary, age 14, had been referred to a clinic for acting out in school and truancy. Her mother, Sandra Bell, is a 31-year-old woman who had her first child, Annie, when she was 15 years old. That child has been raised since birth by her great-aunt, Aunt Mattie, in Georgia. Annie is now 16 and only visits the household for a couple of weeks each summer. Sandra Bell has three daughters who live with her: Mary, Martha, age 6, and Barbara (called "Boo"), age 3. In addition, Ms. Bell's younger sister, a drug abuser, died last year of AIDS. Her two children are now part of the household. Ms. Bell's mother, Pearl Bell (age 49), lives in an apartment upstairs in the same building. She functions as if she were part of the household and frequently babysits and cooks for the family. The therapist did not learn until some time later that Ms. Bell's boyfriend, Sandford Jones (age 38), also lives with the family and that his daughter, Kenya (age 15), visits occasionally on the weekend. Ms. Bell and Mr. Jones have one child together, Aisha (age 1), who is also part of their household.

It is important for the therapist to explore the questions listed earlier in order to obtain this information. The first and often most important question that must be asked is "Who lives with you or who lives in your household?" This question is, in fact, much more appropriate than the typical intake form questions that ask for mother's name, father's name, and number of siblings. It is important to ask if there are any other children who are not living in the home. In this case, the mother had her first child when she was 15 and was unable to care for her. Therefore, her childless aunt raised the daughter. As can be seen from the arrows on the genogram (Figure 11.2), the informal adoption process often creates a very complicated family tree.

Another important question to ask is "Who helps you out?" In this family, the question revealed the presence and role of the grandmother; probing further and asking the mother if she had a special man in her life revealed the presence and role of Sandford Jones. It is not unusual for the degree of a central male's involvement to be minimized initially. Questioning also brought up the mother's church family, including her minister and his wife, and Mary Word, Ms. Bell's best friend and godmother to two of her children.

Asking about Mary's natural father revealed that he lives in another state and has not had contact with Mary in 5 years. Another important question to ask is whether there is any contact with the father's family. In African American families, although individuals or couples may divorce or "split up," one does not divorce grandparents. In many families, the father's parents or members of his extended family may provide an important connection for the children and a tie to a father whom they may not have seen in a long time. This connection is worth exploring, even with families where a cutoff has occurred between the mother and her children and the father's extended family. Children are very important in African American families, and "time heals all wounds." A very isolated and overwhelmed mother with little extended family support of her own might be encouraged to reach out now to the extended

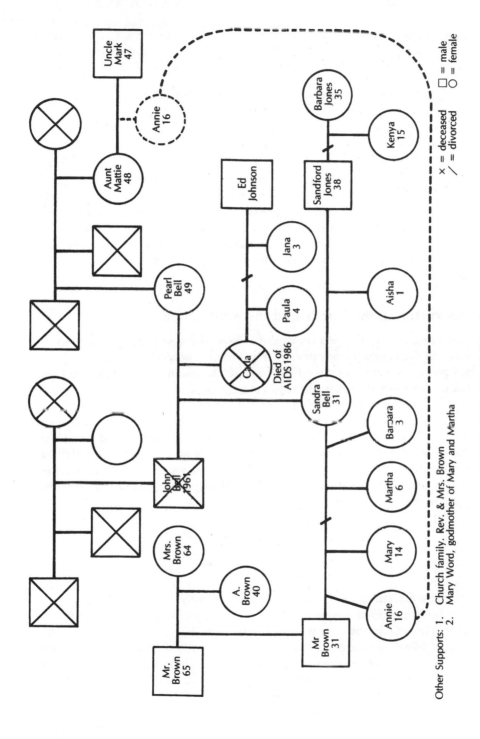

FIGURE 11.2. The Bell family genogram.

Other Supports: 1. Church family. Rev. & Mrs. Brown
2. Mary Word, godmother of Mary and Martha

x = deceased   □ = male
/ = divorced   ○ = female

237

family of the children's father or fathers. This is an important consideration when placement decisions must be made. The father's extended family, although they may still be angry at the mother, may rally to take a child who is about to be placed in a foster home.

Once a complete picture of the family is obtained, the therapist can explore the involvement of the extended family members, friends, and nonblood kin in the family's life. Questions such as "Who disciplines the children?" or "Whom do you ask for advice when Mary has a problem?" are very helpful. If the therapist stays problem-focused he or she can seek the family's advice about who should be involved in a family session regarding a particular problem. "Tribal" or "network" sessions (Kliman & Trimble, 1983), where the entire extended family is asked to be present, are most useful when there is a major family crisis or an emergency problem to be solved. In the following example of the Bell family, the therapist discovered that the mother, her boyfriend, and the grandmother were often in disagreement about how to discipline the children.

Restructuring the Family and the Multisystems

The remainder of this section describes how this disagreement was restructured in the family therapy process. The problem-solving focus and the gradual process of structural assessment become the roadmap in restructuring the family system as well as its interactions with outside agencies.

The therapist began with a subsystem of the family (often a mother and her child or children). In interviewing this family, she discovered that Mary is very oppositional, particularly at home toward her mother and at school toward her teacher. The therapist's assessment of the family was that Ms. Bell has not functioned in an executive, parental role vis-à-vis this child and therefore feels overwhelmed. The following structural diagram represents the first hypothesis about the family structure.

$$\frac{?}{\begin{array}{cc} \text{M} & \text{0000} \\ \text{(mother)} & \text{(children)} \end{array}}$$

This diagrammatic representation shows that the mother and children appear to be functioning as siblings, with no one effectively assuming the parental functioning. In the early sessions, the therapist began to focus on the problem of Mary's acting-out behavior and began restructuring the interaction within this part of the family. She worked gradually to empower Ms. Bell to feel more in charge in her interaction with her children. The family structure of this subsystem would then become:

$$\frac{\text{M}}{\text{0000}}$$

As the therapist began to develop a relationship of trust and credibility with Ms. Bell, she learned that there are a number of important individuals involved in the care of these children, many of whom contribute to the feeling of powerlessness that this mother experiences in raising her children. This information was used to make a more complete genogram.

The genogram segment that clarifies household composition revealed a boyfriend and a maternal grandmother. Both the boyfriend and the grandmother were in fact interfering with rather than supporting Ms. Bell's efforts.

$$\text{GM (grandmother)}$$
$$\text{M} \qquad\qquad\qquad\qquad\qquad\qquad\qquad \text{BF (boyfriend)}$$
$$\text{O} \qquad \text{O} \qquad \text{O} \qquad \text{O}$$
$$\text{identified}$$
$$\text{patient}$$

Upon further exploration, the therapist discovered that the grandmother works while the mother is home (she is receiving welfare payments), and that the grandmother often feels that she therefore has a right to tell her daughter and her grandchildren how to behave. The mother's boyfriend, as the father of the younger child, has been a part of the family system for 4 years. He wants to parent his child but has a very difficult time relating to Mary, the identified patient, because he feels that this girl resents him for assuming the father role.

The therapist then reached out and called the grandmother and the mother's boyfriend to ask them to attend a family session. The conflict between the three adults is very clear:

$$\text{BF} \not\!/\!\!/ \text{ M } \not\!/\!\!/ \text{ GM}$$

In addition, structurally, it appears that in the home the boyfriend and the grandmother assume the parenting or executive role, even though they are frequently in conflict, and the mother is constantly relegated to a child-like role:

$$\frac{\text{BF} \ne \text{GM}}{\text{M: 0000}}$$

The therapist asked that the children be left with a babysitter for the next family session in order to meet with the mother, her boyfriend, and the grandmother alone. She pointed out to all three that their level of disagreement was contributing to Mary's acting out. She told them that they are all important parental figures to her and that they must work together to decide how they will parent her. The therapist asked the mother and grandmother to talk first:

$$\text{M} \leftrightarrow \text{GM}$$

They discussed the fact that the grandmother is angry at her daughter for not doing well with her life and feels that Mary is just like her. The therapist acknowledged this problem and asked the mother and grandmother if they could stay focused on the problem of Mary's acting out and how they will handle it. They came to some agreement that the grandmother will no longer deride the mother in front of her children, but will support the mother's rules for Mary.

The mother and her boyfriend were then asked to discuss their differences around the parenting of Mary. The mother's boyfriend pointed out that the mother has never really allowed him to parent Mary. From his viewpoint, she is "too easy on the girl." He then feels obligated to be tougher on her. They discussed the need for mother to take the lead in being firm with her daughter as her biological parent.

After these individuals agreed on a strategy of setting limits for Mary and the other children, they could be brought together with the children once again to clarify their decisions.

$$BF = = = M = = = GM$$
$$\overline{}$$
$$0 \quad 0 \quad 0 \quad 0$$
$$\text{(children)}$$

Eventually the mother, with the support of the grandmother and boyfriend, spoke directly to Mary and to her other children about the rules that had been agreed upon to curb their acting out. Thus, the mother is supported and empowered in her parental role by the two other significant adults in the home.

We have looked at the dimensions of the therapeutic process as it impacts the family. Now it is important to explore the multisystems levels of Axis II.

AXIS II: MULTISYSTEMS LEVELS

One of the complicating factors in the treatment of many African American families is that data collection is often an evolving process because of their resistance to approaches that collect massive amounts of historical and family data in the first session. Working within the multisystems approach, I have found it much more useful to join with a family, focus on the initial problem in the first session, and save extensive data collection until trust has been established. For many therapists, between session 2 and session 5, it becomes necessary to begin collecting this data. This data may take many forms and encompass many system levels. The multisystems approach provides the therapist with a way of organizing this data so that he or she does not become overwhelmed by it and can use it effectively to produce change.

The multisystems model is a theoretical concept utilized by the therapist to organize complex data and to plan and prioritize intervention. *It does not require that the therapist intervene at all levels.*

Level I: Working with Individuals
in the Multisystems Model

The concept of treating an individual using a multisystems model is not a new one in the family therapy field. My students often ask me if I do individual or family therapy. According to the multisystems model, such a distinction is artificial, unnecessary, and may be counterproductive to effective treatment with many different ethnic groups. The elegance of the multisystems model is that it provides an overall framework that allows a therapist to provide treatment successfully at whatever level or levels (individual, family, extended family, or other systems) that is relevant to the situation at hand. The multisystems model expands the therapeutic frame of reference, and thus the therapist's ability to provide effective service to African American families. Within the multisystems model, the second axis (Axis II) is comprised of the following multisystems levels (see Figure 11.3). (This model is consistent with the work of Bronfenbrenner [1977], Falicov [1988], and Aponte [1994].)

Level I. Individual
Level II. Subsystems
Level III. Family household
Level IV. Extended family
Level V. Nonblood kin and friends
Level VI. Church and community resources
Level VII. Social service agencies and other outside systems

Since therapy is so new to African American families, often only one individual in a family will be sent for therapy. Seeing that individual first can often expedite the process of building credibility with an African American family. Carter and McGoldrick-Orfanidis (1994) discuss the concept of family therapy with one person and Bowen (1976) discusses the concept of "coaching" an individual to produce changes in family relationships without seeing the family (see Chapter 10). Kliman and Trimble (1983) highlight this process:

> Families frequently are reluctant to bring significant network members into direct contact with their therapists and the participation of nonrelatives in psychotherapy may conflict with agency policy. Even when such obstacles are present, the therapist may conclude that coaching the family is the most efficient means of achieving the desired change. (p. 283)

It is important to note that this approach may be very useful with individual clients as well as with families. Once a therapist adopts a family systems orientation, it will permeate all levels of intervention. Even more importantly, it will influence the theoretical construct of change. Family therapists provided with this wealth of cultural information often despair when they cannot engage the significant family members. Coaching provides a model whereby the therapist

Multisystems

Level I	Individual
Level II	Subsystems
Level III	Family household
Level IV	Extended family
Level V	Nonblood kin and friends
Level VI	Church and community resources
Level VII	Social service agencies and other outside systems

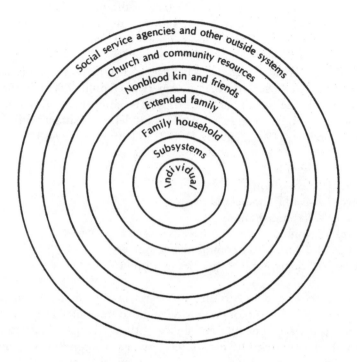

FIGURE 11.3. Axis II: The multisystems levels.

can help the family members present in therapy to begin to rethink and ultimately to restructure their contact, interaction, and involvement with their extended family (see Chapter 10).

Kliman and Trimble (1983) have presented a concise outline of the coaching process:

> The first step in coaching is to introduce the family to the social network concept, through helping family members develop detailed descriptions of their personal networks and teaching some basic principles about the relationships between networks and mental health. The combined family network (i.e., the combined networks of all the family members) is then examined critically concerning both its contributions to the family's difficulties and its strengths and the access it provides to helping resources. Finally, family and therapist develop strate-

gies for changing network patterns, and/or making better use of the network to meet family needs. (p. 283)

The following case example describes an intervention involving the coaching of an individual family member whose family, although living in another state, was interacting in a very dysfunctional pattern.

Joan Miller was a 35-year-old African American woman who entered therapy following a major extended family crisis. Her mother, father, brother (age 19), and two sisters (ages 24 and 30) lived in South Carolina. Joan was living in New York City. Her brother had been abusing drugs for some time. He overdosed and would have died if not for Joan's middle sister's quick intervention by taking him to an emergency room. Joan had been her family's "therapist" for many years and had received a number of calls from frantic family members asking her to come home and "take charge." As was typical of her family's pattern, her parents had each "gone helpless" and abdicated their parental role.

   Joan's first reaction to her brother's crisis was to feel that she should pack her bags and fly to South Carolina immediately. She and her therapist worked together to create a careful family genogram and a network drawing and to discuss family interactional patterns. She was helped to see that she had taken on "parental child" responsibilities in her family as a young child and that her sister had "filled her shoes" since her move to New York City. She explored the issue of her parents' role and their abdication of their responsibility. She decided that instead of rushing home she would call her parents and tell them how upset and angry she was at being called upon to be a parent to her brother. She told them quite directly that he could have died and that it was their choice about whether they got help for him at this time. She suggested that they call her mother's sister, a social worker in South Carolina, in order to find help for him and place him in a drug program. Her parents, frightened by her brother's near-death and by Joan's pulling back, mobilized and insisted that her brother enter a drug treatment program. Joan was at first greatly relieved but then gradually began to feel that she was not doing enough. At times she even became jealous of other family members—such as her aunt—who were now more involved in the latest family crisis.

   The investment in and pull of old patterns is often very strong. A great deal of Joan's work from then centered on her need to take on the role of "helper" and her need to "fix" situations in all areas of her life. As she worked on these issues, she was able to stay involved with her family without becoming engulfed by constant demands and crises.

The concept of working with individual family members within a family systems context is relevant here on a number of levels. First, many African American adults struggle with Joan Miller's dilemma of how to be differentiated and individuated within a close extended family and yet not become either too enmeshed or totally cut off. Many other ethnic groups that have a collective focus, such as some Hispanic and Italian families, also struggle with this concept of finding a balance between cultural and familial expectations and the ability to meet the needs of the individual. For many African American family members, where the tradition of a collective unity or identity can be traced to their African heritage, this struggle can be very intense. This dilemma can appear in the treatment process and may require individual work with a particular family member.

With some African American families who enter treatment, the therapist may make the decision that one or more family members needs individual work for a variety of reasons. Unfortunately, a rigid dichotomy is often made between individual and family therapy in some mental health agencies. In these clinics, different family members may be assigned to different therapists, an administrative procedure that often adds to the sense of feeling overwhelmed and exacerbates the underorganization with which many African American families present. In many of these cases, further systemic confusion can be avoided by a systems therapist who can intervene at many levels, including work with individual family members, the entire household, various combinations of extended family members, and outside agencies.

In my experience, the unnecessary dichotomy between treatment levels and modalities often results in complex treatment case conferences between different therapists, which is not only more time-consuming for the therapist but can actually contribute to the fragmentation of family members. In the worst possible (but very common) scenario, however, overburdened therapists may not have time to communicate with each other and so work at cross-purposes. The multisystems model therefore provides a more efficient method of providing mental health services to many African American families. Once again, the flexibility with which the therapist approaches this model is the key to its effectiveness.

Levels II and III: Discovering the Real Family Network, or Going Beyond the Subsystem

Many African American families present at clinics as they feel clinicians expect them to appear. This often means that the clinician initially meets only a "family subsystem" (Minuchin, 1974), such as a mother and a child or children. This is where the therapist's work begins. After the first few sessions, as trust begins to build between the therapist and the family, the therapist will inevitably begin to learn more details about the extended family network. The therapist must have some knowledge of African American cultural patterns in order to ask the questions that will help to give a true sense of the real "family."

After the problem focus of the first few sessions, the therapist will need to begin to explore the network, since in focusing on a particular problem the question of who else is involved in this problem will have been raised and explored. Speck and Attneave (1973) and Kliman and Trimble (1983) have discussed network approaches.

A basic general question that can be asked in order to explore the support system might be "Who helps you out with the children?" Families will often open up and give many examples, ranging from grandmothers and aunts to neighbors and boyfriends. Another important question is "Who lives in the house?" The answer to this question might well reveal information about many different extended family members. It is also important to ask about who visits regularly and whether there are people who sometimes stay over. Such questions will often reveal informal adoption patterns such as those discussed in other chapters. It may also be the first time that a boyfriend or girlfriend may be acknowledged. One might ask a mother directly after trust has been established, "Do you have a special person or a boyfriend in your life?" Many mothers are initially reluctant to reveal the presence of a boyfriend. Rather than asking the typical intake question "How many siblings do you have?," one may learn a great deal more about complex relationships by simply asking "How many children live in the home or stay over often?" The answer may reveal cousins, nieces, nephews, grandchildren, or neighbor's children who interact daily within the household.

Another difficult area to explore in many African American families is the question of the paternity of the children (see Chapter 3). Children may have different fathers, a fact that may not be shared initially. Once a relationship of trust is established, however, one can ask a mother such questions as "Do the children all have the same father?" or "Who are the children's fathers and do they help out?" Often this will reveal other possible aspects of support or involvement by the biological father(s) or his family. As discussed in the previous section, once a father acknowledges paternity of a child, his extended family may be involved in that child's life even if the father himself is not. Many family therapists make the error of assuming that because a child does not see his or her father, he or she has no knowledge of him or of his extended family. For many isolated families who are cut off from their network, it is important to explore whether these paternal relatives have ever been involved, since they may once again serve as resources. Also, as children approach late childhood (ages 10–14), they often become very absorbed with the question of "who they are," and will often reestablish contact with their father's extended family as a way of discovering a "lost" part of themselves. If this has not occurred, it may be an issue that the therapist can explore with the family.

A more important question in some African American families is not just "Who is your mother and father?" and "What relationship do you have with them?" but "Who raised you?" Given the prevalence of informal adoption in some Black families, this may be very relevant to the current family dynamics. These patterns of informal adoption are often repeated over generations. The genogram can be very helpful in gathering and organizing this information.

Levels IV and V: Extended Family Organization and Nonblood Kin

Once joining has occurred with the family or family subsystem that originally came for treatment and at least one important problem has been addressed, the therapist is in a position to explore extended family organization and nonblood kin. This can be done in a variety of ways. One practical way to begin raising the issue of extended family members is to stay focused on the problem or problems that the family has established as being of primary importance and to ask questions such as:

1. How do other family members feel about this problem?
2. To whom do you go for advice?
3. Have a lot of people tried to give you their opinion about this problem?
4. To whom would you listen for advice on this issue?
5. To whom would your child (children) listen?
6. In the past, to whom would you go when you had something serious like this to deal with?
7. Who helps you out when you have troubles?
8. Have you experienced any recent losses (deaths, moves, divorces, fights, cutoffs, etc.) within the extended family, nonblood kin, or friendship network?

As one begins to gather this kind of information, organizing it in the form of a genogram tends to follow naturally.

Once this process is complete and the therapist has a workable understanding of the family's extended support system, specific questions such as the following can be asked:

1. How do family and extended family members interact?
2. How many people have stayed with you (even overnight) in the last year?
3. Do a lot of people turn to you for help? Who are they?
4. Who gets along with whom?
5. Who fights with whom? (Children love Questions 4 and 5.)
6. Who would you say has the last word on things in your family?
7. Have you told any family members and friends about your coming for therapy? How do they feel about it?
8. Do they agree with what you've been doing here?
9. Of these people, who do you feel contributes to the problems we've been working on?
10. Who do you feel might have some ideas that could help us solve this problem?
11. Who's involved in any way with this problem?
12. How long has the problem been occurring?
13. Have there been any major losses, resulting from deaths, moves, separations, fights, and so on in your family during this time?
14. Have any new people come into your life or your family in this time, from changes such as a marriage, a new boyfriend or girlfriend, a new church or religion, an extended family member or other person who has moved in?

Levels VI and VII: Church, Community, and Social Service Networks

Chapter 7 explored in detail the ways in which religious orientation and spirituality can play a role in the lives of African Americans. This section summarizes the levels at which the therapists may need to utilize this resource in treatment. First, the religious or spiritual belief system is so strong in some African American families that the therapist may find it useful to simply explore it as part of general information gathering. For those families for whom religion is of paramount importance, the therapist will quickly receive feedback regarding that importance. It may then be helpful to make reference to spiritual statements made by family members as a help in reframing family impasses.

In times of crisis, the church becomes a very important social service system for many African American families. A crisis such as a fire, homelessness, hospitalization, illness, isolation, and so forth can often be helped by the support of the "church family." For many African American clients and families who are emotionally cut off or geographically isolated from their biological extended family, helping them find a church family and address their fears about doing so can have a long-term therapeutic effect.

For single-parent mothers who have no particular religious orientation but are feeling burdened, overwhelmed, and isolated, an African American church can provide a social life for mother and children, free childcare, school and after-school programs, and meaningful activities for children to keep them off the streets. For some mothers who have difficulty organizing to seek help, African American churches can provide a structure to help them mobilize. They can also "pass the hat" when a family has lost their possessions in a fire or provide a temporary sanctuary if a family is homeless. Chapter 7 also gives examples of special circumstances in which a minister, pastor, elder, deacon, or deaconess might be included in the treatment process. The key here is that therapists be aware of this level of intervention and utilize it when appropriate in order to mobilize help for some African American families.

Community supports are available on a number of levels, and can range from after-school tutoring services, free lunch programs, daycare centers, or free hospital and clinic care. It is important for therapists to become informed about these supports and keep their knowledge up to date. For example, some therapists make use of transportation services that are available through state, city, and Medicaid/Medicare agencies for transporting children and families to and from therapy sessions. This kind of tapping of available resources is sometimes the single most important interaction in facilitating the possibility of treatment.

The seventh level, social services and public institutions, encompasses an area that, as has been stated, many therapists are not trained to address as part of the therapeutic process. The realm of public agencies and services is central to the treatment of poor African American families, who are often very dependent on these institutions for survival. Such families are also particularly vulnerable to institution and agency intrusion into the functioning of their families.

HOME-BASED FAMILY THERAPY
WITH AFRICAN AMERICAN FAMILIES

A natural application of the multisystems model is the use of home-based family therapy and other community interventions. Boyd-Franklin and Bry (2000) in their book *Reaching Out in Family Therapy: Home-Based, School, and Community Interventions,* have described the value of these interventions, particularly when working with African American and other extended family minority cultures. They have indicated that even for therapists who are primarily office-based, one well-timed home visit can change the outcome of the treatment by engaging powerful family and extended family members who will not come into the office, and who may otherwise sabotage the treatment.

Too often, therapists do excellent office-based treatment with the least powerful members in African American families (e.g., young mothers and children). As a supervisor, I have often noted cases of African American families who come in every week for treatment, but never complete homework tasks and don't experience any real change. In these circumstances, it is important that the therapist reassess the power dynamics in the family. As Chapter 3 and 4 in this book have shown, many generations in an African American family may live in one household. Even in cases where families live in different households, extended family members may still exert a great deal of influence. Grandmothers and grandfathers (often even great-grandparents), aunts and uncles, older siblings, the father, the mother's boyfriend, or the father's girlfriend are all "family members" who may have a considerable amount of power in an African American family. If they are opposed to therapy, they can undermine the therapeutic process. Home visits can allow the therapist the opportunity to meet these key family members, to join with them, and to have the opportunity to observe the family's home environment.

During home visits, Boyd-Franklin and Bry (2000) caution us to "remember our own 'home training'" and to respect the client's home. Particularly for poor, African American families, it can be embarrassing to have a stranger intrude in their home. Many of these families have a legacy of intrusions in the past by welfare workers, child protective services staff, and the police. Given this history, healthy cultural suspicion can be very high initially, especially in cross-racial treatment. It is therefore important that family workers not arrive unannounced and that they take the time to join with and put all family members at ease. In home-based family sessions, therapists will often find family members engaged in their usual household routines including watching television, eating a meal, cooking, feeding or changing a baby, and so on. Boyd-Franklin and Bry (2000) caution clinicians to "learn to 'go with the flow' of the family. Do not be in a hurry on a first visit to impose rules or your own sense of order. Try to relax, fit in, and get to know all of those present" (p. 39). It is also important that therapists from other ethnic and racial backgrounds understand that they may often unwittingly compromise the family's confidentiality by their presence in the community, particularly if they are very different in ethnic or racial appearance from the family.

It is essential that clinicians use themselves effectively to enter the family on their terms (Aponte, 1994; Berg, 1994; Boyd-Franklin, 1989; Boyd-Franklin & Bry, 2000). Because of their past experiences with multisystems agencies, some African American clients may be angry initially. It is important that therapists avoid taking this response personally. Boyd-Franklin and Bry (2000) offer suggestions to therapists on how to convey our ability to tolerate the client's anger and continue the work. They also discuss guidelines to ensure the personal safety of clinicians in home-based work.

CONCLUSION

The multisystems approach expands the "road map" of the therapist in working with African American families, helping to highlight the levels to be explored and allowing the therapist to maintain a problem-solving focus and to address the ways in which each system level contributes to the problem that a particular family is struggling to resolve. Therapists often have to help African American families in therapy establish clear boundaries between the different system levels, and construct ways in which each level involved can be a support rather than a hindrance. As the section above illustrates, even one home visit or a multisystems meeting at an agency can bring together key extended family members or workers from other agencies, who may have the power to support the needs of the family or to undermine the outcome of treatment. The multisystems approach also enables the therapist to explore systematically each of the levels in looking for resources of people and services that might aid in finding the solution to a particular problem.

Chapter 12 explores the public policies of which clinicians must be aware if they are to understand the contingencies impacting many of the families they treat, particularly those living in poverty. Chapter 13 discusses the ways in which multisystemic social service networks can be utilized to function in a more supportive and empowering fashion for poor African American families.

12

Public Policy Issues

A Guide for Clinicians

WHY CLINICIANS SHOULD BE AWARE OF POLICY ISSUES

Burdened by the day-to-day demands of large caseloads, many therapists find it difficult to pay close attention to public policy issues. This is unfortunate because a number of important public policies have changed, especially in the last decade, and these changes directly affect the African American families we treat, particularly those living in poverty. In order to empower and to advocate for families on multisystemic issues, it is crucial for therapists to be aware of current law and policies. An extensive review of all public policy issues effecting African Americans is beyond the scope of this book. Although there are many important issues that effect our clients' lives, this chapter will provide a brief overview of five areas that directly impact our treatment approaches: welfare "reform," the Adoption and Safe Families Act, kinship care, managed care, and affirmative action policies. (Readers should bear in mind that a chapter such as this may be obsolete almost as soon as it is written. Policies are often changed or refined, so staying informed should be an ongoing process throughout our careers. The implementation of these policies also varies considerably from state to state.)

Welfare Reform and Its Effect on African American Families

In 1996, a major process of welfare reform in this country (Hill, 1999b; Weil & Finegold, 2002) began when President Bill Clinton signed the Personal Responsibility and Work Opportunity Reconciliation Act (PRWORA) into law. This legislation ended the 61-year-old Aid to Families with Dependent

Children (AFDC) program, which provided federal aid for open-ended entitlements for dependent children in poor families (Di Nitto, 2000; Hill, 1999a). Under the new legislation, the responsibility for welfare was transferred to the states in the form of block grants. The Temporary Assistance for Needy Families (TANF), the most important of these block grants, was intended to remove recipients from the welfare rolls and to help them to find jobs. Welfare recipients were expected to obtain jobs within 2 years and were given a lifetime limit of 5 years on the welfare rolls (Hill, 1999b).

Welfare reform has brought about a dramatic decline—statistics show a 50% reduction—in the number of families receiving welfare grants since 1996 (Weil & Finegold, 2002). Many of these families have at least one parent who is now part of the workforce.

These statistics may seem encouraging at first glance, but they hide the number of families, particularly single-parent ones headed by women, whose situation has been made worse (Hill, 1999b; Weil & Finegold, 2002). The legislation has, in fact, increased economic hardships for many former welfare recipients and their families (Hill, 1999b). Therefore, the statistical decrease of 50% in the welfare rolls must be examined critically.

Although some of these former welfare recipients are working, they are typically paid low wages, receive few benefits, and often have no health insurance for their families. Weil and Finegold (2002) have pointed out that welfare reform was enacted during a period of unusually high economic prosperity and expressed their concern that many of the most at-risk families will not be able to maintain employment during times of economic slowdown and recession. Many vulnerable families have faced further hardship due to the economic stresses and higher unemployment rates that were consequences of the terrorist attacks on September 11, 2001 (see the unemployment statistics in Chapter 1).

Finegold and Staveteig (2002) found that welfare reform has affected racial and ethnic minority groups differently. They report that the minority share of the caseload has increased and that the White share has continued a decline that had started before the reform legislation was enacted. Blacks also appear to experience many more administrative problems within the welfare system than their White counterparts. There is a statistically significant gap between the wages of White and Black former welfare recipients. Other studies suggest that Black and Hispanic women are more likely than White women to spend at least 5 years on welfare and to reach the lifetime limit of 5 years allowed under this legislation (Duncan, Harris, & Boisjoly, 2000; Finegold & Staveteig, 2002). In addition, "Lack of education and job skills, limited access to transportation and child care, high rates of incarceration, and employer discrimination all make finding and keeping a job difficult for low-income Blacks and Hispanics (Holzer, 2000; Holzer, Stoll, & Wissoker, 2001), and may contribute to other disparities in the effects of welfare reform" (Finegold & Staveteig, 2002, p. 212).

Hill (1999b) has explored other issues for African American families. He has argued:

> This welfare reform legislation had mixed effects on African American mothers. Indeed, a minority of recipients who had high school diplomas and marketable skills were more likely to obtain stable jobs after leaving the welfare rolls. Yet, the overwhelming majority of mothers were not likely to experience such positive outcomes upon leaving the rolls. Many studies reveal that most welfare leavers encountered many barriers, such as low-wage jobs that did not pay enough for food and rent, jobs that provided no health benefits for family members, and the lack of affordable child care which prevented many of them from being able to obtain or keep their jobs. (p. 6)

Despite assurances from the states that they would provide subsidized childcare, lack of affordable childcare is an enormous financial burden and a huge concern for many of these mothers (Hill, 1999b; Weil & Finegold, 2002). Hill (1999b) has documented the difficulty of obtaining affordable childcare: there were long waiting lists; the quality of the available care was often poor; most mothers did not earn enough in their low-paying jobs to even pay for the cost of subsidized childcare for one child, let alone more than one; and for those who worked unconventional schedules (i.e., night shift or weekends), childcare was not available at all. Many of these mothers were virtually forced to leave their jobs in order to ensure that their children were cared for appropriately.

Under the previous AFDC guidelines, children were automatically given health coverage under Medicaid and food stamps. Now that the responsibility for providing for such needs has been delegated to the states, policies vary. Many children of low-income wage earners lack health coverage (Hill, 1999b; Weil & Finegold, 2002). Families in increasing numbers are dependent upon charity programs—such as those conducted by food banks and churches—for food, and emergency services from homeless shelters when they were unable to pay their rent. The numbers of homeless individuals and families have also increased in many cities (Children's Defense Fund, 2000).

In 2000, the Children's Defense Fund, under the leadership of Marion Wright Edelman, released a report entitled *Families Struggling to Make It in the Workforce: A Post Welfare Report* (Press release, 12/14/2000, *www.childrendefense.org /release001214.htm*), which detailed many of the hardships faced by low-income working families who have left welfare since 1996. Their study found that:

- Despite their best efforts, their paycheck did not stretch far enough to feed, clothe, and shelter their children.
- Stable employment was extremely unlikely for former welfare recipients without a high school diploma and those without child care and transportation.
- Nearly a third of the parents who left welfare for work lost their jobs and many had cycled in and out of the workforce. . . .

- Fifty-eight percent of those who were working had family earnings below the poverty line.
- Despite low earnings, approximately half of the families surveyed were not receiving food stamps for which they were eligible.
- Child care was cited more frequently than any other reason for not working.
- Families who were "pushed off" the welfare rolls for non-compliance with the new rules were more likely to be burdened by educational deficiencies and health problems than current recipients.
- More than one in five former recipients who lost a job reported transportation problems.
- The only group likely to escape poverty by their earnings alone was those workers with at least a two-year post-secondary or vocational degree. (Children's Defense Fund, 2000, p. 2)

Marion Wright Edelman made the following plea in a press conference, following the release of this report:

The bottom line is that work should lift families out of poverty. We cannot ignore the hardships many working families and children face. They are playing by the rules but working in dead-end jobs which often do not insure self-sufficiency. . . . Working parents need child care, health care, and transportation help so they can be successful and meet the basic needs of their families. . . . We need to talk about poverty reduction and not just caseload reduction. (p. 2)

Additional barriers to employment often ignored in the welfare reform process include "physical disabilities, mental health or substance abuse issues, limited English proficiency, learning disabilities, domestic violence, etc." (Holcomb & Martinson, 2002, p. 5). Clients coping with chronic mental health and substance abuse issues who have reached the 5-year time limit have been "sanctioned" off the welfare rolls. These clients and their families are at risk for experiencing even more severe poverty and homelessness (Weil & Finegold, 2002).

Therapists working with these families need to recognize that welfare reform had many unintended negative effects on other family and extended family members (Hill, 1999b). One group particularly impacted by these changes was grandmothers who were raising their grandchildren, as is common in many poor Black families. Hill's research has demonstrated that one reason for the decrease in the welfare rolls was that punitive sanctions on mothers for failure to obtain jobs, attend drug treatment programs, or adhere to numerous regulations resulted in the adult portion of the aid being terminated, leaving "child-only" grants. One consequence of "child-only" grants is that many of these children are actually being raised by extended family members, such as grandparents, aunts, or uncles.

In many states, nonrelated foster parents receive higher welfare payments to care for children than relative or kin caregivers (Hill, 1999b). Kin caregivers also often receive fewer social services than foster parents, even when these children have special health and mental health needs (Hill, 1999b). A 1997 study, "Informal and Formal Kinship Care," sponsored by the U.S. Department of Health and Human Services, indicated that over 40% of relatives involved in kinship care are elderly and poor. (See the Kinship Care Policies section below.)

Another tragedy for families is that many working and relatively young grandmothers and aunts are forced to leave their jobs in order to care for multiple dependent children. As a consequence of these problems, many of these African American children, according to Hill, "are experiencing even more severe economic hardships than when they were on welfare" (p. 8).

Implications for Clinicians

Clinicians can empower such families by becoming familiar with the entitlements available in their states for health care (such as Medicaid), food stamps, childcare, and the like, and by helping them to advocate for these services and benefits. The Children's Defense Fund (2000) reported that families who received the supports described above were more likely to maintain stable jobs.

Given these conditions, it is extremely important that mental health practitioners lobby lawmakers for policy changes that will provide real and lasting changes to raise families out of poverty, such as support for these vulnerable, newly employed families during economic slowdowns; subsidized childcare; provisions for families whose substance abuse, health, and mental health challenges make it difficult for them to survive without welfare support; providing Medicaid and food stamps to low-income working families; and giving more adequate stipends to extended family caregivers.

THE ADOPTION AND SAFE FAMILIES ACT

On November 13, 1997, President Clinton signed the Adoption and Safe Families Act (ASFA) of 1997 (Public Law 105-89) into law. This law is widely regarded as one of the most far-reaching laws effecting adoption and child welfare policies since the 1980 Adoption Assistance and Child Welfare Act (Grimm, 1997). This law was intended to address the concerns that some children were being left in or returned to unsafe family situations and that approximately 100,000 children awaiting adoptions were still in foster care (*www.childrensdefense.org*). Grimm (1997) presented a detailed analysis of the ASFA legislation, excerpts of which follow. This legislation:

- shifted the emphasis to the protection of the child as the first priority.
- redefined "reasonable efforts" to prevent foster home placements and to reunite children with their parents.

- [required r]easonable efforts [to] be made to find permanent placements for children for whom reunification with parents is not the permanent plan.
- permitted concurrent planning under which family preservation, legal guardianship and adoption planning possibilities are all pursued simultaneously.
- required a permanency planning hearing within 12 months of a child's placement in the foster care system.
- required the Department of Health and Human Services (HHS) to submit a report by June 1, 1999 on kinship placement. . . .
- reauthorized the Family Preservation Program (now called the Promoting Safe and Stable Families Program) with its aim toward family reunification.
- Authorized state child welfare agencies to file a petition for Termination of Parental Rights if a child has been in foster care for 15 of the most recent 22 months.
- Allowed three exceptions to the termination of parental rights provisions:
  1) For children who are being cared for by relatives, the state may adopt a policy that a termination petition need not be filed.
  2) If the state has documented in the case plan a compelling reason why it is not in the child's best interests, termination need not proceed.
  3) If the parent(s) were not provided with services as part of the reasonable efforts.
- required that biological parents, extended family members and foster parents be notified of the dates of permanency planning hearings.
- eliminated geographic and bureaucratic obstacles to adoption.
- authorized health care coverage for adopted children with special needs (including medical, mental health or rehabilitative services). (Grimm, 1997, pp. 1–15)

Implications for African American Families

This law was well-intentioned. It recognized the need of children in the foster care system for a sense of permanency in their lives when there was little hope of reunification with their biological parents and it set a number of positive goals for children in the foster care system. But Jackson (2002), while acknowledging some of the positive aspects of ASFA, has listed numerous problems presented for African American and other poor families in the years since its implementation:

- The number of children placed in out-of-home care increased from 557,000 children in 1998 to 588,000 children in 2000.
- Although African American children comprise 15% of the population, they continue to be overrepresented in out-of-home placements at 45%. Research shows that African American children are at a greater risk for entering the system. African American families are reported to the formal system at a greater rate than white families, and African American children stay in care longer than white children. African American children are half as likely as white children to return home and less likely to achieve permanency through adoption.

- The national length of stay of children in out-of-home care has not decreased dramatically.
- Placement resources in child welfare are scarcer than ever. Children are placed in mental hospitals in one state, in public agencies in others, and often in over-crowded conditions in most states because there are not enough emergency foster homes to accommodate the placement rate.
- Focus has shifted from reasonable efforts to prevent placement to reasonable ef-forts toward permanency. State policies to meet permanency goals are some-times counterproductive and not always in the best interest of children.
- The Promoting Safe and Stable Families program [created by ASFA] was too rigid to get anything working in the way of prevention, requiring equal spend-ing for family preservation services, community-based and family support ser-vices, time-limited reunification services, and adoption promotion and support services. . . . The United States needs to keep children out of the child welfare system and make significant investments in serving families and children who come to the attention of the system.
- State child welfare directors say they have been successful in increasing the safety of children and moving them toward permanency because of a 28% in-crease of permanent homes in 1999. States were so successful in increasing adoptions that the numbers exceeded budget expectations. Still more than 100,000 children are waiting to be adopted.
- Since the mid-1980's child welfare policy and legislation has tended to view the placement of children with relatives as a type of foster care, which it is not. . . . The practice of placing children with relatives came about not because administrators thought it was in the best interest of children but because of a shortage of foster homes. Kinship care, therefore, was never a planned program. Most of these children are African American and, because of cultural tradition, relatives often struggle with trying to care for their kin.
- Relatives should be applauded and not forced to be a part of an unnatural sys-tem like foster care. Kinship care must be considered a permanent living ar-rangement whenever possible. It is time for the federal government to make clear policy decisions and not place unnecessary restrictions on kinship care as a placement option.
- Perhaps a more appropriate funding stream should be through the Promoting Safe and Stable Families program, because kinship care is family preservation as well as community-based family support and family reunification. (Jackson, 2002, pp. 1, 5)

See further discussion below of issues related to kinship care.

Implications for Clinicians

Clinicians working with families whose children are in care due to a parent's substance abuse have raised concerns about ASFA's time limits for the initia-tion of termination of parental rights. Grimm (1997) states that "recovery can be a long process and even for those who are able to recover from drug and al-cohol addictions, it can be a difficult process that generally involves periods of relapse" (p. 7). Clinicians can advocate for more substance abuse services in their communities, particularly those that provide for the placement of "children and parents together in residential treatment facilities" (Grimm, 1997, p. 7). Clinicians can help parents identify extended family members who can provide kinship care for their children while they are enrolled in programs for substance abuse. This can prevent placement of their children in the foster care system.

ASFA has other implications for African American families. Many African American preadoptive parents, foster parents, and kinship and extended family caregivers are faced with a cultural conflict when informed of the "termination of parental rights" provision of the law. This process is in direct opposition to the cultural values of many Black families. For generations, African Americans have engaged in informal adoption without the termination of the parents' rights. In addition, children who are old enough to have had a relationship with their parents prior to placement in foster care often experience loyalty conflicts at proposed termination. Clinicians are advised to discuss these issues carefully with all children, family, and extended family members involved.

States vary considerably in the ways in which they have chosen to implement this law. Some states have interpreted it to require adoption by kinship caregivers. While this can keep the child within his or her extended family (Satterfield, 2002), it can also cause cultural and familial conflicts, as described above. An alternative to adoption that does not require termination of parental rights is for the kinship (extended family) caregivers to petition for legal guardianship. One difficulty for kinship caregivers outside of the foster care system who provide permanency by assuming legal guardianship is that support payments are considerably lower than those for foster parents. (See further discussion in the "Kinship Care Policies" section below.)

Clinicians who are aware of the policy implications of this law and the areas in which it can be made more flexible, such as those described above, can best advocate for their clients and empower African American families to intervene on their own behalf.

THE CHALLENGES OF SPECIAL NEEDS ADOPTIONS

Many children in the foster care system have medical, behavioral, emotional, and psychological problems, which have complicated the adoption process, especially prior to ASFA when there was no guarantee of Medicaid coverage for these children. ASFA now provides health insurance for special needs adopted children. Clinicians working with these families need to familiarize themselves with other entitlements available to adoptive families in their state.

Adams (1998), of the South Carolina Department of Social Services, discussed the theoretical change inherent in the adoption process:

[Historically] the belief prevailed that adoption would magically alleviate or modify the problems so a single family could function successfully and independently. Agency involvement after finalization was considered to interfere in a family's integration.

Experience has shown that adoption is not an end in itself, but rather a beginning. Many of the principles that previously governed the program have proven false. Therapy can be viewed as one preventive service that can help with the child's and the family's adjustment. While most difficulties can and should be handled by families, some problems are so serious that a family must reach out for support. In such times of crisis, the [child welfare] agency must be seen as a resource to assist in preserving the adoptive family unit. Agency services must be viewed as preventive in nature, i.e.[,] focusing on the avoidance of a child's possible reentry into the foster care system. (p. 4)

Clinicians can help adoptive families to understand that children who have been in the foster care system have often experienced multiple losses (Henry, 1999). When faced with the possibility of adoption, these children experience paradoxical emotions. They are often thrilled with the possibility of permanency, but may be conflicted about the loss of their biological family. In addition, they may have had so many experiences of loss, change, disruption, and rejection that they are afraid to trust that their adoptive parents will keep them. They often act out just prior to the adoption or in the first year in an attempt at self-protection, essentially conveying the message that it would be preferable to be rejected by an adoptive family at the start, rather than be rejected (which they often regard as inevitable) after they care about their new family. A therapist who is aware of this process can help to prepare an adoptive family and the adoptive child to be aware of these issues and can avoid a failed adoptive placement. Hughes (1999), in his discussion of the challenges of adopting children with attachment problems, gives additional guidelines for clinicians working with these families.

KINSHIP CARE POLICIES

African American families have historically informally adopted or "taken in" children whose parents could not effectively care for them (Billingsley, 1992; Boyd–Franklin, 1989; Hill, 1972, 1977, 1999a; Hines & Boyd-Franklin, 1996; Logan, 2001; also see Chapter 3). This process was also common in African tribal societies when death or loss of the parents occurred (Hines & Boyd-Franklin, 1996). "Kinship care" is the term that has been used in recent years to describe this informal adoption process (Hill, 1999a).

It is only within the last 20 years that child welfare agencies have begun to recognize the value of kinship care, particularly for those children where family reunification is not an immediate alternative (Hill, 1999a). Hill (1999a) attributed the creation of a new foster care category, kinship care, to the shortage of available foster homes, the rising number of children needing care, and the dramatic increase in the number of children living with extended family members (Berrick & Barth, 1994; Wilson & Chipungu, 1996). The rise in the number of children needing care has been ascribed to increasing rates of parental drug and alcohol addiction, AIDS, and incarceration. Prior to 1980, public policy was not culturally sensitive, and many African American children were removed from their homes and placed in foster care when viable extended family placements were available (Boyd-Franklin, 2002; Hill, 1999a).

Hill (1999a) has demonstrated that the majority of these kinship care arrangements are still informal:

> Of the one million black children currently living in the households of relatives without either parent, 80% are informally adopted by kin, while the remaining 20% are in foster care. While child welfare agencies find it difficult to obtain permanent homes for 200,000 black children in foster care, the black extended family has succeeded in finding homes for 800,000 black children. (p. 126)

As with many public policies impacting the poor, the implementation of kinship care policies varies considerably among the states.

Given the need for research on the policy implications of kinship care, the U.S. Department of Health and Human Services was directed by the Adoption and Safe Families Act of 1997 (ASFA; P.L. 105-89) to convene an expert advisory panel (Report to Congress on Kinship Foster Care, 2000). In its analysis, the report of the panel used the term "non-kin foster care" to describe traditional, nonrelative foster homes and separated kinship care into two categories (Report to the Congress on Kinship Foster Care, 2000, p. iv). The first category, which is informal and occurs without outside agency involvement, is termed "private," and the second category, a formal arrangement in which children in the custody of a state child welfare system are officially placed with extended family members pursuant to a formal licensing process, is termed "public."

People who wish to become licensed foster care providers are required to undergo a thorough background investigation to determine whether any members of the family household have criminal records or a history of abuse. There are also requirements mandating a minimum living space, a separate room in the home for the child, and a certain income level. Some requirements may be waived, unless they are related to safety concerns; again, states vary in terms of policy (Report to the Congress on Kinship Foster Care, 2000).

Many extended family members are not aware of the licensing process. In some states, the requirements are reduced for kinship foster parents. Beyond a minimal TANF payment (described in detail below), no further help or public funding is available to nonlicensed kinship caregivers. There are enormous discrepancies between the foster care payment rates and payment rates for informal or private kinship care providers. The Report to Congress on Kinship Foster Care (2000) pointed out that while all kin caregivers are eligible for "child–only" grants under the TANF program, these are significantly lower than payments given to foster parents. The report gives the following example, about a licensed foster parent in the state of Maryland:

> [This foster parent] would receive $535 to $550 a month for care in 1996 (APWA, 1998), whereas a child being cared for by a welfare-assisted relative would have received only $165 a month in a basic child-only grant. These differences become even greater when there are multiple siblings in care, since the welfare payment is prorated on a declining scale and foster care payments remain constant regardless of the number of children in the household. . . . Two children [living in a home] . . . licensed by the foster care system would have received $1,070 to $1,100 a month in 1996; two children financed by that State's AFDC program [living with unlicensed relatives]would have received $292 a month. (Report to Congress on Kinship Foster Care, 2000, p. 21–22)

Clinicians must recognize that despite the figures presented above, the majority of informal kinship care providers or relatives in most states receive *no* financial support for the children in their care. This Report to the Congress also demonstrated that there are other major discrepancies in terms of the services provided to licensed foster families and private kinship families. For example, children in foster care are given counseling services and other health and mental health services at no cost. Extended family members who become private kinship care providers must pay for such services themselves (Report to the Congress on Kinship Foster Care, 2000).

Hill (1999a) has discussed the consequences of these burdens for many extended family members who informally adopt children:

> The low income aunts or grandmothers who care for their kin receive the lower AFDC grant for child care and are denied or discouraged from obtaining the higher foster-care stipends. In addition, many of the kinship care families are not provided important social services. Such lack of social support increases the social stress, economic hardships, and excessive burdens for these grandmothers, because many of the children in kinship care have more severe health needs than other foster placements, especially those who were born to alcohol addicted, drug addicted, or HIV-infected mothers (Burton, 1995). Research reveals that children in kinship care families have more stable placements than children in nonrelative foster care (Le Prohn, 1994; Wilson and Chipungu, 1996). Thus, kinship families should be viewed by public and private agencies as vital foster care resources for quality, long-term placements for children who are not able to return to their biological parents (Burton, 1995). (p. 127)

Implications for Clinicians

Many therapists are unaware of the burdens incurred by African American families involved in kinship care. As Hill's (1999a) statement above indicates, many of these grandmothers and aunts are poor, elderly, and often have serious health concerns. Family crises, such as a son or daughter who is on drugs, dying of AIDS, or incarcerated, often place these caregivers in an impossible situation. Culturally they are expected to care for their grandchildren, nieces, or nephews, and they may already be caring for one or more grandchildren. They often struggle with their ambivalence about accepting the burden of taking in still another child with no monetary help from the state.

There is a critical need for major federal and state legislation to provide funding to support viable kinship care for African American families (Boyd-Franklin, 2002; Hill, 1999a). The policies in this area are changing rapidly. Because states vary considerably in how they license kinship foster parents, it is essential that therapists become aware of the current laws in their state and keep abreast of federal policies. It is also important for all of us to work to change the laws and to push our state agencies to adopt a more compassionate interpretation of the guidelines to allow relatives providing informal kinship care to receive more equitable stipends.

MANAGED CARE AND SERVICE DELIVERY ISSUES FOR AFRICAN AMERICAN CLIENTS

Frank and VandenBos (1994) have indicated that with rising costs, access to adequate health care has been eroded for many people in the United States. African Americans, along with other ethnic minority groups, have traditionally been underserved by health and mental health services, and that gap—although prevalent among all socioeconomic levels—is especially significant for poor clients (La Roche & Turner, 2002; U.S. Department of Health and Human Services, 1999).

Racial and ethnic group differences are evident in private insurance coverage; public programs, such as Medicaid; and among the uninsured. For example, a U.S. Department of Health and Human Services report (1999) indicated that while 78% of Whites were covered by private insurance, only 56% of Blacks and 45% of Hispanics were so insured (La Roche & Turner, 2002). These figures may even understate the discrepancy, given the economic slowdown and higher rates of unemployment in the years after the study was done.

La Roche and Turner (2002), in their discussion of this report, indicated that ethnic minorities are overrepresented on Medicaid: "More than 15% of all ethnic minorities compared with only 5% non-Hispanic Whites are enrollees." Since Medicaid recipients are, by definition, poor, such restrictions will place a great burden on poor clients in need of health and mental health services.

The discrepancy in the rates for those with no health insurance are even more striking (La Roche & Turner, 2002). A report issued by the Kaiser Family Foundation and the UCLA Center for Health Policy Research (2000), entitled *Racial and Ethnic Disparities in Access to Health Insurance and Health Care*, indicated that among Whites, 14% are uninsured; among African Americans, 25%; and among Hispanics, 37%.

According to La Roche and Turner (2002), African American and other ethnic minority clients have historically experienced limited access to mental health services. These limitations have only been exacerbated under managed care. Researchers (DeLeon & VandenBos, 1995; La Roche & Turner, 2002) have defined *managed care* as both private and governmental health care delivery systems that are partially funded and partially controlled by a third party.

La Roche and Turner (2002) have identified both financial and cultural barriers to access to mental health services for African American and other ethnic minority clients: They state:

> Low income and lack of health insurance are the major constraints that contribute to lower health service utilization (U.S. Department of Health and Human Services, 1999). . . . Uninsured minority individuals often lack access to preventive care, particularly mental health services, and often delay seeking treatment for many conditions until they become so severe that emergency care or hospitalization is required. . . . Despite these adverse consequences, the federal government has reduced funding for health care programs, especially mental health services that serve low-income individuals. (pp. 190–191)

Vega and Rumbaut (1991), in their discussion of the National Medical Expenditure Survey, indicate that Blacks are only 61% as likely as Whites to receive mental health care. Many mental health providers have the mistaken belief that barriers to mental health care access under managed care are limited to poor African American and other ethnic minority clients. But La Roche and Turner (2002) have shown that "even when socioeconomic differences are controlled, minorities continue to have greater difficulties accessing mental health services" (U.S. Department of Health and Human Services, 1999, p. 191).

A part of the issue of access to care for African Americans is that under managed care, the primary care physician (PCP) is responsible for referrals to mental health providers. Many PCPs and mental health clinicians are not culturally sensitive to indications of mental health distress. For example, somatization is common among African American and Latino clients (La Roche & Turner, 2002; U.S. Department of Health and Human Services, 1999), and spiritual references to pain and mental health distress are quite common especially in older African American women (see Chapter 7).

Inadequate screening procedures are further compounded by the lack of continuity that many minority clients encounter (La Roche & Turner, 2002; Sue & Sue, 1999), particularly in large urban hospitals. The building of a relationship and the use of self are often crucial to the development of the trust necessary to help African American clients overcome the "healthy cultural suspicion" (Boyd-Franklin, 1989; Grier & Cobbs, 1968) many bring to their interactions with medical and mental health service providers.

These time pressures can affect the quality of care for many clients. The time constraints inherent in managed care inhibit a relationship of trust, thus presenting a particular challenge for clinicians of a different ethnic or racial background working with African American clients. Another complication of managed care arises when case managers refuse to pay for any sessions beyond a set number. The number of sessions allowed is often insufficient (La Roche & Turner, 2002; Miller, 1996; Murphy, DeBernardo, & Shoemaker, 1998; Seligman & Levant, 1998). Many therapists who work primarily with minority clients struggle with an ethical dilemma (La Roche & Turner, 2002; Murphy et al., 1998; Phelps, Kohout, & Eisman, 1998): do they continue to work with the client and charge according to the client's ability to pay (which would mean virtually donating their services or working pro bono), or do they abandon the client or his or her family? This ethical dilemma can exist for clinicians in agency work as well as those in private practice who treat African American clients.

Managed care decisions are often based on policy manuals that prescribe short-term treatment for individuals. A "one size fits all" approach does not take cultural differences into account and may sometimes feel too rigid or restrictive to African American clients (Austad & Berman, 1995; Dana, 1998; La Roche & Turner, 1997). Managed care interventions frequently focus solely on the individual (Cushman & Gilford, 2000), which is incompatible with the more collectivistic, family, relationship, and community orientations of many African Americans. Some managed care companies do not pay for family or couple therapy sessions at all (La Roche & Turner, 1997, 2002; Triandis, 1994). These obstacles may perpetuate already existing distrust by African Americans toward mental health services and cause their high number of premature therapeutic terminations (Sue & Sue, 1999). There is a critical need for research on specific treatment approaches that are effective with African American and other ethnic minority families (Chambless et al., 1996).

Culturally sensitive practices, such as home visits to reach extended family members who will not come to an office for treatment (Boyd-Franklin & Bry, 2000), are often not funded by managed care. Family therapists have been forced to become creative in their interventions with multisystems and other agencies on behalf of their clients (see Chapter 11). For example, when regular meetings are not possible because of pressure for "billable hours," clinicians have effectively used e-mail, phone calls, conference calls, and case management coordination conferences.

In periods of economic downturn, unemployment rates among African Americans are often high due to their position as the "last hired and the first fired" (Boyd-Franklin, 1989; Hill, 1999a). This increases the number of African Americans with no health insurance. Therapists who began treatment with clients who had jobs with good health insurance benefits can now find those clients unemployed, uninsured, and, understandably, in great distress. La Roche and Turner (2002) have discussed the dilemma in terms of low-income patients, but their suggestions that therapists in clinics and agencies "develop a sliding scale of fees or a long-term payment system"(p. 196) also apply to clients who are unemployed or who have lost their health benefits during a period of a job transition. Some clinicians and agencies are able to carry a small number of "pro bono" cases where they will treat a client for a specific limited period of time (e.g., 10 sessions) at no fee. The timing of the sessions can be flexible so that therapy can be done in a shorter, time-limited manner or sessions can be spread out over a longer time period. In order for such treatment to be effective, clinicians need to be familiar with short-term, time-limited approaches (e.g., structural or strategic family therapy; see Chapter 10).

Implications for Clinicians

Whenever possible, therapists should lobby managed care companies and legislators to provide reimbursement for more mental health services such as family and couple therapy and home-based interventions, which are often not covered under these plans. It is extremely important that clinicians be proactive and advocate for legislation and policies at the state and national level that endorse national health care policies that provide quality health and mental health care and culturally sensitive services to all clients, irrespective of their socioeconomic or income level and employment status. Frank and VandenBos (1994) and La Roche and Turner (2002) describe this as an ongoing debate fueled by ambivalence within the U.S. health and mental health care system. It is yet another example of the conflict between a Euro-Western mental health policy based on individualism, which argues that the individual must pay his or her own way, and a more compassionate health and mental health policy based on need and ability to pay (Frank & VandenBos, 1994; La Roche & Turner, 2002). Such a compassionate policy would be far more consistent with the more collectivistic cultural beliefs of many African Americans who value caring for others in the family, extended family, and the larger community (Hill, 1999a).

AFFIRMATIVE ACTION POLICIES

It would be very difficult in this brief section to do justice to as complex and controversial an issue as affirmative action. It is essential, however, that clinicians working with African American families understand the importance of this issue in these communities.

In order to understand the issues that are relevant to affirmative action policies today, it is important to first explore the original purpose of these programs. As Allen (2001) has indicated, African Americans had experienced the dual oppression of slavery and "Jim Crow" laws, which relegated them to separate but unequal educational facilities and lack of employment opportunities for more than 400 years. Throughout this book, I have emphasized the ways in which more covert examples of racism and discrimination persist to this day

(Hill, 1999a). Allen (2001) has provided the historical context in his discussion of the view of President Lyndon Johnson, who launched affirmative action and equal opportunity programs in the 1960s in an attempt to rectify past and present examples of racism in U.S. history:

> He invoked the powerful metaphor of a people in chains for 350 years being required to race another people who were and had been free of restraints. Thus, Johnson declared, it wasn't enough in 1965 to merely unchain African Americans and declare the competition an even one from that point on. " You do not take a person, who, for years, has been hobbled by chains and liberate him, bring him up to the starting line of a race and then say, 'You are free to compete with all the others,' and still justly believe that you have been completely fair." (p. 89)

Affirmative action, therefore, began as an attempt to redress almost four centuries of racism and negative treatment against African Americans in this country. In the 1970s, however, affirmative action policies were expanded to include other groups, including Latinos, Asian Americans, and women. Ironically, as Allen (2001) has shown, "the outcomes of their adoption have been skewed; white women have by far been the greatest beneficiaries of affirmative action. They increased their college enrollment by 26 percent between 1978 and 1994, compared to increases of 1 percent for African Americans, 3.6 percent for Asian Americans, and 2.9 percent for Chicano/Latino Americans (Wilson, 1998)" (p. 89).

Allen (2001) has demonstrated that affirmative action programs "brought hope and promise and real gains to the disenfranchised" (p. 88) and "dramatically expanded opportunity in American society that systematically prevented the full participation of Blacks, people of color, and women" (p. 89). Ironically, despite the advances achieved by many African American individuals and families, Blacks as a group benefited less than the other groups discussed above.

In the 1990s, however, affirmative action programs came under a major attack in this country. As Allen (2001) has indicated, California was in the forefront of the efforts to reverse the benefits of affirmative action gains. It ended affirmative action programs in 1995. Sadly, this movement was led by an African American man, Ward Connerly, the chair of the University of California Board of Regents (Allen, 2001), who was used by conservative elements within the state to reverse these benefits. Erroneously, Connerly and his counterparts argued that "affirmative action had served its purpose and was no longer necessary; or that it was 'reverse discrimination'" against Whites (Allen, 2001, p. 89).

In recent years the controversy regarding affirmative action has led to the dismantling of many of the gains for African Americans, as Allen (2001) has shown:

> This is the history that brings us to the present, a moment where American higher education is in the process of resegregation. For African Americans in par-

ticular, low rates of college enrollment and degree attainment had caused concern. Since the rollback of affirmative action in 1995, black and Latino and Latina enrollments at the University of California's most prestigious campuses, Berkeley and Los Angeles, have dropped by roughly 50 percent. At these institutions, the gains for blacks in college enrollment and earned degrees are now being reversed.

More generally, since the early 1960's, African Americans had made significant gains in enrollment and degree attainment at the university level. The percentage of African Americans who completed four years of college or more rose from 4 percent in 1962 to 15.5 percent in 1999 (U.S. Census Bureau, 2000). However, the representation of African Americans in this category compared to other racial groups remains relatively poor. Although undergraduate enrollment for African Americans increased 8.3 percent since 1993, the rise is less than half the rates of increase for Chicano/Latino, Asian Americans and Native Americans during the same period (Wilds, 2000). (p. 91)

Other concerns are evident as well:

Compared to their white counterparts, black disparities in enrollment are even more alarming. Most recent data show that African Americans comprise less than 12 percent of the total undergraduate enrollment nationally, whereas whites make up 71 percent of the student population. Moreover, among bachelor's degrees awarded in 1997, African Americans received only 8.1 percent, though they represented more than 11.2 percent of all undergraduate students (Wilds, 2000).

At the same time, whites were awarded 77 percent of the bachelor's degrees with 71 percent undergraduate enrollment. If the disproportionate contributions of Historically Black Colleges and Universities [HBCU's] to total Black student enrollment and earned degrees were removed, these figures would be even more lopsided. (Allen, 2001, pp. 91–92)

Challenges to Affirmative Action

Affirmative action policies have been the subject of ongoing debate in the United States for over 30 years (Bowen & Bok, 1998; Cross, 2003). Springer (2003) has shown that one of the earliest, "the Supreme Court's 1978 ruling in *Regents of the University of California v. Bakke,* 438 U.S. 265 (1978), stated that a university could take race into account as one among a number of factors in student admissions for the purpose of achieving student body diversity" (p. 1). Affirmative action was seen as a national commitment to rectify the "effects of past discrimination" (Springer, 2003, p. 1), "historical injustice," as well as "current institutionalized discrimination" (Anderson, 2002, p. 18), and to increase diversity in institutions of higher education and in the workplace (Springer, 2003). In recent years, there have been a number of states in which affirmative action practices in college admissions have been banned, including California, Texas, Georgia, and Florida (Cross & Slater, 2003). All of these states, with the exception of Texas, have had dramatic declines in the numbers of African Americans enrolled at major state universities (Cross & Slater, 2003).

Since that time, there have been a number of court cases challenging affirmative action. Recently, there have been a number of cases at universities in Texas, Georgia, Michigan, and Washington (Springer, 2003). On December 2, 2002, the Supreme Court announced its historic decision to hear two cases, which challenged the affirmative action policies at the University of Michigan. Springer (2003) described these lawsuits:

> In the fall of 1997, two class action lawsuits were filed by the Center for Individual Rights on behalf of White students denied admission to the University of Michigan's undergraduate and law school programs.(*Gratz v. Bollinger et al. and Grutter v. Bollinger et al.*). The suits allege that the University utilizes different standardized test score/grade-point average standards for White and minority students, but the University counters that race is only one among a number of factors taken into account in its admissions processes (p. 5).

As of this writing, it is expected that a decision will be made by Summer, 2003 (Springer, 2003). The outcome of these two cases will have a major impact on the educational future of African American youth and families.

Implications for Clinicians

Affirmative action has had a tremendous impact on the lives of many African Americans. Since the late 1960s, many Black people have benefited from the educational and employment opportunities offered through these policies. While Wilson (1987, 1996) has argued that primarily middle-class African Americans have benefited from these policies, Hill (1999a) has demonstrated that many poor and working-class Blacks benefited from these gains as well, particularly in the 1970s and 1980s. Nevertheless, there are a growing number of African Americans who are still trapped in poverty and who feel little hope of attaining the "American dream" (Wilson, 1987, 1996). Allen (2001) argues that if affirmative action policies are reversed nationally as they have been in California, a resegregation process will occur.

Clinicians should be aware that both poor, working class, and middle-class African American families have already begun to feel the impact of the negative reactions to affirmative action (Bowen & Bok, 1998) and the reversals in states such as California, Florida, Georgia, and Texas (Cross & Slater, 2003). Many African American parents fear that they will be unable to pass the educational and socioeconomic gains of the 1960s and beyond on to their children. Because of declining numbers, many African Americans who do go on to predominately White universities often find themselves even more in the minority than they would have been in the 1970s. It is not unusual for African American parents to express concern in therapy about the reality that the decision to send their children to these institutions may result in their children's isolation and loss of their sense of racial identity. In my own practice and those of many of my colleagues, we have treated a number of African American clients and families who have been psychologically damaged by the negative messages these students have received at these institutions. For some, the price of a higher education has been a marked decrease in self-esteem and a sense of social isolation. This has led to an increase in the numbers of African American students choosing to attend "Historically Black Colleges and Universities" (HBCU's). Still other families worry that by the next generation, African American children will no longer have even the limited degree of access to predominately White colleges and universities that they have today.

Clinicians will have many opportunities in the next decade to voice their opinions to their legislators and to address this reversal of affirmative action policies. As stated above, the U.S. Supreme Court will soon decide landmark cases regarding affirmative action. Some clinicians have had to struggle with their own ambivalence about affirmative action policies, particularly when they affect their own children. It is very important that clinicians working with African American families carefully examine their own feelings and counter-transference on these issues. Allen (2001) has reminded us that "affirmative action inclusiveness and diversity have the power to enrich the higher education experience for all involved (Hurtado, Milem, Clayton-Pederson, & Allen, 1999)" (p. 97). It will also become an even more important issue discussed in treatment by African American families. It would be tragic for the advances of the civil rights movement to be reversed in this next generation.

III

SOCIOECONOMIC CLASS ISSUES AND DIVERSITY OF FAMILY STRUCTURES

13

Poor Families
and the Multisystems Model

The multisystems model provides the family therapist with an approach for moving beyond the structure of the individual, the family, and the kinship system. It allows the therapist to assess, clarify, and ultimately restructure and change the interaction between poor African American families and the outside systems and agencies that intrude in their lives. These systems include schools, courts, child welfare agencies, housing offices, welfare departments, police, hospitals, and health care and mental health providers. It will often be important for the family therapist to help the family "navigate the system" by meeting with representatives from these various agencies and to assess the boundary, alignment, and power issues involved. Often the family therapist may find it necessary to restructure or help the family to renegotiate and clarify its relationship with a particular agency.

Because of the number of social systems involved, often intrusively, in the lives of poor African American families—many of whom feel completely overwhelmed by life's demands and socioeconomic realities—these families often find that they cannot interact effectively with agencies. It is not unusual for a therapist to discover that a number of these agencies are working in opposition, and that the family has been triangulated by them. Many African American inner-city parents report that they feel manipulated and condescended to by these agencies. This sense of powerlessness when faced with "the system" is often a metaphor for a more general sense of defeat that many of these parents feel in relation to societal institutions. When assessing family dynamics, family therapists must be willing to examine the impact of these external structures on the family and help to support the family in their interactions with these other institutions and agencies.

271

THEORETICAL CONTRIBUTIONS
TO THE MULTISYSTEMS MODEL

Aponte (1994) has made the most significant contribution to the theoretical and clinical development of this model. Building on his foundations as a structural family therapist, he developed the "ecostructural" model, which examines the role of the family therapist vis-à-vis outside agencies working with poor families. Bronfenbrenner (1977) utilized an ecology of human development to illustrate these different levels and their impact on the family.

The ecostructural model and the multisystems model offer important contributions to the treatment of poor African American families. First, they provide the therapist with a conceptual framework within which to organize the large number of agencies and institutions that are involved in the lives of their patients. Second, they offer a clear path that the therapist can use to assess the structural issues not just *within* the family but *between* the family and these organizations. The therapist can then expand the structural concepts of boundary, alignment, and power to assess accurately these broader system interactions (Aponte, 1994). Third, as Aponte (1994) has stated, the ecostructural model allows the family therapist to organize and integrate other treatment modalities and methodologies within one coherent approach.

Henggeler and Borduin (1990) and Henggeler et al. (1998) have utilized a multisystemic approach to the treatment of these families. Hartman and Laird (1983) and Holman (1985) have described an "ecological approach to family assessment . . . [that] acknowledges that families do not exist in a vacuum" (Holman, 1985, p. 18). Recognizing the interaction between families and their environment, they present a model that describes the complex interplay of organizations and individuals that may have an impact on a family system.

Before we proceed further in exploring specific treatment aspects of this approach, it is important to examine the issues of concern to families that are Black and poor. This will offer the therapist an understanding of the needs of this population and the advisability of adopting a multisystems approach.

THE REALITIES OF BEING BLACK AND POOR

We have already established that the impact of racism creates a burden that is unique for African American families in this country. This burden is particularly heavy for low-income African American families who also struggle with the oppression of poverty. These are the families whom Wilson (1980, 1987) describes as the Black "underclass" or the "truly disadvantaged." Parents live not only with the financial burdens of doing without and with the inability to provide for the basic needs of their families, but also with the seemingly endless cycles of unemployment, poor housing, and inadequate community services. When one adds this information to the national statistics that indicate unemployment among Black people to be the highest in the country, one can understand more fully the feeling of hopelessness in many African American communities.

To be Black and poor is to live in fear. Families are constantly afraid for their children and are well aware of the location of the local "crack house" or the neighborhood "pusher." Children can be enlisted by the "drug culture," first as "runners" and later as "pushers" or "users." When disillusionment grows strong, drugs and alcohol can often lure youth. The process of educating their children is another "minefield" for African American parents (Boyd-Franklin, et al., 2001). Inner-city schools are often not responsive to children's needs, and can be viewed by many African American parents as just another hostile, overwhelming system, one more impossible wall to scale. It is not difficult to understand therefore why Black youth have one of the highest dropout rates in the nation.

There are fears on many other levels for African American families living in poverty. Street crime is extremely high in inner-city neighborhoods. The discrepancies between African American inner-city communities and the rest of the nation increase the desperation of these families. The rage that this process causes often erupts in domestic violence, child abuse, and "Black on Black" crime. In many Black inner-city neighborhoods, many African American families are struggling to survive and feel that they have no protection. Experience has taught them not to trust the police or the courts to deliver justice. Thus they avoid these systems at all costs.

PAST EXPERIENCE WITH WELFARE AND OTHER SYSTEMS

One of the issues that has led African American families to resist mental health services arises from their confusion about the relationship between clinics and other agencies (e.g., welfare, courts, schools) (Hines & Boyd-Franklin, 1996). Many African American families that have a history of involvement with the welfare system, for example, report experiences of intrusiveness and prying by these agencies in the past. It is noteworthy that even though welfare reform has occurred and past practices have been changed, many African American families have a long memory and continue to distrust the system. (See the section Welfare Reform and Its Effect on African American Families in Chapter 12). The welfare system had the power in the past to drop families from its rolls and leave them with no financial security if the father of the children (or another man) was proved to be living in or contributing to the household.

In the past, prior to welfare reform legislation, if the father of a child contributed a small amount to that child and his or her mother, even if the parents were not living together, he could have compromised the family's right to receive financial help through welfare. This, coupled with the tragic unemployment rates for African American men and the "last hired, first fired" policies in this country, has contributed to the breakup of many African American families in past generations and the fragile nature of some family units today (see Chapter 5).

Many of our inner-city families are referred for therapy by the courts. For example, this is a frequent recommendation in child incorrigibility cases. In family dispute assault cases, both police departments and courts often refer a family for therapy. This creates a difficult dilemma for the therapist and the family on at least two levels. First, African American families in these situations are not self-referred. They feel forced to come; indeed, they are often forced to come for treatment by probation officers and courts. Second, Black families in these situations are extremely suspicious of the therapist and are dubious about the confidentiality of their treatment. They are well aware, often before the therapist him- or herself is aware, that the courts or referring agencies will require a report or evaluation of their progress in treatment. Therapists in these situations frequently find themselves asked to make difficult decisions or recommendations regarding the lives of their clients. These realities must be discussed frankly, honestly, and realistically with African American families if trust is to develop.

Schools are one of the most frequent referral sources for African American children and families to clinics and community mental health centers. In keeping with the multisystemic view of the child or identified patient as the person whose symptoms reflect distress in the family system and the need to get help for the whole family, it is not surprising that these symptoms or problems often manifest themselves at school. Poor African American families place a very high value on the education of their children; educational orientation is therefore a focus of strength for these families (Hill, 1999a; McAdoo, 2002). Such families, however, are often so overwhelmed by survival demands that they are not able to monitor or intervene effectively in their children's education process.

FOSTER CARE AND CHILD WELFARE SYSTEMS

Social service agencies also have a great deal of power in poor African American communities. Hill's (1999a) research demonstrated that African American children are disproportionately overrepresented in foster homes and child welfare systems. Child welfare agencies have the power to remove children from their houses if they suspect abuse or neglect. They have the power to divide the children in a family by placing them in numerous foster homes and to petition the courts for "termination of parental rights." Once a child has been removed from a family, the regaining of custody is often a long and difficult process. Poor African American families are often very frightened and resentful of this power. Given this context, it is not surprising that an African American family who is referred for therapy by one of these agencies would tend to be suspicious of the therapist's role. Many fear that they will be "reported" to these agencies if they share personal information. As mentioned in Chapter 9, even African American therapists are sometimes surprised to discover that they are perceived as part of "the system" and are not trusted initially.

Prior to 1980, it was less common for children to be placed with relatives. In response to research and lobbying efforts by the National Urban League (Hill, 1977), that process has begun to change (see Chapter 12). Today, a greater effort is being made by some social service agencies to locate extended family and to place children with their relatives. However, often these efforts have not been sufficient: many children "fall between the cracks." Today kinship care has become much more common, but these kinship providers are often given little or no financial assistance as compared to nonfamilial foster homes (Hill, 1999a).

The complex interaction of social agencies and poor African American families makes it important to return to a discussion of the multisystems approach and to describe its basic principles, strategies, and interventions. The next sections explore four basic principles of this approach: (1) the therapist's own values and assumptions; (2) the family therapist as system guide or facilitator; (3) concrete problems as a legitimate part of the family therapy process; and (4) the concept of empowerment in the treatment of poor African American families.

EXPLORING THE THERAPIST'S OWN VALUES AND ASSUMPTIONS

One of the hallmarks of the multisystems approach is that it forces the therapist to examine and clarify his or her own values and explore his or her own belief systems (see Chapter 9). Therapists must examine their own families and their own cultural identification, as well as their own beliefs about poor African American families. In the process of doing this kind of clarification of values with trainees, the author has often heard statements based on class biases such as "The poor are lazy," "They want to live that way," and "They like getting welfare." Some clinicians deal with such issues by ignoring the racial component, preferring to state that the issue is one of "class not race."

Once the therapist has explored his or her own beliefs, biases, and values about what it means to be Black and poor, he or she is in a very different position to work with these families. One of the most important issues therapists must handle within themselves is the tendency to "blame the victim," or to see poverty as the "fault" of the person. The approach to treatment presented in this book is based on the concept of empowerment. Parnell and Vanderkloot (1989) have emphasized this point: "Blame is counter to empowerment. It paralyzes everyone, families and therapists alike" (personal communication,

1989). Thus, the model of looking for and building upon strengths is essential to our work with poor African American families.

Parnell and Vanderkloot (1989) have demonstrated how to join very effectively with poor African American families around the issue of "wanting something better for themselves and even more importantly for their children" (p. 46). This allows the therapist to reframe the familial position for him- or herself and for the family: "You desperately want things to be better for you and your child and you are struggling against great odds to get there" or "As I listen to your statements I sense that you desperately want things to be better for your children than they were for you." Parnell and Vanderkloot (1989) have elaborated further on this issue:

> We have presented a clinical model which is basically non-blaming and non-pathological for working with poor people. We have shown that in helping the parents of poor children to do well what they most want to do has a powerful effect on the children and the family. *We have searched for that part of the parent that fiercely wants life to be better for his children than it was for them.* We have validated the totality of the person's experience and thereby formed a powerful bond with the parent and children. We are seen as "we" rather than "they" when we work in this way. As one of our patients stated (a convicted rapist) when he asked himself what was different in our treatment of him, "All the other people were nice and helpful, but it is as if I were out in a canoe in rough water. Everyone else is standing on the shore calling out directions. You dove into the water, swam out, got into the canoe and showed me a new way to shore." (p. 461)

THE FAMILY THERAPIST AS SYSTEM GUIDE OR FACILITATOR

Poor African American families often depend on outside agencies to provide very basic needs and services. With these government services, families must contend with an enormous bureaucracy. Often each agency is perceived as a baffling maze of individuals who do not give clear answers or show respect. Therefore, in addition to helping families to learn to structure their involvement with these agencies, the family therapist is frequently faced with the task of helping families learn how to effectively navigate the social service system. In this role, the therapist often has the task of becoming a system guide or facilitator for the family. In the traditional medical model, this was the role of the social worker. However, family therapists of all disciplines who work with poor African American families have commonly found that the therapist's willingness to assume this role (irrespective of discipline) is an essential part of joining with such a family and building trust.

The concept of a facilitator is important here. It is crucial that the therapist not take over the central role for family members but rather support the parents or parental figures in assuming their respective executive roles. The distinction between help and empowerment is an important one to understand. As Boyd-Franklin and Bry (2000) have demonstrated, our ultimate job as therapists is to empower our clients to successfully advocate for themselves in the multisystems bureaucracy.

As an important component of their role as facilitators, therapists should have at their disposal files of information on social service agencies that can provide their clients with vital social services. It can be very useful for clinics or community mental health centers to establish files containing this kind of information and to request that each staff member contribute new ideas to their files. It is also very helpful if such clinics find contact people in key agencies who can serve as resources and expedite the process of obtaining services for a family.

Poor African American families often expect active involvement from us as clinicians, often waiting for us to take the first step and being afraid to trust us as agents of change. It is thus extremely important for therapists to convey a willingness to get involved and to "roll up their sleeves" and get to work. Parnell and Vanderkloot (1989) have framed this issue as follows:

> If we as clinicians are not prepared to "dive in," difficult as that may be, it will be hard, if not impossible to capture the attention of poor children and their families. They are so busy struggling just to stay afloat that there is little energy left to focus on anything that is not immediately useful in the resolution of those struggles. (p. 461)

In conveying this involvement to the family, it is important for the therapist to "take the family where it is," starting with the problems that seem most overwhelming to them.

CONCRETE PROBLEMS AS A LEGITIMATE PART OF THE FAMILY THERAPY PROCESS

A major fact of life for some poor African American families is that they enter treatment with an overwhelming array of life problems. Survival issues such as money, housing, food, and safety are ever-present realities. What role if any do these issues have in the process of family therapy? In truth, most major schools of family therapy have not even addressed these concerns. This is a serious error in working with poor Black families. My experience as a supervisor of beginning family therapists working with poor Black families has taught me that it is not unusual for a family to present their housing problems, for example, as their first priority in family therapy. Many beginning family therapists will ignore this kind of concrete problem and search instead for problems related to family structure or dynamics. I have supervised therapists who feel frustrated by the presentation of these kinds of issues and ask, "When do we get to the *real* family problems?"

This a very serious error in working with these families for four reasons. First, families who are homeless or hungry are often so overwhelmed by these realities that they have no energy left to focus on other issues. Second, therapists who ignore these issues miss a primary opportunity to join with and engage these families. Working with them on these survival issues establishes the therapist as a "helper" and a person who can be trusted.

Third, family therapists often miss the opportunity to observe the structure of the family firsthand by asking them to discuss their presenting problem with each other or to discuss ways of resolving the problem together. Such observation can provide an opportunity for a clear enactment of the interactions that occur routinely at home. The therapist can then observe these interactions and note where the process breaks down. The ways in which a family discusses and handles these concrete problems also function as indications of their more general communication and problem-solving strategies. By asking a family to interact and discuss one of these concrete issues among themselves, a therapist can gain important data about such issues as family boundaries just by observing whether the children or the adults lead this discussion. The assessment of concrete problem considerations also provides the therapist with an opportunity to evaluate the family's support system. Questions such as "Whom do you have that you can talk to about this problem?" are often very revealing.

Fourth, the feeling of powerlessness or hopelessness in the face of a racist society is often overwhelming for many poor African American families. It has an impact on many structural levels. Often a mother who feels powerless to solve her housing problem also feels powerless to discipline her children. Empowerment of the family and the parental system is a major task of family therapy in general, and is particularly important in working with poor Black families. Empowering a single-parent mother to contact the housing department and begin to get help in finding an apartment for her family can become an empowerment to be utilized in other areas: her willingness to take charge can then be stated clearly for the family and redirected to the setting of disciplinary rules and structure for her children. The next section discusses the role of empowerment in this treatment process.

EMPOWERMENT AS AN ISSUE IN THE TREATMENT OF POOR AFRICAN AMERICAN FAMILIES

Throughout this book, the concept of empowering African American families has been emphasized within a number of frameworks. It is important to give this concept careful consideration because it is particularly central to the process of providing therapy to poor African American families. Many of these families have a multigenerational history of victimization by poverty and racism. Unlike other cultural or ethnic groups who can "blend in" or become part of the "melting pot," Black people by virtue of their skin color are visible reminders of the inequities and racism of society. With this experience of victimization comes a sense of powerlessness and, for many African American families, a sense of entrapment. This sense of being unable to make and implement basic life decisions in their own lives and the lives of their children often leads to a sense of futility. Empowerment most often involves helping parents to regain control of their families and to believe that they can effect important changes for themselves. This is very threatening to many family therapists because it often requires them to take a stand on a decision made by another agency, forcing them to abandon their fantasies of "neutrality" in therapy. As many of the chapters of this book indicate (see especially Chapters 9, 10, and 11), family therapy in general and family therapy with African American families in particular is an active therapy that insists upon the examination of the therapist's political, cultural, and religious beliefs and biases and demands active intervention.

Empowerment can revolve around the seemingly innocuous issue of encouraging a mother to call her child's teacher rather than having the therapist make the call. If the mother needs further support, the call might be role-played with the therapist first and even made from the therapist's office so that it can be discussed at a later point. Or empowerment may mean deliberately not acting to quiet the children at the beginning of each session and instead allowing the mother to begin doing this herself with the therapist's support.

When many outside agencies are involved, it is also necessary to hold meetings with representatives from the different agencies or schools and the family. When these occur, it can be very useful for the therapist to role-play in advance with the executive or parental figures in the family the process of raising issues that they want to clarify at such a meeting. The goal of this therapeutic process is to provide them with a sense of personal control, and to encourage the executive figures to take this kind of active role when confronted by these life events (Boyd-Franklin & Bry, 2000).

It is often a very dramatic and powerful moment in family treatment when a mother who has presented as feeling overwhelmed by her children and perceives herself to be at the mercy of child welfare agencies and schools can come into a session with her therapist and the representatives of these agencies with her list of issues, needs, and questions that she wants to address. This scenario represents a very effective restructuring. Moreover, it communicates the structural message to the children that their mother is "taking charge." This is true empowerment.

It is through this kind of examination and the therapist's ability to convey respect for the families she or he treats that she or he creates an atmosphere in which empowerment can occur. This holds true whether we reestablish generational boundaries and put the parent or parents in charge or empower a poor African American family to reestablish the external boundary around itself and set limits on intrusion by outside agencies.

STEPS IN THE MULTISYSTEMS APPROACH WITH OUTSIDE AGENCIES

As indicated in Chapter 11, the building of trust between therapist and family is often a prerequisite to exploring the involvement of other system levels. The processes of joining and engaging, assessing, and problem solving are ongoing and should be addressed early on. The following are a number of crucial issues and steps that should be addressed in the multisystems approach.

1. Many low-income African American families are not self-referred. They are sent or forced to come to treatment by outside agencies such as the police, courts, schools, hospitals, child welfare agencies, probation officers, and so on. These families are well aware that agencies will expect verbal and sometimes written reports from clinicians regarding the family's progress in therapy. Issues of confidentiality should be addressed openly with the family and done so early on in treatment.

2. It is important for the therapist to distinguish him- or herself from these outside agencies as much as possible and to clarify these distinctions for the family. Therapists should pay attention to referral sources and get permission from the family to contact them early in the treatment process. Families often expect that a therapist will speak to referral sources. Contact can often help clarify the agenda of the referring agency, which might be quite different from the needs or wants of the family. The clarification of the referral source's expectations regarding the treatment process can help prevent the frequent dilemma of many well-meaning therapists who become triangulated in a battle between the referral source and the family.

3. Once trust has been established with a family, it is often helpful to do a more complete "eco map" (Holman, 1985) with a family in order to assess more carefully the role of outside agencies. The eco map is a drawing of the different outside systems and agencies that have an impact on the family. Hartman and Laird (1983) and Holman (1985) discuss this technique for diagramming the interconnections between a family and its ecological system.

Holman (1985) gives the following summary of the data collection process.

> As an eco map is developed with the involvement of family members, it provides the workers and the family with an understanding of the stresses on the family system as well as the available supports, and family members are likely to feel more comfortable and less defensive about providing information (Hartman, 1978). Using a structured map simplifies the procedure for the worker and clarifies for the participating family members how various systems in their ecological field relate to their family. (p. 63)

Holman uses arrows to signify a flow of energy or resources and different kinds of lines to illustrate the nature of connections: a solid line for strong, a broken line for tenuous, and a broken line with slashes through it for stressful connections (see the eco map for the Kelly family, Figure 13.1).

An eco map might indicate that there is considerable friction between this particular family and the school, the social welfare system, and the extended family. The therapist can then choose to explore these issues further and to intervene if necessary in these systems.

The eco map can help not only to clarify the structural involvement of outside agencies, but also to determine which agencies are helping the family to resolve problems and which are creating or contributing to the family's difficulties. Sometimes eco maps also provide a quick, efficient method for discovering which crucial social services the family is not receiving.

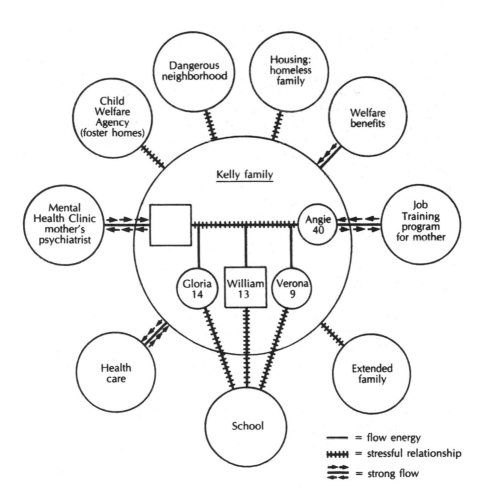

FIGURE 13.1. Eco map for the Kelly family.

4. Many African American families present with multiple problems. A therapist should spend early sessions helping the family to identify the most urgent problems. He or she should remain focused on these problems until they are solved. Many families are so flooded by needs and problems that they quickly become immobilized. Therapists will begin to feel helpless too if they attempt to address too many problems at once. It is important to start with a problem that can be addressed and solved quickly in order to establish the therapy process as helpful.

5. As much as possible, family therapists should become facilitators of the process and should avoid taking over the family's executive role. Enactment and role playing should be used with family members to help clarify their roles with outside agencies. Family sessions should be used to empower family members to delegate tasks and design strategies for dealing with specific agencies.

6. The therapist should function as a source of information for the families he or she treats. It is very important for therapists and agencies working with this population to set up a resource file or to designate some person who can be consulted by the family to locate the particular services they need.

7. The therapist should be prepared to call for and to attend meetings with the family with outside agencies or schools. Often the therapist then becomes the system's therapist and must assess the boundary, alignment, and power issues between the therapist, the family and outside agencies. Sometimes this process involves calling for meetings of numerous social service agencies involved with a family. A joint plan can then be designed so that the family does not become overwhelmed by multiple forms of output.

8. Once again, it is important to stress the necessity of going outside the clinic to meet with other agencies, make school visits, and meet with significant family members at home when necessary.

The following case example illustrates this process.

The Kelly family consisted of Angie, a 40-year-old Black schizophrenic woman, Gloria (age 14), William (age 13), and Verona (age 9). The family was supported by welfare benefits. The family was referred by a local child welfare agency because all three children were truant from school, experiencing academic difficulties, and had been repeatedly placed in foster homes over the years. In the first session, Angie Kelly and her three children were transported by their caseworker. Angie looked particularly helpless in the session. Her oldest daughter Gloria took charge and described the family's concerns. She stated quite bluntly that they lived in a "hell zone" in which they could not sleep at night. Their apartment had been broken into a number of times but was "better than nothing." The family had in fact been living in shelters for the homeless prior to finding this apartment 6 months earlier. The child welfare worker reported that the family had been homeless a number of times because the children often vandalized the buildings in which they lived. She also reported that the youngest sister had been placed in a foster home the previous week because her mother had burnt her head with a curling iron when fixing her hair. All of the children had been removed and placed in foster care a number of times. Gloria had been placed in a foster home but had recently run away and returned home. Angie Kelly expressed a helpless feeling of not being able to "get these children to act right." She was herself seeing a psychiatrist in the adult clinic at the community mental health center, and had been maintained on 300 milligrams of thorazine daily for 2 years. She had not had a hospitalization in that time.

The therapist listened to everyone's input and thanked the child welfare worker for her support in bringing the family. She then asked if she might meet with them alone briefly. She felt strongly that the family was very guarded and careful in their statements and she wondered if the presence of the child welfare worker might be adding to their reluctance to discuss their family.

The worker understood and waited in the waiting room for the family. The therapist had created a boundary between herself and the child welfare agency. The atmosphere in the session changed considerably after she had left. William immediately jumped in and stated that he wanted his family "back together." Gloria made clear that she felt that their housing situation was urgent. The therapist noted that the children had assumed a "parental role" and began mobilizing the mother by asking her what she wanted. She very passively agreed with her children. The therapist became very concerned about her passivity and was afraid that the generational role reversal in this family would be a permanent one because of the mother's diagnosis and the limitations on her functioning.

The therapist used future sessions to explore the limits of the mother's capabilities and to empower her to take responsibility for her own family. To accomplish this, the therapist worked with the mother individually as well as in family sessions with her children. In an individual session shortly after Gloria was again placed in a foster home, Angie admitted that she really did not feel that it was in the best interests of her children to live with her at that time. She felt that she needed to find a new apartment in a safer neighborhood. She was also required by the Welfare Department to pursue job training opportunities for herself. In a subsequent family session, Angie Kelly was able with the therapist's help to explain this plan to her children. She told them that she wanted them to behave in their foster placements and that she would begin the process of meeting with the child welfare agency to make plans for bringing them together in the future. Family therapy sessions became a regular meeting place for the family. The therapist arranged for the caseworker to transport the two girls who were in foster homes.

After a number of attempts, Angie reported that she had been unable to find a new apartment. The therapist suggested a meeting of Angie, her children, the therapist, the child welfare worker, and a parent advocate who had been assigned the task of helping her to find a new home. The therapist and Angie had role-played her involvement prior to the meeting. Her children were obviously impressed and surprised to see their mother take charge in the meeting and to clearly state her needs and the difficulties she faced. The two outside agencies agreed to offer her concrete help with finding an apartment, and the parent advocate offered to accompany her on a number of the visits to view possible apartments.

During this period, Gloria again ran away from her foster home. Her mother, with the therapist's help, was able to explain to her in front of the other children that they must work together as a family and stick to the original plan if they were to bring about change. There was a marked sense of empowerment in Angie; the helpless individual of earlier sessions was less in evidence.

William, who was still living with his mother, had been truant from school for an extended period of time. The therapist met with William and his mother to discuss this problem and learned that he was often afraid to leave his mother alone when he went to school. The therapist helped Angie to discuss this fear with her son and to tell him about her own plans to enter a vocational rehabilitation program. He agreed with his mother to explore a number of special programs for children who had experienced difficulty in attending classes regularly.

This was an extremely difficult family to treat. Nevertheless, despite constant crises, the therapist managed to help the family identify their most pressing needs and empowered the mother to assume a parental role, involving the social service agencies but drawing a boundary between her own work and theirs.

The process of working with outside agencies can be very complex. Often it takes time for the therapist to visualize the entire terrain and to understand the network of interrelationships. The following case is an example of a situation in which both the therapist and her supervisor missed an essential component of the dynamics between the family and an outside agency. The case involved a number of serious mistakes. But these mistakes provided the therapist and her supervisor an opportunity to learn and to grow.

Mrs. Brent, a 40-year-old Black woman, brought her "son" Carl (age 7) for treatment. They were accompanied by Carl's child welfare worker, Mrs. Black, who had made the initial referral for treatment. Mrs. Brent explained that she was planning to adopt Carl officially as soon as possible. Her child welfare worker had recommended treatment because he seemed withdrawn, depressed, immature, very dependent, and was experiencing academic problems in school. She also produced a number of reports by psychologists that questioned the degree of psychological bonding that had occurred between Mrs. Brent and Carl.

The therapist then learned that Mrs. Brent's family consisted of four children: Carol (age 21), Evelyn (age 18), Ella (age 15), and Rashan (age 5). The family was supported by public assistance. There was a great deal of competition and tension between Carl and Rashan, which often resulted in Carl bursting into tears and withdrawing.

Mrs. Brent had been a babysitter for Carl for brief periods of time during the first 6 months of his life. When he was approximately 1 year old, his natural mother, who was reputed to be an alcoholic and a prostitute in the area, left Carl with Mrs. Brent and asked her to care for him. She had never returned. This "informal adoption" arrangement continued for many years until an eviction created a housing crisis for the Brent family and the child welfare department became involved. They designated Mrs. Brent an official foster mother for Carl at age 4.

Two years later, when Carl was 6, Mrs. Brent was informed that under the law of the state a permanent adoptive home had to be found for Carl. She was told that if she did not agree to adopt him a new home would be found. Because Carl's natural mother had not contacted him in many years, the child welfare agency was pushing for a procedure known as "termination of parental rights."

The therapist, a psychology intern, worked very hard to engage this family in treatment. She had a number of sessions with Carl and Mrs. Brent in which she attempted to clarify the boundaries between them and to reinforce Mrs. Brent's parental role. She also attempted to schedule sessions with the entire family, which were always cancelled. Finally, Mrs. Brent, who suffered from asthma and a cardiac condition, was hospitalized after a severe asthma attack. During that period, Carl's child welfare worker continued to bring him for treatment. The therapist began to lose contact with Mrs. Brent and to become increasingly angry at her for her resistance to treatment. She was preparing to terminate their case.

Learning from Our Mistakes

The family had pulled back from treatment. Mrs. Brent felt increasingly threatened by what she perceived as observations of and judgments about her mothering. The therapist and her supervisor realized rather late in the treatment process that Mrs. Brent was resistant because she saw the therapist as an extension of the child welfare agency, which she perceived as having the power to remove "her child." A session was arranged in which the therapist and her supervisor met with Mrs. Brent and explored this issue. The therapist asked Mrs. Brent how she saw her role. She also shared with Mrs. Brent that many families in her situation had told her that they weren't sure they could trust the therapist. Mrs. Brent burst into tears. She shared for the first time that she had been terrified for more than a year that Carl, whom she thought of as her child, would be taken away.

Mrs. Brent was also very conflicted about the adoption process in other ways. She and her family were attached to Carl and wanted to keep him. They would have gladly continued in their "informal" arrangement throughout his life. She was very anxious, however, about the process to "terminate" his mother's rights. In her view, which reflects Black cultural values, one never terminates a mother's rights to her child even if someone else raises him and becomes his de facto mother. In a variety of ways she communicated this conflict and ambivalence to Carl, which he interpreted as her hesitancy about keeping him. She was so conflicted that she had difficulty setting limits for him. He was treated very differently by the entire family and was infantilized by them.

In addition, the formal adoptive process brought with it a number of evaluations, which are routine and are designed to evaluate the quality of the psychological and emotional bonding of the parent, child, and family. These procedures were never explained to Mrs. Brent, and she therefore felt that everyone was judging her mothering of Carl and finding problems.

She explained to the therapist that she had read a report that said that Carl was more bonded to her daughter Evelyn than to her, and she was therefore afraid to let the therapist meet the rest of her family.

The therapist was then able to help Mrs. Brent to separate her role from that of the child welfare agency. Poor Black families feel very much at the mercy of these agencies and truly do feel that they could "lose their children." The therapist encouraged Mrs. Brent to ask for a meeting with the therapist and the child welfare worker to discuss her concerns about the adoption process and her fears of losing Carl. The worker explained that the evaluations were a "routine" part of the assessment process. At this meeting a child welfare worker was able to help her to see that in her particular case, there was no danger of losing her child but that there were some problems that could be helped by family therapy. She was then able to "begin again" in treatment. Unfortunately, as so often occurs in our training programs, the psychology intern was completing her internship and leaving at this point. She was, however, able to help Mrs. Brent "clear the air" and recontract for treatment for Carl and her family.

The Brent family "started over" with a new therapist with whom Mrs. Brent was now able to develop a bond of trust. She met regularly and involved her other family members. By the time treatment was completed, Mrs. Brent and her other children had learned how to work together to provide clear, consistent limits for Carl, instead of setting up a good mother/bad mother dynamic between Mrs. Brent and Evelyn. All family members were helped to verbalize their fears and anger about the protracted nature of the adoptive process, and Carl was able to talk about how jealous he was of Rashan because Rashan was a "real family member." Once these issues were out in the open, they could be addressed, and Mrs. Brent could be helped to take charge of handling them with Carl instead of ignoring them or delegating them to one of her daughters.

The therapist also supported Mrs. Brent in calling regular meetings with the child welfare agency in order to get clarification about the lengthy and complex adoptive process.

Although the complexity of the formal adoptive process gives an added dimension to this case, Mrs. Brent's reactions are not atypical of many poor African American families who feel judged and intruded upon by outside agencies. The therapists and supervisor who worked with this family learned a number of important lessons from their early mistakes. They learned to pay close attention to how families perceive therapists. Particularly in cases where a family is brought in or referred by another agency, it is important for therapists to create some distance between themselves and the outside agency and to clarify their differences in roles. This is a difficult process at times because the therapist does need to have contact with and to work closely with the agencies involved. As in this case, however, it is important for the therapist to help empower the parental figures to call meetings with agencies when necessary and to voice their own concerns. If this is not done, therapists become parental surrogates or create a false dependency on both themselves and the therapeutic process.

In this case the therapists also learned not to minimize or fail to address the very real fear of many poor African American mothers that their children will be removed by child protective agencies. Most have either had this experience themselves or know of other families in their communities who have had similar experiences.

14

Single-Parent
African American Families

The startling increase in African American female-headed families within the last three decades parallels a similar trend in all U.S. families. In the last 30 years the number of single-parent households in the United States has more than doubled. These single-parent households include a diversity of family structures (e.g., single never-married, single divorced or separated, and single widowed).

FUNCTIONAL SINGLE-PARENT FAMILIES

Clinicians typically work with families who are in trouble or in crisis. It is important therefore to keep a clear perspective on what constitutes a "well-functioning" family. This is particularly important when one is dealing with African American single-parent families because so much of the early literature was derogatory (e.g., Moynihan, 1965). One must avoid the tendency to see families whose structure may be very different from that of the clinician as "deviant." Therefore, it would be helpful to begin the discussion of single-parent African American families by describing what constitutes a well-functioning African American single-parent family.

Single parenthood does not necessarily make a family dysfunctional. Many African American single parents who have never been married function well as parents, and their children grow up to be capable adults. Many divorced or separated Black single parents—a population that is increasing in numbers, similar to the White population—are functional as well.

The first characteristic of functional African American single-parent families is a clear understanding of who is in charge of the family. As Minuchin

(1974) has illustrated, all family members know precisely their roles and responsibilities in the family. The functional family has well-delineated, but flexible boundaries and all of the children have easy access to the parent (Nichols & Schwartz, 1998). Whether the parent is working or on public assistance, the children are well cared for and their basic needs are met. Emotionally, both parent and children feel free to give and receive nurturance and communicate their own needs.

In some functional single-parent families, there may be a parental child who helps the mother care for younger children. This may be an economic necessity: an older child may care for his or her siblings when a parent works to support the family. Once again, the mere presence of this structure is not dysfunctional in and of itself. A single-parent family with a parental child can function quite well as long as the parent does not abdicate parental responsibilities or overburden this child in an inappropriate way. A parent who delegates certain responsibilities to her oldest son or daughter while she is at work but who assumes leadership when she is at home can often support the development of a sense of responsibility in her child. The parental child must also have access to other age-appropriate peer activities and not feel that the total responsibility for the care of the family is on his or her shoulders. In these functional African American families, single parents keep an open dialogue with each of their children and are sensitive to issues such as the ones described here. Parental children in these situations receive praise and nurturance along with responsibility.

Another feature of well-functioning African American single-parent families is that they have and utilize a support system. This might include blood and nonblood extended family, church members, friends, and community supports. They are not cut off and they are not afraid to ask for help when it is needed. If a father (or fathers) is (are) not involved, other men in the extended family or the broader network are utilized as male role models. Children have a sense of "belonging" to a family. The other extended family members are involved with the children in a constructive way and do not undermine the mother's role or authority with them.

The final aspect of these well-functioning families is that the parents (usually mothers) have a life of their own apart from their children. Among Black single-parent mothers, this life can take many different forms. It might involve having a job or a career or having a boyfriend. For many Black women, the church serves a very important social function and often constitutes their only time for themselves apart from their children.

TYPES OF PROBLEMATIC SINGLE-PARENT FAMILIES

Because of the significant numbers of single-parent families mentioned above, it is very important for family therapists who are working with single-parent African American families to be aware of the common issues in these families and the different ways in which they may present. The following section discusses the clinical implications of a number of different presentations of single-parent families: (1) the underorganized family; (2) the overcentralized, overwhelmed mother; (3) the dysfunctional parent; and (4) the boyfriend, or hidden family member.

The Underorganized Family

One clinical presentation of African American single-parent families is that of the underorganized family in which children seem out of control and mother appears totally overwhelmed. Aponte (1994) describes this type of family as one in which

> power is loosely distributed . . . the power of any one individual is not effectively woven through the various operations in which he or she is involved, nor is it balanced flexibly. . . . In the underorganized family, a parent may not be able to take for granted his/her power and may be able to exercise it only when he/she asserts it with exceptional force. In such a household, one is likely to see a mother repeatedly yelling or striking her children to obtain some order. (p. 438)

Boundaries in this type of family are usually very vague. There is no clarity as to the rules and responsibilities of the members. Alignment patterns in this type of family tend to be extremely inconsistent and chaotic, with different family members siding with each other randomly and inconsistently. Power is weak and force is inconsistent: excessive sometimes and nonexistent at other times. If one visits the home of such a family, one is met with a sense of underorganization at the front door. Family members often function in a manner reminiscent of "bumper cars," colliding with one another and interacting briefly but never really relating. Mothers in these families tend to be totally overwhelmed, often having "stairstep" children very close in age and being unable to manage the pressures and burdens they face.

In some underorganized African American families, there is inconsistent extended family involvement; when it occurs, it is usually erratic, unpredictable, and destabilizing rather than supportive. In other families of this type the family is very emotionally cut off (Bowen, 1976) from extended family supports and there is no one who supports the parent in assuming executive parental responsibilities. The degree of dysfunction in these families is often directly related to their degree of isolation or lack of utilization of their supports.

On the continuum of family involvement described by Minuchin (1974), these families can be characterized as "disengaged." The feelings of being overwhelmed cause underorganized families to be "in crisis" all the time and to present with one or more children in serious trouble at home, in school, and/or in the community.

Overcentralized Mothers

The second type of a single-parent African American family that often presents at clinics is characterized by Aponte (1994) as "overcentralized," or having power overconcentrated in one person, usually a very overwhelmed and overburdened mother. She is in fact the "switchboard" for family communication:

> A single or a few family members may possess an inordinate amount of control over all operations, regardless of function. Since any single person, or even an exclusive few can never, by the force of their talents, make every family undertaking work, this kind of overconcentrated power is inefficient. If a mother holds on to all the family controls, her young children may be very well-behaved in her presence, but very disorderly and negligent about carrying out household duties whenever she is out of the home. (p. 437)

On the continuum of family boundaries described by Minuchin (1974), these families are often on the "enmeshed" end of the scale. While this structure may function adequately with young children, it often leads to difficulty in adolescence, when this rigid, mother-dominated structure is challenged by her teenagers. Behavior problems in adolescent children usually present at this time, including stealing, lying, running away, and oppositional behavior at home and in school. Often other children or family members collude to undermine the power of the overly central mother. Aponte, in a masterful videotape, has illustrated the strategy of working with such a family.

The R. family was an African American family composed of a mother, age 38, and four children, girls ages 17, 16, and 12½, and a son, age 18. The mother and the three daughters attended the session. The mother began by characterizing herself as "overprotective" of all of her children. She was the central force at home and usually "preached to" her kids rather than talked with them. She expressed particular concerns about the lying and behavior problems of her 12½-year-old daughter and the school problems of her 16-year-old. With careful questioning, the therapist learned that the mother had kept a very high degree of control over her children when they were young, but as they reached adolescence each became more oppositional in school and at home. In focusing on the acting out and the lying of the youngest child, he learned that the two older girls often protected their younger sister from their mother's censure and "took her off punishment." The therapist relabeled the entire family's involvement as "loving her too much" and helped the mother to ask for the help of her older children in working together to provide limits for her younger child. He helped her to learn how to delegate responsibility when she was at work and to involve her adolescents appropriately in the decision-making process.

The therapist then encouraged the mother to talk about the reasons for her "overprotectiveness" and her own experiences of growing up. He helped her to see that a part of what she must teach her children is how to be strong and stand on their own two feet as she does. By helping her to involve the older children in this process, he facilitated her move to decentralize herself and delegate responsibility appropriately.

The Dysfunctional Parent

Another type of presentation in single-parent African American families is that of an obviously dysfunctional parent whose children are actually "running the family." Often this is characterized by an overburdened parental child. This can occur for a number of reasons. The mother may have (1) a medical illness, (2) an emotional or psychiatric disorder, (3) a drug or alcohol addiction, or (4) a low intellectual level or mental retardation. In some of these families, a highly functional parental child essentially runs the household. The family often does not present until this role conflicts with the developmental thrust toward age-appropriate independence in the adolescent.

Frequently, however, these families resemble the first category of underorganized families, in which the mother presents as a member of the sibling group rather than as the head of the family. The strategy outlined in the first example applies here also. The therapist's task is to help build a family structure that can function predictably and help meet the needs of all its members. In this case, however, the family therapist is faced with the dilemma that the executive member may in fact be dysfunctional and unable to assume those responsibilities. The therapist must first assess the mother's capabilities and support her in exercising what power she has. In some cases the therapist's task will be to seek support for her outside of the family in order to help her function in her role and relieve the burden on her children.

A more extreme example of this type of parental-child-controlled/dysfunctional parent system is that of the alcoholic single-parent family. Often as the mother becomes increasingly incapacitated by her alcoholism, an older child will assume the parental child role for the mother as well as for the other children. In some African American alcoholic families this child is often female and becomes what Brisbane and Womble (1985–1986) call the "Black female family hero." These "family heroes" assume total responsibility but receive little or no nurturance. Brisbane and Womble state that in alcoholic families there is "a greater possibility that [the family hero] will not receive nurturing which is necessary if she is to pass through the various stages of her own development with a sense of fulfillment and mastery" (p. 254). This pattern can also be seen in families where a parent is drug-involved.

Because of her central role, the involvement of this "family hero" is crucial in the treatment of such families. It is also important to note that these families come to our attention via two main routes: (1) by extreme acting out in the younger children and/or (2) a threat by an outside child welfare agency to remove the children. Often the latter is necessary to produce a sufficient crisis for the family to mobilize and for the alcoholic member to even consider a treatment program. The following case example illustrates this process.

The Glenns were an African American family referred for treatment after Ms. Glenn, the mother, was reported to the local child welfare agency by neighbors for neglecting her children. The family consisted of Mary (age 15), the "family hero" who cared for the younger children; Brian (age 6); Nikki (age 4); and Kenya (age

2). As her mother's alcoholism worsened, Mary took on more and more family responsibilities and ultimately became frustrated and unable to cope. She gave up and began neglecting the younger children. The child welfare agency removed the three younger children and placed them in separate foster homes pending an investigation. Mary was sent to a group home for adolescents. As often occurs in these cases, the referral to our clinic was made for Brian, the 6-year-old, who became aggressive in the foster home and at school. When he was first seen, he was extremely angry and frightened at being separated from his family. The family therapist mobilized the child welfare agency to transport all family members including the mother to a session at the clinic. The mother had been given an ultimatum by the agency to enter an alcoholism treatment program or her children would not be returned. She was very frightened of losing them and expressed that fear in the session. Mary, true to her role, quickly moved in to comfort her mother.

The therapist emphasized the love and caring in this family and the desire of the mother to be with her children. The mother discussed her fears about the alcoholism treatment program. With the support of her children and that of the therapist, she agreed to enter an inpatient alcoholism treatment program at an affiliated hospital. The therapist was able to arrange for her to participate in family sessions during this time. In the initial detoxification period, Ms. Glenn was extremely irritable and "snappish" with her children. Mary again tuned in to her mother's distress and tried to quiet the other children. The therapist talked with Mary and her mother about this impossible job that she had taken on of trying to be "supermom." This theme was stressed for a number of sessions. As Ms. Glenn became more functional, the therapist encouraged her to take more responsibility for talking directly to the children and planning for their return. As she soothed and talked with the children, Brian's aggressive behavior decreased in the foster home and at school. Mary was initially blocked from intervening by the therapist. The mother was helped to talk openly with her daughter about the burden that had been placed upon her. In these discussions in subsequent sessions the mother was surprised to learn how serious Mary's neglect of her own needs had been. She had been truant half of the school days in the last year. Because of her alcoholic haze, the mother had been oblivious to her daughter's distress. In one very tearful session, she expressed her sadness and sorrow about this to her daughter.

After discharge, the alcoholism treatment program required a long-term follow-up and intensive outpatient and AA (Alcoholics Anonymous) involvement. During that time, the therapist worked with Ms. Glenn and her children to discuss carefully how things would be different when the children returned home. Although Mary and the other children were still in foster homes, Ms. Glenn (at the therapist's urging) arranged to go with Mary to school and to discuss her needs. At the mother's request, the therapist accompanied her on this first visit. The mother also made a visit to Brian's school and was pleased to learn that his aggressive behavior had decreased. For the first time in many years, she was assuming appropriate parental responsibilities.

As the time for the children's return home approached, the therapist helped to arrange for a homemaker from a social service agency to care for the younger children and help with some household chores while Ms. Glenn attended her AA meetings and treatment sessions. Family therapy continued throughout the first year of the return home. The focus was on emphasizing and reinforcing the mother's competence and helping Mary to give up the "family hero" role and become involved with her school and her peers. Ms. Glenn became directly responsible for the care of Brian and the two younger children. Brian's aggressive acting out stopped completely within the first month of his return home. At the time of completion of treatment, Ms. Glenn had been abstinent from alcohol for over a year and was an active member of AA.

The Boyfriend: The Hidden Family Member

Some single-parent African American families that include the mother's live-in boyfriend function extremely well, with the boyfriend considered as a viable member of the family. In others, the mother's boyfriend is a "hidden" family member. The mental health field has been in a dilemma as to how to label this "family member's" role in Black families. He has been referred to by a series of derogatory terms, such as the "paramour," and, in more long-term unions, as the "common-law husband." In other cases where a marriage eventually occurs and he has been absorbed into the children's lives, he may be referred to as the "stepfather." The role of the boyfriend is a complex one in Black single-parent families because it is often "hidden" when the family initially presents for treatment for a number of reasons discussed in previous chapters.

This section focuses on the three major ways in which the boyfriend can become an important focus in family therapy: (1) secrecy about his presence; (2) his involvement in the treatment process; and (3) the definition of his role in the family.

Secrecy about the presence of a boyfriend is an issue that many family therapists must address in the treatment of these families. Often, the mother presents initially with her children as a family unit and makes no mention of her boyfriend, or his presence is so minimized that his involvement with the family is at first very unclear. Because African American families often do not trust clinics and therapists initially and are dubious about confidentiality, the issue of the boyfriend is usually not available for discussion until trust is developed. Once the family, particularly the mother, trusts the therapist, the boyfriend will often be mentioned much more openly. Sometimes the children in the family will begin discussing this person. Many African American mothers initially deny such relationships even to their own children. Indeed, these boyfriends might be called "uncles" by the children. The entire family often colludes to deny the true relationship. Once a family raises the issue of the boyfriend, the therapist should definitely pursue discussions of his role and function in the family and consider including him in a session.

One of the most helpful ways in which to raise the issue of the boyfriend with a single-parent mother is to ask her frankly, "Who helps you out?" This can be pursued by a question such as "With all of these responsibilities for taking care of everyone else, who takes care of you?" Asking a mother if she dates or goes out herself can help focus attention on her role as a woman apart from her role as a mother. This is a very important intervention with Black single-parent mothers. If the therapist has communicated support and not censure, these issues can then be discussed more openly.

Once the boyfriend's presence can be discussed, the family therapist can begin to explore his role and the amount of time that he has been involved with the mother and with her children. The answers to both these questions tend to vary because many African American women choose not to involve their boyfriends in their children's lives unless a clear commitment has evolved between the partners.

At this point, it is often helpful to include the boyfriend in the treatment process. The first task is the issue of engagement. It is often helpful for the therapist to contact the man directly by phone or letter and to try to talk or meet with him alone before bringing him into the family sessions. If a man is living as part of a household or even "visiting" or "staying over" on a regular basis, he has an impact on the family alignments, boundaries, and roles within the home. It is often necessary to state how important he is to the family and to let him know that his input will be valued and respected.

The role relationships that boyfriends develop within such situations vary considerably. Some are essentially peripheral to the running of the household and the care of the children, visiting primarily for sexual encounters with the mother. Still others may "stay over" regularly, eating meals at the home and keeping clothes there. In other cases, there is a long-term "live-in" relationship from which there may be children. In many states, if this persists for 7 years or more, it is considered a "common-law marriage." There are also situations that begin as one of the above and eventually evolve into a marriage. Although this situation would officially qualify as a "stepfather" relationship, some of the issues are similar to those discussed above. Despite the label or the surface description of the relationship or the period of time involved, one must carefully clarify the degree of involvement that the man has with the children and the amount of his responsibility for parenting, childcare, and discipline.

One of the most common issues in the involvement of boyfriends in African American single-parent families is the protectiveness that many Black mothers exercise in the involvement of their men with their children. Often, even if a man has been living in a home for many years and expresses a desire to be involved in parenting, the mother in this situation will create a "buffer" between her children and the man. This may continue to be true even after the relationship evolves into marriage. The case of the Jacobs family illustrates this point.

Ms. Jacobs, an African American woman in her 30s, initially presented at the clinic with her three children, ages 16, 15, and 2. She was very careful to avoid mentioning her boyfriend of 6 years. The identified patient was her son Anthony, age 16, who was having academic difficulties in school and who would often have loud arguments with his mother. He refused to follow her rules and often came home long after his curfew in the evening. He had been suspended from school after having been picked up by a truant officer outside of school during class hours. The therapist worked initially to help the mother to set clear limits for her son and to be consistent in her discipline with all of the children. She had great difficulty in doing this, and eventually shared with the therapist that John, her live-in boyfriend, was always "after her" to discipline Anthony. She stated that her boyfriend felt she was "too soft on the boy." They often got into arguments in which the mother would tell her son to do one thing and her boyfriend would criticize her openly in front of the boy. The therapist, recognizing the triangulation that was occurring in this process, called the boyfriend and asked him to join a family session.

In the session, the boyfriend sat on the periphery of the family. Ironically, the family member seated closest to him was Anthony. During the course of the session, it became clear that Anthony had had a rather good relationship with his mother's boyfriend until 2 years ago when his little sister had been born. At that point, the boyfriend had begun to live with the family. He had attempted to take over some of the disciplinary responsibility but was always blocked by the mother, who would yell "Don't you touch my son!"

The therapist asked the mother and her boyfriend to sit together. She then asked them to discuss the question of the parenting of Anthony and who should do it. The mother stated that she didn't feel her boyfriend should take over and was very fearful of this. Her boyfriend stated that he just wanted to help and became angry when she allowed her son to "talk back" to her. The therapist helped these two individuals to discuss a consistent policy for handling Anthony, including the establishment of clear rules and consequences. They agreed that Ms. Jacobs would present these to Anthony with her boyfriend there to support her statements. They agreed, for example, that if Anthony was truant from school or was late coming in the evening, he would not be allowed out with his friends for a week. They were able to reinforce the rules together.

The therapist also helped Ms. Jacobs to create a regular time when she could talk with her son alone about his needs, and she was able to encourage him to spend some "man time" working on the car with her boyfriend.

Often the therapist's role is one of helping a family in transition to negotiate the inclusion of a new member. This transition is often made more difficult by the mother's own ambivalence, and possibly by her earlier experiences with men. For example, a woman who has had a number of painful relationships may find it very difficult to trust a new man and allow him to become involved with her children.

In other situations, the family therapist's task is to help a young single mother to place a protective boundary around her children and separate them from her transient relationships with men. The case of Laura Tate and her children illustrates this situation.

Laura Tate was a 25-year-old Black single parent who came into treatment after a referral by a sexual abuse unit at a local hospital. Her 5-year-old daughter, Imani, had been raped by her mother's boyfriend. This boyfriend, although he did not live in the home, had visited frequently. The therapist learned that the mother had in fact been raped as a young child by her "uncle," but had never discussed the experience with anyone. Imani was having night terrors since the experience and would frequently have angry outbursts at her mother. She had also been involved in some sexual play at school.

A strategic "pretend" strategy (Madanes, 1981) was utilized in which Imani was asked to pretend to be frightened of an assailant and her mother would pretend to protect her. The mother would then pretend to be frightened of an assailant and Imani would pretend to protect her. This scenario was prescribed every night before bedtime. Imani's symptoms disappeared within a few weeks. Her mother was able to talk about her own unresolved experience of sexual assault as a child and to discuss ways in which she would protect her daughter in the future. Ms. Tate was able to create a protective boundary around her child and to discuss openly the need to be careful about exposing her daughter to her male relationships. Most importantly, however, she began to establish a relationship with her daughter such that the daughter could feel safe in speaking to her mother. A channel of communication that had been closed was opened between them. This was the beginning of trust.

Lindblad-Goldberg and Dukes (1985) have compared "functional vs. dysfunctional Black single-parent families" and have made the following observation regarding boyfriends:

> Mothers of less adaptive families more frequently relied on boyfriends to help with their family's functioning. These network males may be a less stable type of support for the single-parent mother in that their role definitions and functions within the family might not have been clearly defined.

This observation is certainly a challenging one. It is particularly relevant in families in which the mother continually changes boyfriends or has very short-term relationships and has either very negative interactions with her extended family or is cut off from them. In these situations, she and her children may rely too heavily on her current boyfriend for emotional and financial support, which may result in his overload or a burnout of that relationship because of the premature burden of caring for a family. In these circumstances, it may be the task of the therapist to help the mother resolve her issues with her own extended family and/or to create other supports for her family that are not dependent on the survival of her relationship with a current boyfriend.

EXTENDED FAMILY AND NETWORK INVOLVEMENT FOR AFRICAN AMERICAN SINGLE-PARENT FAMILIES: POSITIVE AND NEGATIVE CONSEQUENCES

The importance of the extended family as a strength for African American families was clearly documented in Chapter 3. However, many Black single-parent families that present at clinics may have experienced a breakdown in the support function of the extended family. In some cases, the presentation of a child as the identified patient may in fact be a symptom of a dysfunctional structure or pattern of relationships within the extended family. This is a complicated issue for many clinicians and family therapists. As therapists, we have often been trained to take the "single-parent family" at face value when they appear at our clinics. Too often, however, this is a serious error because the family that presents may well be a subsystem of a much more complex extended family. The presenting problem brought by a member of an African American single-parent family may well be a symptom of a dysfunctional pattern or an emotional cutoff in the extended family.

Lindblad-Goldberg and Dukes (1985) make the following observation in their study of functional and dysfunctional African American single-parent families:

> One primary implication to be drawn for ecostructural therapy with low-income female-headed families is not to assume that an extended kinship network necessarily operates as a support system. In working with these families it is important to assess how the presenting problem relates not merely to dysfunctional structure within the nuclear family but rather to the dysfunctional structure(s) in the extended kinship system of both blood and non-related persons. Thus, the definition of the "family" becomes the definition of the extended kinship system.

Findings such as those of Lindblad-Goldberg and Dukes are very relevant to our clinical assessment of these families. The primary concern of these researchers was "to discover if there were differences in the social networks of functional and dysfunctional African American low-income female-headed families." In looking at a clinic and a nonclinic population of African American single-parent families in Philadelphia, they found the following results: (1) there were no significant differences in the numbers of family members involved; (2) more female than male network members were reported for both groups; and (3) the importance of support categories were reported in the following order: "family," "friends," and "relatives." The three categories were described to the interviewers as: (1) family—mother's children, mother's siblings, mother's parent(s); (2) friends, both female and male; and (3) relatives—grandparents, aunts, uncles, cousins (female and male), nieces, nephews, and inlaws (p. 9).

Lindblad-Goldberg and Dukes (1985) and Lindblad-Goldberg, Dukes, and Lasley (1988) identified other variables including those described by Pattison (1977) in the "neurotic type" of network. "Less adaptive" mothers more frequently listed people who were deceased as important to them. They also tended to list more people who were important because they were disliked or because they caused these mothers difficulty. This type of network can be impoverished and isolating (Pattison, 1977). The unresolved mourning and subsequent longing for a lost object may prevent these mothers from interacting meaningfully with those available to them. In addition, real-life interaction may be limited by avoidance of contact, especially when there are negative emotional influences in some of these relationships.

This distinction is important because sometimes these families present with severe problems, especially after the loss of a very significant family member such as the mother's mother or grandmother who may have "held the family together" or been "Big Mama" to everyone. This often leaves a very real emotional and executive vacuum in the family, which the single-parent mother who has suffered such a loss may feel that she is unable to fill. The case of the Wilson family illustrates the emotional impasses that can arise in such a situation.

The Wilson family entered treatment when Vernette, age 12, began fighting with her peers and acting out in school. The teacher reported that when she was not fighting she appeared isolated from other children and somewhat withdrawn. The teacher encouraged Vernette's mother, Ms. Wilson, to take her to a local mental health center for treatment. The Wilson family consisted of Ms. Wilson (age 26), Vernette, Willy (age 9), and Paula (age 7). When asked by the therapist when Vernette's problems had begun, all the family members became very quiet. Finally Ms. Wilson stated that they had started a year earlier. When the therapist explored what had been happening in the family at that time, at first all of the family members looked puzzled. The therapist then asked if there had been any changes in the family at that time, whether anyone had died, left, and/or entered the family. Ms. Wilson then reported in a very tearful voice that her mother had died about a year ago. Vernette had been very close to her grandmother and took her death "hard." All of the family members looked very sad and found it difficult to talk about her death. The therapist very gently helped them to talk about that period. She learned that the grandmother had been the real "mother" in this family. She had been the family switchboard and most of the family's communications had passed through her. She had "held the family together." When she died suddenly of a heart attack, Ms. Wilson found herself alone raising her children, and she felt completely overwhelmed. At the time of her mother's death, Ms. Wilson's sister, Martha, and her two children, who had also been living in the grandmother's apartment, moved in with Martha's boyfriend. Ms. Wilson felt betrayed and abandoned and had not spoken to her sister since then. Ms. Wilson had become more depressed in the last year and had withdrawn from her children. She had begun to stay in her bed, frequently for much of the day, leaving the care of the younger children to Vernette. No one in the family had mourned the grandmother's death, and both Vernette and her mother were feeling sad, overwhelmed, and abandoned.

The therapist's first task was to help this family mourn. In a number of very emotional sessions, Ms. Wilson talked with her children about their sadness. Vernette and Ms. Wilson were able to talk about their feelings of being alone and having to take on all the family responsibilities. The therapist had a number of sessions with Ms. Wilson during this period and placed her on antidepressant medication. As Ms. Wilson felt given to or "fed" by the therapist, she was able to give to her daughter.

It became clear that Ms. Wilson's mother had held all the decision-making power in the family and that Ms. Wilson needed help to evolve into her role as "mother." A number of sessions were held with Ms. Wilson and her children in which the therapist supported her in assuming a parental role with her children. Therapy focused on such concrete issues as (1) a planned visit to Vernette's school, (2) homework, and (3) discipline at home.

As the family's depression began to lift, the degree of isolation in which they functioned became increasingly clear. A number of sessions were spent in helping the family construct its genogram and look at its former support system. The emotional cutoff of Ms. Wilson from her sister was very loaded for her because they had been very close. The children were very close to her also. In an atmosphere of increasing trust, the therapist was able to challenge Ms. Wilson's assumption that her sister had left because she "didn't want to live with her anymore." In the discussion of her possible reasons for leaving, Ms. Wilson was able to acknowledge the possibility that her sister may have felt freer to live with her boyfriend after their mother's death and that her move had not been related to her sister at all. The therapist, with the children's support, encouraged Ms. Wilson to go talk to her sister about this. After many weeks of discussion and coaching (following Bowen, 1978), she was able to call her sister. Their reconciliation was a major step in reconnecting with the rest of the extended family.

Both Vernette and Ms. Wilson were not depressed at the completion of treatment and Vernette had shown significant improvement in school.

There were a number of other areas of difference between functional and dysfunctional single-parent families that Lindblad-Goldberg and Dukes (1985) have identified in their study. One key area was an imbalance of reciprocity in the extended families:

> Being able to count on someone for concrete assistance such as helping with domestic tasks, finances, child care, is a critical factor for all low-income families. A significant difference found between these successful and non-successful families was that perceived help from family network members was less for families in trouble than for those doing well. The groups did not differ in the amount of help they felt they gave to network persons.

This is an important piece of information for the family therapist who is working with such families. An imbalance in the reciprocity loop or "kin insurance" (McAdoo, 1981, 1996) can give rise to a situation in which the usual, culturally prescribed patterns are not occurring in a particular family. The task of the therapist with a broader systems perspective is to help the family or the individual single-parent mother find a way to balance the scales. This might involve renegotiating relationships in her extended family and/or helping her to find other sources of support. In some families this support may exist, but the single mother and her children may not be benefiting because of an emotional cutoff that has occurred. In other situations the single mother may have become overcentral and overburdened, but because she has been playing that role for so long she has never learned how to scream for help or how to accept it when it is given.

15

Middle-Class
African American Families

The numbers of African American middle-class families have increased dramatically in the last 30 years (see Chapter 1; Billingsley, 1992; Hill, 1999a; Landry, 1987; Pattillo-McCoy, 1999; Daniels, 2001). Moreover, there has been a small, but growing, cohort of upper-income African Americans (see Chapter 1; Billingsley, 1992; Collins, 1997; Graham, 1999; Hill, 1999a).

Billingsley (1992) discussed the reasons therapists should not assume that income levels are a decisive measure of African American progress or that the same income level has the equivalent meaning for Blacks as for Whites:

> Most middle-class blacks are still first-generation middle class. In the foreseeable future, they may continue to be characterized by their precariousness, as more dependent than independent, more employees of others than owners and managers, and with relatively little accumulated wealth. Moderate and even high salaries and income will not automatically translate into wealth, which refers to the net value of assets over liabilities. (p. 287)

Whites of comparable income levels have as much as 10 times the wealth and assets of Blacks (Anderson, 1994; Hill, 1999a; Oliver & Shapiro, 1995), whose status is largely the result of Blacks living in traditional families where both parents work and contribute two incomes. Despite these cautions, as Billingsley (1992) has stated, "the black middle class is a major achievement sustained by education, two earners, extended families, religion, and service to others" (p. 287).

Mental health professionals make a mistake when they assume that middle- and upper-income Black families have "made it" and are now free of the burdens of racism (Wilson, 1987). Successful Blacks actually experience a more covert form of personal and institutional racism (Collins, 1997; Coner-

300

Edwards & Spurlock, 1988; Cose, 1993; Feagin & Sikes, 1994; Hill, 1999a; Landry, 1991; Staples & Johnson, 1993)—stressors that often lead them to seek therapy.

The majority of the literature on African American families has focused primarily on low-income families. In recent years, however, a number of researchers have begun to explore patterns of upward mobility and middle-class status among Black families (Bagarozzi, 1980; Billingsley, 1992; Collins, 1997; Coner-Edwards & Spurlock,1988; Cose, 1993; Daniels, 2001, 2002a; Feagin & Sikes, 1994; Graham, 1999; Hill, 1999a; Landry, 1987; McAdoo, 1981, 1996, 2002; Stack, 1974; Staples & Johnson, 1993; Watkins, 2001).

McAdoo (1978, 1981) discusses two different views of the role that the extended family or the kin network may play in the upward mobility of African American families. The first view describes a positive impact of the African American extended family on upward mobility and states that Blacks have moved up the economic scale because of the help of their kin network (Billingsley, 1968, 1992; Hill, 1972, 1999a). The second viewpoint, represented by McQueen (1971) and Stack (1974), states that although Black families have developed patterns of mutual help and kin support that aid them in the struggle to cope with poverty, the extended family becomes a liability once a Black individual or family become middle class (McQueen, 1971). McAdoo (1978) summarized this viewpoint as follows:

> McQueen and Stack seem to indicate that only by cutting him/herself off from the family can the black of poorer circumstances move up to a more stable level of living. This isolation does not exclude casual visiting and joint holiday and ritual celebrations. It also does not exclude support of aging parents or occasional help. It does mean that to some degree, upwardly mobile blacks separate themselves from the draining process of dealing with the everyday needs of their families of orientation. (p. 764)

In contrast, McAdoo's (1978, 1981, 1996) and Billingsley's (1992) results indicate that African American families in the middle-income group in general maintained their close ties to their extended families and did not have to avoid these ties in order to become upwardly mobile. The data from such findings challenge the notion that economic well-being is achieved at the cost of denying bonds of family, extended family, race, and culture.

CLASS AND SOCIOECONOMIC DIFFERENCES WITHIN AFRICAN AMERICAN FAMILIES

Therapists should be aware that, because of the involvement with extended family members in many African American families, there may be considerable variability in income and class level among family members. This phenomenon can be illustrated by the following case.

The Daniels family was composed of three adult siblings: one male, Robert (age 38), and two females, June (age 39) and Pat (age 32). Their parents were deceased. Robert was a lawyer, living with his wife and children in a Chicago suburb. June, who was the parental child, was a teacher and divorced mother living with her two children in New Jersey. The youngest sibling, Pat, was an active crack addict whose one child, Chandra (age 7), had been living in foster homes for 2 years. Pat was often homeless and difficult to locate.

Child welfare services informed Robert and June that their sister's parental rights were being terminated. The siblings were confronted with the possibility that their niece would be adopted by someone outside the family. Robert and his wife were not willing to take Chandra in, but June, consistent with being the parental child, felt she had the obligation to adopt her niece and give her a home.

June sought therapy because of her ambivalence about her decision to adopt Chandra who had been born with fetal drug syndrome, was diagnosed with attention-deficit/hyperactivity disorder (ADHD), and was engaging in acting-out behaviors in June's home. Even though June earned a good salary as a teacher, providing for Chandra was extremely stressful. The small stipend provided by the special needs adoption services pursuant to the Adoption and Safe Families Act of 1997 (see Chapter 12) was not sufficient to obtain the help Chandra required and paying for these services out of her salary made June feel that she was depriving her own children. Her anger at Chandra for acting out, and at her sister for putting her in this untenable position due to substance abuse, left June deeply troubled, depressed, and overwhelmed.

These types of presenting problems are quite common among African American clients, particularly women, who are very connected to extended family members. It is important to remember that even if your clients are financially successful, they often contribute to the financial or emotional support of family members who are less-well-off.

DIFFERENT TYPES OF AFRICAN AMERICAN MIDDLE-CLASS FAMILIES

Four different mobility patterns evident in African American families have been identified by McAdoo (1981, 1986, 1996).

1. In the first group are individuals who were born into the working class and are newly upwardly mobile. Generally, they became middle class by acquiring professional degrees and moving into higher status jobs.
2. The second group is composed of those who have been upwardly mobile over three generations from lower class, to working class, to middle class.
3. The third group was born into middle-class status but had less educational achievement than their parents.

4. In the fourth group of families the grandparents, parents, and the current generation had all maintained their middle-class status.

One disturbing aspect of Black family upward mobility, which does not tend to have the same effect when it occurs in White families, is the difficulty Black families have in maintaining their middle-class status in subsequent generations. McAdoo's (1978, 1981, 1996) research indicates that some families may experience a decline in future generations, with educational achievement—and the ability to achieve a particular socioeconomic status—having peaked in the generation that was upwardly mobile. McAdoo hypothesizes that being born into middle-class surroundings may reduce the success drive that motivates those in lower socioeconomic brackets. Middle-class status and financial security can provide the freedom to pursue a career path based on individual interest rather than economic need (McAdoo, 1978, pp. 767–768).

Although this "downward mobility" exists in the mobility patterns of other racial and ethnic groups, the impact that such a change in status has on Black families differs significantly. The most obvious disadvantage for African American families is that they rarely have the level of financial security sufficient to cushion a subsequent generation with diminished educational attainments and careers. Because the only way a nonachieving generation could assure the maintenance of a middle-class lifestyle would be through inheritance, the lack of accumulated wealth—even in successful African American families—prevents such continuity of status (Billingsley, 1992; Daniels, 2001; Hill, 1999a; McAdoo, 1981). For many Black families, a failure to maintain economic stability jeopardizes not only their own middle-class status but ultimately their sense of personal and family security (Billingsley, 1992; Hill, 1999a; McAdoo, 1981, 1996).

BICULTURALISM AND AFRICAN AMERICAN MIDDLE-CLASS FAMILIES: LIVING IN TWO WORLDS

Although the problem of living in two worlds is an issue for all African American families, it has even greater salience for families in the middle class because their contact with people of different cultures is increased.

Pinderhughes (1982) maintains that "values from all three value systems—African, American, and victim" (p. 110) are found in African American families. The attempt to incorporate a solid African American identity within the multicultural scenario that characterizes U.S. society requires an ability to adapt. The flexibility necessitated by this biculturality serves in some families to strengthen their sense of cultural identity and to increase their tolerance for cultural difference and ambiguity. In other families, the sheer difficulty of both adapting to different systems and forging an identity leads to a confusion of values and roles and a sense of powerlessness in the face of cultural complexity.

This has often given rise to a self-defeating cycle: identity confusion, role and power conflicts, and rigidity in relationships reinforce one another in a process by which powerlessness begets more powerlessness (p. 114). This struggle to maintain one's own cultural identity while living in a bicultural world has a unique impact on African American middle- and upper-income families.

Irrespective of the socioeconomic level of the family, however, the therapist must be keenly aware of the impact of racism and oppression on the lives of Black people. Pinderhughes (1982) states that: "as long as racism and oppression maintain the victim system, the goal of family treatment must be to enable the family to cope constructively with those stresses and to counteract their pervasive influence" (pp. 114–115). Ultimately our goal is to empower families to reverse the effects of this racism and produce changes in their lives.

DIFFERENCES BETWEEN BLACK AND WHITE MIDDLE-CLASS FAMILIES

Black middle-class families differ from their White counterparts in a number of areas that are important to consider if one is to attempt to understand the intricacies of Black family functioning (Bagarozzi, 1980; Billingsley, 1992; Hill, 1999a; Hines & Boyd-Franklin, 1996). First, although many White middle-class families do not themselves fit with the family life-cycle model that some sociologists have proposed, the life cycles of Black middle-class families often diverge sharply from the proposed model. An example given by Bagarozzi of this divergence is the fact that the "launching phase" of a family life cycle is often marked in Black families by the entrance into the household of children of the extended family. Such children may be those of relatives who are teenage mothers, who are divorced working parents, or who are otherwise unable to provide care. Thus, at a stage in which a couple is, under "normal" circumstances, engaged in adjusting to an empty house and to refocusing on each other, the house of an African American family may be quickly filled with children, extending the time period in which the spouses fill parental roles.

Another area of difference is the character of male–female power structures in each racial group. Prior to the 1970s, many White middle-class families tended to exhibit a male-dominant power dynamic, while Black families showed a greater incidence of a structure in which power is shared more or less equally by the spouses. Some sociologists (e.g., Scanzoni, 1971) have hypothesized that this greater egalitarianism may often be the result of the fact that Black wives were more likely than White wives to be employed—and often to contribute substantially to the family income. This difference in power dynamics has decreased in recent years as both Black and White women have entered the labor force in increasing numbers, a fact that supports the connection between working wives and the balance of power in the family structure. Black families, however, have a longer history of finding this type of balance.

Family boundaries constitute another area in which race functions as a difference in family dynamics. African American family boundaries have been considered by many scholars (e.g., Hines & Boyd-Franklin, 1996; McAdoo, 1978, 1981, 1996, 2002) to be more permeable, more open to outside influence—be it from the extended family or from the African American community. Many White families, in contrast, are relatively closed to such influence, tending to maintain more of a nuclear family focus. It should be noted, however, that Black family boundaries may be unusually impermeable where input from the White community is concerned (Grier & Cobbs, 1968).

THE VULNERABILITY OF AFRICAN AMERICAN MIDDLE-CLASS FAMILIES AND ITS IMPACT ON TREATMENT

Racism, Discrimination, and African American Middle-Class Families

Over 20 years ago, Bagarozzi (1980) examined the issues related to therapy with Black middle-class families. He found that Black middle-class parents shared some similar goals and expectations for their children with White middle-class parents. Bagarozzi states, however, that "[w]hile their basic goals do not differ significantly from their White counterparts, Black middle-class families find their attainment more difficult because of discrimination and prejudice which is inherent in many social, cultural and economic institutions in the United States" (p. 161).

In the last 40 years, strides have been made in giving equal opportunity to Blacks in various fields. However, some African American middle-class families are becoming disillusioned as they increasingly find that the roads of access stop short of widespread, high-level equality, where they are obstructed by more subtle forms of the racial injustice they faced decades ago.

This disparity is evident for what McAdoo (1981) originally called the "golden cohort" of Black male and female professionals who were the first generation to have access to White institutions in significant numbers. Although they entered the job field at much higher levels than their parents, as they climbed the occupational ladder they were sometimes viewed by their White counterparts as products of affirmative action, and hence as "second-class citizens." As they attempted to enter higher management and executive levels, many African Americans became victims of the "glass ceiling" and were frustrated and disillusioned when they felt unable to realize their true potential. Cose (1993), Pattillo-McCoy (1999), and Feagin and Sikes (1994) have explored the issues faced by Blacks working in corporate America.

The inequities of the social system felt by African Americans across the socioeconomic spectrum have clear consequences for family life. Most African American middle-class parents struggle with the knowledge that although more doors have been opened for them, their children and grandchildren may have to struggle to find the same opportunities.

Some of the Black middle-class families whom I have seen in treatment have talked openly to me about the insecurity they feel. Although they may have well-paying jobs, they fear that their positions in large White corporations or institutions are tenuous and that the advantages they have worked for and want for their children will disappear.

These fears are not without a basis in reality. Although written over 15 years ago, Williams's (1987) *New York Times* article about African Americans in corporate America is still strikingly accurate today. One particularly depressing aspect of this article featured a Black network executive who lost her job because of "last hired, first fired" practices. Many Black professionals were hired by White companies to fill jobs in human resource areas or affirmative action and equal opportunity programs. In times of cutbacks, these jobs are the first to go.

Williams (1987) described a work scenario in which African American employees in both public and private industry are still inhibited in their professional advancement due to the color of their skin. This situation creates a very real internal pressure for Black employees, a pressure to constantly prove themselves in a system that may never recognize their efforts. Many aspects of the sense of alienation that Williams describes are in fact subtle indications of racial barriers that clearly add to the emotional burden of African American employees and interfere with the development of good mental health and self-esteem. The specifics of this subtle racial bias are described by African American professionals in various ways. Some tell of the "glass ceiling" sensation, that "invisible but very real" barrier that prevents the Black professional from reaching the top of his or her field (Williams, 1987, p. A16). Others describe instances of obvious prejudice, such as indications that their White coworkers believe Blacks to be lacking in intelligence, while others speak of having the sense of being always monitored and judged. Williams's interviewees also mention as a factor the sense of "social and professional estrangement . . . among White colleagues" (p. A16).

In relation to this first factor, Williams notes that the level of "integration" in the workplace is also deceptive. Her section entitled "Integrated Offices, Segregated Lives," is also still very relevant in the 21st century:

Specialists in black advancement say that more than 50 percent of black executives are graduates of predominantly black universities, and black executives are frequently the first from their families and neighborhoods to move into the upper echelon of American society. While they may work in integrated offices, the lives they lead outside the office are in many ways segregated. (p. A16)

UPPER-INCOME AFRICAN AMERICAN FAMILIES

There is a small but growing upper-income group of African Americans who earn over $100,000 per year (see Chapter 1; Billingsley, 1992; Collins, 1997; Daniels, 2002a; Graham, 1999; Hill, 1999a). In addition, Billingsley (1992) identifies a group of "very wealthy" African American families, such as the Johnsons of Chicago, the Russells of Atlanta, and the Llewellyns of New York, who amassed their fortunes through entrepreneurial endeavors. Even in the days of segregation and "Jim Crow" laws, a tiny segment of African Americans became very wealthy as a result of entrepreneurship—the most prominent of whom was Madame C. J. Walker, who invented and marketed hair care products and cosmetics for African Americans in the late 1800s (Graham, 1999).

In the past half-century, a number of African American entertainers and athletes have also become very wealthy. Some of these, such as Oprah Winfrey, Bill Cosby, Magic Johnson, and Michael Jordan, have become successful entrepreneurs as well. Additionally, African American professionals, such as doctors, dentists, and lawyers, who served the African American community often became financially successful. It should be noted, however, that the standards for White and Black "wealth" are not comparable, and that a family considered "wealthy" in the Black community would likely be considered "upper middle class" among Whites.

Many upper-income African Americans are corporate executives. Navigating corporate America has been a complicated process for African Americans. There is a small, but visible group of powerful executives—and even CEOs—of major companies in the United States. In an article for *Fortune* magazine, Daniels (2002a) surveys this group, which includes Stanley O'Neal, COO at Merrill Lynch; Ken Chenault, CEO at American Express; Richard Parsons, CEO of AOL Time Warner; Franklin Raines, CEO at Fannie Mae; Thomas Jones, CEO of Global Investments at Citigroup; and Bruce Gordon, president of retail markets at Verizon. It is noteworthy that there are no African American women on this list. The African American women whom Daniels acknowledged in her article attained their status through starting their own companies, continuing the strain of entrepreneurialism that has been the traditional route to financial success for African Americans (Daniels, 2002a).

More often than not African Americans in white-collar executive positions have found themselves reaching a "glass ceiling" beyond which they could not advance (Cose, 1993). Others have found themselves in "racialized jobs" (Collins, 1997), such as executives in human resources, diversity training, or affirmative action programs. These positions are outside of the corporate mainstream with no bottom-line responsibilities, and hence no ability to generate profits. These executives find themselves with few possibilities for advancement and their departments are the first to be downsized or eliminated during difficult economic times (Collins, 1997).

Cose (1993), in his research with high-achieving African Americans in top jobs throughout the country, noted the following concerns: the inability to fit in; exclusion from "the club"; low expectations by coworkers and supervisors; shattered hopes; faint praise or the "you are the exception" messages; presumption of failure; coping fatigue; pigeonholing; identity troubles, or the fear of being forced to shed one's racial identity in order to succeed; self-censorship and silence; defending the lack of racism in a company that promotes itself as "color-blind" when the truth is far different; and being treated like a criminal because one is Black. Many of these experiences with racism can be very subtle and thus easily denied by the perpetrators.

Clinicians should be aware that these experiences with racism and loss of position or changes in status can lead to rage (Collins, 1997; Cose, 1993) or depression, which can not only effect the family member but can have repercussions throughout the family and the extended family. Children and adolescents often act out in order to distract their parents and loved ones from this depression or to mirror and enact their rage. There is a need for more research on the experiences of African Americans in these upper-income categories.

RAISING AFRICAN AMERICAN CHILDREN IN PREDOMINATELY WHITE SCHOOLS AND COMMUNITIES

More African American families have moved to suburban areas in recent years (Billingsley, 1992; Hill, 1999a), some to predominately Black areas—such as Stone Mountain or Lithonia outside Atlanta, or Prince George's County, Maryland—others to predominately White communities. Families sending their children to predominately White schools in the suburbs have been very surprised at the level of cultural, racial, social, emotional, and often educational challenges that their children face (Boyd-Franklin et al., 2001).

In the early elementary school grades, these children often find some degree of acceptance from their peers that dissipates as the children get older. By age 9 or 10, they may find themselves beginning to be excluded from social activities, although this can occur even earlier, particularly for girls. I can still remember a 5-year-old African American girl stunning her mother in a family session when she said "The other kids don't like me 'cause I'm Black." Therapists should be aware of these possibilities and inquire about the children's experiences. Well-meaning parents, who work all day outside the community, may be unaware of what their children or adolescents experience.

These children may grow up as "the only one" in many settings (Boyd-Franklin et al., 2001). As adolescents approach the high school years, and dating becomes an issue, exclusion can become even more pronounced. Many Black parents become disturbed by the cross-racial dating practices of their children. Since more African American males date cross-racially, some African

American high school girls report having very little or no social life in high school. Some White parents (as well as some Hispanic and Asian parents) are opposed to interracial relationships because they "project their fears, often sexual in nature, onto African American male teenagers" (Boyd-Franklin et al., 2001, p. 113). These issues can create major conflicts for African American adolescents and their families.

Another challenge for Black teenagers and their parents in predominantly White schools arises when teachers and school officials bring their own stereotypes about Blacks into the classroom. When children receive negative messages about their abilities, strengths, and performance, this can become a "self-fulfilling prophecy."

Many Black parents whose children attend predominantly White schools struggle with the lack of African and African American history being covered in the curriculum and issues surrounding their children being assigned books that these parents consider degrading to Africans or African Americans. Parents who take the initiative and raise these issues with teachers, librarians, and school officials often risk getting themselves (and their children) labeled as "troublemakers."

Often African American children face conflict with the school administration on cultural differences such as hairstyles, clothing, music, and speech. Black children have been suspended from predominantly White schools for wearing their hair in dreadlocks or for dressing in a way that is perceived as "gang-related."

Black children who have spent their entire lives in predominantly White communities may not have spent any time with Black peers, other than relatives, until adolescence. For parents who are concerned about their son's or daughter's development of a positive Black racial identity (discussed below), his or her exclusively White peer group may present a problem, especially when their son or daughter begins dating. Black males often begin to experience subtle and not-so-subtle experiences of being singled out because of their skin color—for example, by being followed in stores or through "racial profiling" by police (Boyd-Franklin et al., 2001). (See Chapter 8.)

RACIAL IDENTITY ISSUES FOR AFRICAN AMERICAN MIDDLE-CLASS CHILDREN AND ADOLESCENTS

The struggle to promote positive racial identity and self-esteem presents complications for upwardly mobile families who may live in all-White areas. Black children often feel very isolated, particularly as they enter their preteen and adolescent years. Some of these children may identify as White (see Chapter 2). Some African American parents, in an effort to address this dilemma, have begun "networking" with other Black parents and families in neighboring communities. Some have arranged informal groups and activities for their children.

Others have used more formal social groups such as "Jack and Jill" clubs, as described by Boyd-Franklin et al. (2001).

> Jack and Jill is a national black family organization with chapters in most areas of the country. New members need to be nominated by a family that has children in Jack and Jill. It was started by African American parents wanting to ensure that their children could have a black peer group who valued African American history and culture, educational achievement, and the spirit of giving back to the community. Prior to the 1960s and 1970s, Jack and Jill had a reputation for being restricted to blacks with light skin color as well as education and professional status.
>
> In recent years, however, the organization has become more inclusive and has developed a more positive black focus (although this may not be true of every chapter). Many younger African American mothers have brought a more Afrocentric focus to their Jack and Jill chapters. Although the organization was started when schools and communities were racially segregated (whether through Jim Crow laws in the South, or restrictive housing policies in other locations), it has particular relevance today for African American children who live in predominantly white communities.
>
> For some black teens where the black community is defined by "how many black folks you can drive to in a half hour," Jack and Jill has provided a social lifeline of black friends and activities. It has helped in the development of racial identity for some black adolescents. For others, it has provided black peers, dates, and prom escorts. Some kids, particularly teenage boys, may resist participation in activities when young (early teenage years and younger), but this may change as they enter their late high school years and begin to benefit from the social networking opportunities the organization offers.
>
> In today's mobile society in which families often move because of job demands, Jack and Jill has sometimes provided friends for kids in a new community. Jack and Jill is still primarily run by mothers, although many chapters have made an effort to involve fathers. Family activities, talent shows, dinners, and "black family" celebrations are a part of most chapters. The organization provides many Jack and Jill parents with other black parents to talk to about your worries about your kids. For single parents, this can be a particularly important support in a predominantly white area. It can also be an opportunity for black parents and adolescents to develop their leadership and organizational skills. (Boyd-Franklin et al., 2001, pp. 117–118)

Some families take their children back to their former African American communities for their social life. As discussed in Chapter 7, Black churches have served an important social as well as spiritual function for many of these families. Black families will often travel a great distance in order to attend a Black church for the feeling of belonging and support.

Some families with strong Afrocentric beliefs have begun Rites-of-Passage programs, based on traditional African beliefs, in their communities and churches to initiate boys and girls into "manhood" or "womanhood." Therapists interested in learning more about this movement should read

Boyd-Franklin et al. (2001), Harvey (2001), Hill (1992), Kunjufu (1985), and Warfield-Coppock (1992).

In their efforts to achieve upward mobility, some African American families have adopted a "color-blind" attitude in which they deny the impact of racial differences. Their children often suffer the brunt of the cultural isolation such attitudes engender. In recent years, I have seen an increasing number of Black adolescents and their families struggle with this dilemma. One of the most important tasks for therapists working with these families is to help them open up communication between African American parents and their children on the issue.

The following case example illustrates this point.

Dwayne Carlton, age 15, the only child of professional parents, was growing up in a suburban community in which Black people had always lived. His family was one of the first to live in the predominantly White section of town, rather than in the "other-side-of-the-tracks" Black neighborhoods.

Dwayne felt caught between White kids who saw him as different for racial reasons and Black kids who saw him as different in regards to class and as "stuck up." His father, a banker, rigidly maintained that he had always operated in a color-blind way and that he felt that his son should just "ignore" these issues. Ms. Carlton, a college professor, took a very passive role, attempting to placate her husband and her son. They often sent messages to each other through her. It was quickly apparent in the first session that Mr. Carlton "preached" to his son through his wife. In subsequent sessions, the therapist worked with the father and son to open up communication and to help the son share his dilemma openly with his father For a number of sessions the therapist had to block the father from "preaching" and help him to just hear his son's concerns. He was finally able to recognize his son's struggle and to discuss ways in which Dwayne might find his own way in this difficult situation. Gradually, with his parents' support, Dwayne was able to find his own friends in school.

The Emotional Price Paid for "Advancement"

Both subtle and overt forms of discrimination can cause persistent feelings of low self-esteem and constant anxiety. These feelings effect more than just the individual. The stress engendered by such treatment is often displaced onto spouses, children, and other family members. Since it is typical for both spouses to work in African American families, both partners are at risk for bringing these issues home.

It is not uncommon for individuals who feel powerless in their work situation to abuse power in their home environment, since this feeling of powerlessness can result in intense anger that gets acted out in a sphere where the individual can exercise some amount of power. The following sections address the issue of handling this anger in treatment with African American families.

The Theme of Power

The influences of racism and discrimination greatly affect African American family and couple relationships at all class and educational levels, particularly in terms of the misuses and abuses of power. The following case example clarifies the existence of this struggle in an upper-middle-class Black family.

Mr. and Mrs. Smith, a Black couple in their 50s, entered treatment following an incident in which Mr. Smith had come home from work as an upper-level manager in a major White corporation and had yelled at his wife and knocked the food she had prepared off the table. Mrs. Smith became frightened and took their three children (ages 14, 10, and 6) to her mother's house. It was during this brief separation that she called to make an appointment for marital therapy.

When they appeared for the first session, both Mr. and Mrs. Smith looked very uncomfortable and somewhat rigid. Mrs. Smith reported that for the first time in her 18-year marriage, she had been very frightened of her husband. Mr. Smith, threatened by this crisis in his marriage, had agreed reluctantly to come in for treatment.

As the work with the couple progressed and both members became more comfortable with the therapist, Mr. Smith shared the root of his concerns. He was being considered for a promotion to vice-president that he expected to get because of his qualifications and positive performance reviews. When a White colleague received the promotion, Mr. Smith was devastated. His corporation had never had a Black vice-president and he was convinced that he had been passed over because of racial discrimination. He was in a rage but felt impotent and powerless to change the system.

He was intensely embarrassed by this and had not been able to discuss it with Mrs. Smith until this particular couple session. She was very surprised at the intensity of his anger and shame, and for the first time she began to understand the reasons for his angry outbursts. The therapist was able to help both members of the couple see that as a Black man, Mr. Smith felt angry and that he had passed on this anger to his wife and family. As he felt more powerless and out of control on the job, he had more of a need to exert his power at home. The process between them was reframed as the need to support each other in spite of the racism from the outside world.

As this example demonstrates, this experience of racism cuts across class levels for Black people. Because of this issue, the impact of the pressures of racial discrimination plays a very significant role in the treatment of African Americans. Often Black individuals, couples, and families feel themselves to be without recourse in the face of this racism. Therefore, the issue of empowerment is a very prominent one in the treatment process.

The Theme of Anger in Middle-Class African American Families

The sense of vulnerability, of powerlessness in the face of entrenched racism, thus gives rise in many Black people to an anger that must be discussed in therapy if one is to treat African American families effectively. The contradictions that arise from the position of the Black middle-class family in a social structure dominated by White culture often serve to obscure the sources of such anger. Also, the increased social and economic similarities between Black and White middle-class families run counter to the often unexpected experiences of prejudice (Bagarozzi, 1980; Billingsley, 1992; Hill, 1999a). Thompson (1987) stresses the need to help African American clients distinguish between racism and neuroticism. Family therapists who treat African American middle-class families need, therefore, to aid these families in the process of recognizing the extent to which their problems are influenced by their involvement in the external racist social structure and when they result from their own personal issues:

> The family therapist . . . must help family members become aware of how anger at societal injustices may be displaced and acted out within the family context. He/she also should help families determine how much of their difficulties stem from the effects of discrimination and how much they result from personal dysfunctional behavior styles, faulty communication patterns, unverbalized expectations or coercive interpersonal behavior change attempts. (Bagarozzi, 1980, pp. 163–164)

The following case vignette illustrates one example of the types of anger that therapists often sense in African American families. It often surprises therapists that Black middle-class families who appear to have "made it" still have a tremendous amount of rage in reaction to the subtle injustices and racism that they encounter.

Earl Owens was a Black 40-year-old executive at a major White corporation. He was director of human resources. There had been a series of cutbacks and "job abolishments" at his organization for the last 3 years, and he had lived in constant fear of losing his position. He was married to Martha Owens, who had been a homemaker for many years and was in her first year of a master's program in social work when the family entered therapy. They had three children, Leticia (age 16), Amena (age 10), and Earl Jr. (age 6).

The family came into treatment originally around the issue of Leticia, who was acting out in school. Moreover, the school had reported the family to the state bureau of child welfare because there had been large welts on Leticia's legs, arms, and face. The bureau had investigated and discovered that Mr. Owens frequently flew into rages and abused Leticia.

When the family entered treatment, it was clear that they were embarrassed by the referral. The father was angered, feeling that he was being forced into treatment. Mrs. Owens described herself as feeling both hopeless and helpless to intervene in the struggle between her husband and her daughter.

Leticia was an attractive adolescent who spoke extremely well and was assertive in communicating her ideas. The entire family agreed that until 3 years previously, Leticia and her father had had a wonderful relationship. She even described herself as a "daddy's girl." Then three events occurred virtually simultaneously: Mrs. Owens went back to school to complete work on her BA, Mr. Owens's job became more unstable, and Leticia began reaching out to her peer group more, asserting her independence and becoming more involved in age-appropriate activities.

It became clear in subsequent sessions that Mr. Owens had begun to feel very threatened at work and abandoned by his wife and favorite daughter at home. He had always been verbally volatile, but as pressures increased he became more physically abusive of his daughter, even hitting her with a belt. Initially, Mr. Owens tried to dismiss his actions as related to the cultural norm of spanking children in many Black families. The therapist was able to challenge this idea, eventually helping Mr. Owen to reach a point where he was able to acknowledge that he was so angry and out of control at these times that he had far exceeded the accepted level of "spanking." He began to talk about how everything in his life felt out of control: his work, his home life, his children. He couldn't make anything go "his way."

It became clear that Leticia had become a scapegoat and a focus for all of his anger. The therapist acknowledged Mr. Owens's pain and anger. She helped him to talk to his daughter about why he "flew off the handle" with her. The therapist had a number of sessions with the couple alone in which Mr. Owens's pain and pressures were normalized and the couple was encouraged to address the distance between them and their increasing inability to support each other. The therapist pointed out that Leticia, who was asserting herself as a normal adolescent, had become the target of that anger.

Mr. Owens was able to tell his wife how he had felt abandoned by her at a time when he was feeling very vulnerable at work. This was hard for him because he repeatedly stated that he did not want to "appear weak" in his wife's eyes. Mrs. Owens was able to tell her husband that she had felt his withdrawal from her, was very angry, and as a result had immersed herself increasingly in school.

As the couple worked out some of their own issues they were able to honestly discuss the feelings of vulnerability, castration, loss of control, and rage that Mr. Owens experienced at work. He was able to get his wife's support and the therapist's support for looking at other options that would allow him to take back his sense of control.

The couple was then able to have a number of sessions with their children and the therapist in which they were able to set clear limits regarding curfew, study time, chores, and so forth with clear consequences. Mr. Owens was able to begin to tell his daughter how angry her acting out made him, rather than displacing his rage from the work situation on to her.

THE EMPHASIS ON "KEEPING UP APPEARANCES"

For many African American middle-class and upper-income families there is a tremendous pressure to "keep up appearances" and not let the outside world know the difficulties they face. Children of Black professionals frequently report a "fishbowl" type of childhood in which they were constantly expected to behave and bring honor to the family. "Respectability" becomes an important theme for many of these families and "shaming the family" is viewed as one of the most negative acts. Clearly, this is not totally unique to African

American families, but it often takes on a more intense form because Black middle-class and upper-middle-class families are often held up as examples by other members of their communities. Children of doctors, ministers, or other professionals in African American communities tell of growing up with the sense of having to live up to being the "preacher's kid" or the "doctor's kid."

There is often a tremendous sense of shame and guilt when families who are viewed as the pillars of their communities or the backbone of their churches seek help. For them, it is to admit failure—the failure to live up to community perceptions.

As has been noted, many middle-class African American families live essentially in a bicultural or multicultural world. They often raise their children in integrated neighborhoods and send them to integrated schools, and the parents work in predominantly White job settings. In the cities of the Northeast, for example, Black families who move up the socioeconomic scale often find themselves living in predominantly White suburbs. This creates many levels of stress for African American families as parents struggle to give their children a sense of their racial identity and yet prepare them to survive in a bicultural world.

Sometimes the struggle to maintain middle-class status is so great that parents may work double shifts or juggle more than one job. Time with children may be sacrificed and a family can be torn apart. The following case example illustrates this situation.

The Ross family came for treatment when their son Jeremy (age 13) was referred by his school. The family consisted of Mr. and Mrs. Ross (ages 34 and 35), Jeremy, and Melanie (age 7). Mr. and Mrs. Ross had been married for 14 years. Both were hard-working Black parents who had civil servant positions. Mr. Ross often worked overtime in his job as a postman, and Mrs. Ross was a teacher who was also attending graduate school to get her master's degree in education. Jeremy's school reported that Jeremy, although an above-average student, was failing three of his subjects and was not working up to his potential in others. His parents reported that he often did not obey them and would stay out long hours with his friends without telling the family.

The first key to the structural problems in this family came when the therapist tried to arrange a time for the first family session. It became clear that the parents were so busy that they were seldom available to each other or to the children. Time on a Saturday in which the whole family could be seen was finally arranged. In the first session, the parents very angrily told the therapist about their confrontations with their son. They explained that they were working very hard to give their children a better life but that their son was "ungrateful."

Many middle-class African American families, aware of the subtle forces of racism, put great pressure on their children to achieve. In more enmeshed families, this pressure can become intrusive. The Blackman family serves as an example.

The Blackman family was a middle-class African American family consisting of Mrs. Blackman (age 38), Mr. Blackman (age 49), and their children, Karen (age 16) and John (age 9). They came for family therapy at the suggestion of their minister after Karen's grades became poor in high school and she became increasingly oppositional with her family. She had stopped attending church—a major issue in her family.

Family sessions revealed that John was labeled the "good" child and Karen the "difficult" one. Her parents were first-generation middle class and had both worked hard at educational and career goals. Karen expressed a considerable amount of anger at her parents, which dated back to her earlier junior high school experience in which her parents had moved her from a local neighborhood school into what she called a "White private school." She had felt very isolated and had tried to express this to her parents, but they had been so anxious for her to have a "good education" that they minimized her complaints. When her peers began dating in high school, she felt total social isolation and was resentful of her parents.

The therapist first joined with the parents in their well-intentioned struggle to find quality education for their child. She labeled their struggle as normal, typical of "good parents," and common among Black parents trying to give the most well-balanced education to their children. She then helped Karen to express her concerns directly to her parents and to help them understand the social isolation she felt.

This process uncovered a basic disagreement between the parents in terms of their philosophy of education. Mr. Blackman reported that he felt strongly that Black kids should go to "the best schools." Mrs. Blackman argued for a school with other Black children. As the work with the family continued, it became clear that the Blackmans had basic disagreements on many lifestyle issues, including where and how they should live. They were helped to renegotiate these issues and in turn to help their daughter find a school where she could feel less alone. Gradually, with her parents' understanding, Karen was able to improve her grades and by the time the transfer was made, she was passing all subjects.

The pressure exhibited by the Blackman family on their children grows out the pressure to "make it." There is a very real fear on the part of African American middle-class parents that the gains they have made in education and occupation will be "snatched away" from their children. It is very important to these struggling African American parents that their efforts be recognized. Therapists should be balanced in their responses and sympathetic to the issues facing the parents in this situation as well as the child.

KINSHIP NETWORKS AND AFRICAN AMERICAN MIDDLE-CLASS FAMILIES

Mutual Aid

Unlike the isolation observed in some White middle-class families, Black middle-class families tend to maintain closer ties with their kinship networks. Mutually helpful involvement—both in economic and in emotional terms—

with family members often provides the nuclear family with a sense of dependable support. McAdoo's (1978) study gives detailed descriptions of the kinds of help that upwardly mobile, middle-class Black families received from their kinship network. In 66% of the cases she studied, these families felt that they received a great deal of kinship help. This financial and emotional aid from extended family—comprising substantial outlays in these areas on the part of the network—often continued to be given even after the subjects had achieved a level of financial security that exceeded that of their kin. McAdoo pinpoints family crises and major monetary outlays (e.g., the purchase of a home) as times when kin were most likely to be called upon for help. She further observes that "emotional support was an important element mentioned repeatedly by the parents. In times of stress, they turned to family members for help and felt confident that help would be available when needed" (p. 772).

Childcare was another area in which these families gave and received help from their kinship network (McAdoo, 1978, 1996, 2002). There are many ways in which this exchange might occur. For example, a grandmother may live with her daughter and care for her children while both parents work; on the other end of the exchange, a middle-class Black couple who are "doing well" may take in a nephew or niece so that he or she might attend a better school.

When Help Becomes a Burden

For upwardly mobile families, the close involvement that middle-class African Americans often maintain with their extended family can sometimes be an issue. In many African American families, the first person to attain a college degree is a source of pride for the entire family. If that person has been helped by extended family support, including financial contributions (as is often the case), the extended family believes that he or she has a responsibility to help others with their education. This may result in a financial burden just when the person is ready to start a family.

Many African American professionals find themselves at the center or hub of a complex extended family network, all of whom turn to them for emotional support, advice, and financial help. For many of these professionals, the issue becomes one of how to remain a part of their extended families without becoming overwhelmed by their demands. The following case example illustrates this issue.

Marcia (age 26) was a young African American woman who worked as a teacher in a special education program. She sought treatment because she was feeling overwhelmed, anxious, and unable to sleep at night. Her parents had divorced when she was 12, and she had been a "parental child" to her younger sisters. Marcia's family had been lower middle class during her early years. They had struggled to send her to college, and she had worked her way through. Her current anxiety stemmed from a crisis concerning her younger sister (age 19) who was in her second year of college. Her parents, who had been very hostile toward each other since their divorce, refused to pay for the sister's schooling. Marcia, in a typical gesture, had attempted to take on this burden. She became so overwhelmed with anxiety that she sought therapy. After some initial work with Marcia around her own need to control and take over, the therapist asked for a family session. Marcia's parents and both of her sisters agreed to attend. With the therapist's help, Marcia was able to share with her parents the burden that she felt for her sister's education. The therapist asked the parents if they had been aware that Marcia felt this pressure. They both reported that while they knew that Marcia was "helping" her sister, they had no idea of the strain this was causing her. The therapist then asked the parents to discuss the ways in which they would handle this situation. They were able to work out a reasonable payment schedule.

In a follow-up session, the therapist instructed Marcia to ask her parents if they needed her to continue the job of "parenting" the family. They were rather surprised by this question and emphatically told Marcia that they no longer needed her in that role. The therapist talked at length with the family about how divorced parents can still continue to function as a team on parental issues even if they don't choose to live together.

Marcia was helped to make clear "I" statements about her own needs in her family for the first time. She was able to continue to contribute to her sister's education without feeling obligated to take over the total responsibility.

EMOTIONAL CUTOFF
FROM THE EXTENDED KINSHIP NETWORK

A number of authors have discussed the fact that for some middle-class Black families, "the achievement and maintenance of middle-class status may lead to an emotional cutoff from the family of origin" (Hines & Boyd-Franklin, 1996). Staples and Johnson (1993) and Pattillo-McCoy (1999) discuss this kind of problem for the Black middle-class professional, which McAdoo (1978) illustrates by discussing the case of a young Black professional whose extended family has sacrificed to help him achieve middle-class status. This dilemma is centered upon the expectation that the professional, now that he has achieved middle-class status, will in turn help his family. The expected aid necessitates that he limit his upward movement in order that his resources—financial, psychic, and physical—may remain available to his family. McAdoo summarizes his choices as follows: "The mobile individual has two alternatives: (1) he must either continue his participation in the obligatory reciprocity stream, or (2) he must isolate himself and his family of procreation from his family of orientation" (p. 78).

This either/or choice for African American middle-class individuals and the psychological consequences of the isolation that can result from assuming the burden of responsibility should be an issue of concern for all therapists working with Black families. Often it seems that the Black individual who seeks upward mobility can do so only at the expense of close ties to his or her family of origin. While this may not mean the sacrifice of family holiday and ritual times, the break in day-to-day involvement with the family of origin can give rise to what are essentially class tensions (McAdoo, 1978), which are still evident in some African American families today. These tensions and the sense of disjunction they cause tend to make for even greater feelings of emotional cutoff:

> Probably one of the greatest dilemmas facing the upwardly mobile group is their relationship with blacks left behind. This isolation, while a crucial factor in coping with significant life changes that cause stress, increases the need for supportive therapy that must come from persons outside of the family sphere. Blacks newly arrived in the middle-class, or fighting to remain at working-class status, are often too vulnerable, economically and psychologically, to extend themselves for blacks who have been left behind. (McAdoo, 1978, p. 78)

The role of family therapy here is to help African American middle-class and upper-income families to achieve a balance of contact and involvement with their extended families without drowning or cutoff. The stresses and strains on these families, as demonstrated by some of the case examples, can seriously impinge upon the family system as a whole. The next chapter will explore the implications for training and supervision.

IV

IMPLICATIONS FOR SUPERVISION, TRAINING, AND FUTURE RESEARCH

16

Implications for Training and Supervision*

As this book has demonstrated, there is a tremendous need for more exposure in our graduate schools and training programs in the mental health field to issues of ethnic, racial, cultural and socioeconomic diversity. Without this training, clinicians arrive at our clinics, agencies, hospitals, and mental health centers unprepared to cope with the realities of service delivery to African Americans and other ethnic minority populations. In order to accomplish this goal, these training programs must go beyond the "one course process" and infuse this material throughout the curriculum in all courses.

For many years in the mental health field, formal training in multisystems work with agencies and institutions has been limited to the field of social work. For family therapists of other disciplines to treat African American families effectively—particularly poor, inner-city families—this exposure must be incorporated into all training programs. A formal course that focuses on key multisystemic agencies within the community is essential. These might include welfare, child welfare, housing, courts, police, schools, special education and child study teams, hospitals, or other health and mental health services.

THE NEED FOR AFRICAN AMERICAN AND OTHER ETHNIC MINORITY FACULTY, SUPERVISORS, CLINICAL STAFF, AND TRAINEES

In order for this training process to be both real and effective, psychology, social work, pastoral counseling, nursing, psychiatry and family therapy programs, internships, practicum sites, and residencies must include African American

---

*I would like to acknowledge the contributions of Brenna Hafer Bry, PhD; Paulette Hines, PhD; Rozetta Wilmore Schaeffer, ACSW; Gloria Steiner, EdD; and Beth Hill, MD, to this chapter.

and other ethnic minority professors and supervisors. These individuals can then serve as role models and bring a wealth of the kind of firsthand cultural experience that is so valuable to those in training in this field. Community members and other professional colleagues of different ethnic and racial backgrounds can also be brought in as consultants on specific topics.

In addition, many training programs have found that it is necessary to make a special effort to recruit African American and other ethnic minority clinical staff and trainees. This will help ensure for the future a larger number of ethnic minority professionals specifically trained to work with these populations. This also provides an opportunity for trainees from many different ethnic and racial groups to learn from each other about diverse cultural experiences and values. Moreover, it gives a clear message to the community that the training program, clinic, or agency cares enough to provide staff who reflect their cultural diversity.

EMPOWERMENT OF CLINICIANS THROUGH SUPERVISION AND TRAINING

Thus far, this book has focused on the process of empowering African American families through treatment. Just as empowerment is a concept of great importance in treatment, it is a component essential to training programs for all family therapists and other mental health disciplines. One cannot empower others if one feels powerless. Within this context, supervision and training need to provide a supportive environment in which the trainee can feel free to experiment, to acknowledge successes and failures, to risk, and to struggle with the complex process of treatment. The task of supervision and training should therefore be a gradual empowerment of clinicians by helping them to (1) feel more confident in their ability to treat; (2) understand their own culture, values, and familial background; (3) learn about the cultures of the families they treat; and (4) provide a multisystems framework within which they can view their work.

The initial experience of clinicians of all disciplines who learn to work with African American families, particularly at inner-city clinics, hospitals, mental health centers, and agencies, is that of feeling overwhelmed, helpless, ineffective, and powerless to effect change. These families are definitely a challenge even for the experienced therapist. For the novice, such common circumstances as initial resistance and suspicion, failure to keep appointments, and inability to follow through on issues, can be exceedingly demoralizing and can create a feeling of inadequacy on the part of the therapist, particularly if his or her training has not prepared him or her with strategies for addressing these realities.

Throughout this book the role of the therapist has been described as a very active, supportive one. Not surprisingly, the role of the supervisor is similar. Supervision provides a life line for the clinician in training. There is a definite multilevel relationship between the support that trainees receive from their supervisors and their ability to "be themselves" in the area of joining, so crucial to effective work with African American families. It also involves having supervisors on the "front lines" in clinics and available to the training clinician on site or by phone when emergencies develop.

THE CULTURAL COMPONENT: THE THERAPIST'S OWN CULTURE AND FAMILY

A very important part of the process of training clinicians to work with African American families requires that they explore their own culture and family, including beliefs, values, and biases (see Chapter 9). Early in their training, students are asked to construct their own genograms. This is an important catalyst in their own development as clinicians.

On a very personal level, it can help the therapists and their supervisors to be aware of their particular areas of vulnerability when working with families and of their own countertransference. The sharing of the therapists' own cultures is, in my experience, the most exciting and vibrant way to dispel stereotypes and to convey the notion of cultural diversity. As each trainee presents her or his own family, the concept that there is no such thing as *the* African American family, *the* Jewish, Irish, Italian, Asian, or Hispanic family becomes extremely clear. Again, this is an active, involved model of training. It is most effective if the professors and/or supervisors begin by sharing their families and cultures with their trainees.

Helms and Cook (1999) addressed the issue of helping clinicians to learn to think culturally in their therapy training. McGoldrick et al. (1996) have summarized a number of questions that are salient to this process:

> In training groups we often ask participants to (1) describe themselves ethnically, (2) describe who in their family experience influenced their sense of ethnic identity, (3) discuss which groups other than their own they think they understand best, (4) discuss which characteristics of their ethnic group they like most and which they like least, (5) discuss how they think their own family would react to having to go to family therapy and what kind of approach they would prefer. (p. 24)

BEYOND THE IVORY TOWER: TAKING TRAINEES OUT ON HOME VISITS AND INTO THE COMMUNITY

Another aspect of training clinicians to work in minority communities, particularly inner-city ones, is the need to expose them to these communities. It is important that new therapists, especially those from middle-class backgrounds, who will be working with poor families, be taken to visit and see the communities where their clients live. In the treatment of African American families, particularly extended families, the willingness of therapists to make home visits can be crucial (Boyd-Franklin & Bry, 2000; see also Chapter 11). This is particularly important given the reluctance of many key members of these families to enter clinics. As I discussed in Chapter 11, office-based clinicians should be aware that even one well-timed home visit can engage extended family members in the treatment process. Without this intervention, many well-meaning therapists often find that their efforts are sabotaged when the family members return home after their therapy sessions.

Trainees need encouragement and active training in the process of utilizing effective home visits (Boyd-Franklin & Bry, 2000). Many express fears of entering homes in inner-city neighborhoods that they perceive as dangerous. This perception may be accurate, and it needs to be discussed and respected. Precautions need to be taken for the therapist's safety. New staff should be trained in safety measures. (See Boyd-Franklin & Bry, 2000, for a thorough discussion of these precautions.)

It is often helpful for the trainees' learning and safety for supervisors or more experienced staff members to accompany them initially to help model the appropriate way to enter and respect a family's home. This is particularly important with Black families, who may be sensitive to the issue of a White therapist entering their home or community (Boyd-Franklin & Bry, 2000). When this is openly discussed with the family before the home visit, it can increase the therapist's credibility and convey that he or she is sensitive to the family's concerns. Often this is the most positive approach and can help to facilitate the joining between the therapist and the family.

SUPERVISION, ADMINISTRATIVE SUPPORT, AND TRAINING AS ANTIDOTES TO STAFF BURNOUT

In many training programs within clinics, hospitals, medical schools, internships, residencies, and practicum sites, great emphasis is placed on educating trainees of various disciplines. Often, however, the clinical staff who provide the backbone of an agency, hospital, or clinic are neglected in the training process.

Family therapy is a field in which a body of clinical knowledge and literature has evolved substantially in the last 30 to 40 years. This evolution of family therapy as a field of research and practice makes it all the more essential that clinicians working in the field have access to ongoing support, supervision, learning, and exposure. Many clinicians discover that after rich in-depth training during their graduate school years, internships, practicum placements, and residencies, they are left to "fend for themselves" as staff clinicians—this pattern is particularly likely after they have obtained their professional licensure. This is not only unfortunate but also counterproductive because working with

African American extended families and various other systems requires an active clinician who expends a great deal of energy in the process. The work can be overwhelmingly demanding and draining if the staff is not sufficiently supported.

Staff burnout is a frequent complaint of staff members in inner-city agencies, clinics, and mental health centers. As an antidote to this process of burnout, staff must be provided with seminars and training opportunities that update their knowledge about cultural issues, family therapy, and systems approaches. The ongoing process of clinical supervision is also an extremely important form of nurturing for staff, faculty, and trainees. If training is to provide the antidote to burnout described above, it must occur on a regular basis with clear administrative support within the clinic setting. There is no doubt that it can keep a staff energized and highly productive in this work.

To do this kind of work, however, clinicians require other types of administrative support. For example, the home visits, outreach, and multisystems involvement described in this book can take a very personal toll on staff clinicians. Hines (1999) recommends other ways in which administrative support can be used to counteract staff burnout. She suggests flexible administrative support that takes into account the hours a clinician devotes to a particular case rather than simply requiring that a number of cases be seen. There must also be administrative support for outreach. There is also a need for flexible schedules and staff comp time so that clinics can be open for working families who can only come for treatment in the evenings.

The multisystems model has major implications for the ways in which we provide services to African American and many other minority populations. One of the most important is the need for a more flexible intake process. This process allows time for joining and connecting with families who are very new to and often suspicious of the treatment process. Clinicians often find themselves in conflict with their clinic administration if they postpone information gathering until the joining and problem-solving stages have been addressed. There must be an understanding on the part of administrators that our intake forms may have informational gaps until trust has been established with a family. We lose a large number of African American families, particularly in inner-city clinics and agencies, because of the rigidity of our intake policies.

EMPOWERMENT THROUGH SELF-DETERMINATION

In my experience, clinicians often become overwhelmed and discouraged when we discuss the need for administrative interventions and reorientation in university-based and on-site training programs. The focus must be kept on the obligation of these programs to provide training and support. However, it is important to remember that you do not have to wait for this training to "trickle down" from the top. Empowerment begins with you. The training process described herein grew out of the efforts of a number of faculty, supervisors, clinical staff, and trainees. We tried new ideas, acknowledged our successes and failures, learned from our mistakes, and sought to support each other through this process. We went to conferences and learned and shared our ideas. Do not wait to be given this training: create it. Find a support system of other peers and begin working on change. Try out this approach with the African American families you treat and test its relevance with other ethnic groups.

This book is intended as a beginning. It summarizes my own clinical experiences and those of clinicians whom I have supervised. To the degree that it gives each of you the right to insist upon and to create your own training process, to develop your own intervention strategies, to network with clinicians at other agencies, to explore your own theories, and to follow your own cultural hunches, it has more than accomplished its task.

17

Conclusion and Implications for Future Clinical Work and Research

In the first edition of *Black Families in Therapy,* I closed with a discussion of the book's key themes. Foremost among these was the process of empowerment of both African American families and the clinicians who treat them. This has remained a central focus in this book. In this second edition, I have also introduced many new and expanded topics relevant to the treatment of African American clients and families. The current edition has increased our knowledge of these families and it has also identified areas for future clinical work and research.

The earlier edition was one of the first clinical texts in the scholarly literature that provided extensive case material on the treatment of African American families and couples. With the proliferation of cultural information on African Americans in recent years, I was surprised to discover the relative paucity of in-depth clinical case material in the literature, particularly in scholarly journals. Upon reflection, this is not surprising, given the preference in academic departments and some peer-reviewed journals for empirical rather than case-focused publications. This is highly unfortunate in that it diminishes the importance and the contribution of clinical scholarship in the field. In the worst-case scenario, it can potentially discourage some of our brightest clinical scholars from pursuing this venue, particularly in their quest for academic promotions and tenure. There is definitely a need for a reexamination of these priorities, particularly in the fields of psychology, social work, and family therapy. It would also be very important for clinicians in all disciplines in the mental health field to begin to publish their therapy cases. The infusion of this clinical material on African American clients and families is central to the training of future generations of therapists.

A major contribution of this book has been its comprehensive discussion of the inclusion of spirituality and the religious strengths of African American families and clients in therapy. It has been particularly gratifying for me to witness the inclusion of my original book in schools of theology, divinity programs, and pastoral counseling training. There is a need, however, for a much more inclusive dialogue between these fields and the disciplines of psychology, social work, psychiatry, and family therapy. We have a great deal to teach each other about the incorporation of these central values into our work with African American families.

The focus of the 1989 edition was primarily on Black and White clinicians working with African American families. In the ensuing years, the field has expanded to include many more clinicians from other ethnic minority backgrounds. As I indicated in Chapter 9, this has been a very necessary change, given the increasing number of families from all ethnic minority backgrounds who are entering our clinics. There has been relatively little clinical material or research on the special dilemmas experienced by these Latino and Asian clinicians and those from other ethnic and racial groups in their work with African American families. This is one of the most important new research and clinical directions.

Interest in Afrocentricity and the Afrocentric movement has increased among African American scholars in recent years (Akbar, 1984; Ani, 1994; Asante, 1988; Azibo, 1996; Hilliard, 1990; Kambon, 1998; Karenga, 1997; Nobles, 2003). Similarly, many African American families in this country have adopted Afrocentric principles as core values in their family life and in their childrearing practices (see Chapter 8). Many therapists who are not African American have very little knowledge of how Afrocentricity can affect the treatment process. Afrocentric family therapists such as Aminifu Harvey (2001) have begun this work. This book has contributed to that discussion. However, there is a need for more comprehensive exploration of these issues in the clinical and research literature.

Gender issues in Black families are another major area that is often misunderstood by White clinicians and those from other ethnic and racial groups. This book has presented the issues, particularly as they are impacted by the experiences with racism by African American women and men. The "invisibility syndrome" has affected both Black men and women, albeit in different ways (see Chapter 5). There is a need for further research and clinical scholarship on the way in which this can impact African American families, gender roles, socialization of male and female children, and male–female relationships. Given this disparity, it is very important that Black therapists, researchers, scholars, and feminists continue to clarify the differences between their perspective and that of their White colleagues, particularly on the dual oppression of racism and sexism and its impact on Black family life.

This edition has explored the experience of racism at different class or socioeconomic levels in even more detail and depth. It has placed the discussion of clinical issues within the context of the current demographic trends in African American communities today. While this is an important beginning, there is a need for even more attention in the clinical and research family therapy literature on these topics. If we are to work effectively with African American families, we must confront the issues of racism and the crippling poverty of many African Americans. We cannot pretend that these racial issues are not part of the treatment process or that they disappear as an African American family moves up the socioeconomic ladder. We cannot take refuge in a class, not race, approach. We must recognize both. It is important to remember that even if the therapist does not perceive race or racism as an issue, it is certainly an ever-present reality for many African American families. This has been true in many ways also for African American middle-class and upper-income families. Our acknowledgment that racism and class issues still exist in spite of the tremendous gains of the last 40 years allows us to empower ourselves and the African American families we treat to fight against them and to counteract their effects.

The discourse on the clinical implications of the impact of racism on African American families must be expanded. This book has addressed the issues of racism, racial identity theories, and skin color concerns in some African American families. These differences in attitudes about racial identity and racial socialization have often been "hidden" issues in some African American families, of which some therapists have been unaware. Carter (1995) and Helms and Cook (1999) have written excellent accounts of the role of racial identity in psychotherapy. Jackson and Greene (2000) have explored these issues (as well as problems related to skin color and hair) in the treatment of Black women. There is a need, however, in the family therapy field for more research and case discussion of the role of these issues in the treatment of African American families.

In the last 15 years, there has been a dramatic increase in the separation, divorce, and remarriage rates in this country. This has been true for African Americans also. This edition has presented a chapter devoted to these issues. But there is a need for more discussion in the literature on the impact of these experiences on the lives of African Americans, especially those with complex extended family networks.

Another important theme that this book has stressed is that "there is no such thing as the African American family." Far more work needs to be done to document the diversity among African American families and the range of attitudes, behaviors, and cultural values. More work is necessary to clarify geographic, religious, and cultural differences. As I mentioned in Chapter 1, the case examples in this book are drawn primarily from northern urban and suburban samples of inner-city and middle-class African American families. Further discussion of urban versus rural differences and northern versus western versus southern distinctions by therapists from other parts of the country would be useful. In addition, as indicated in Chapter 8, Caribbean families are a group of Black families that have settled in large numbers in the United States—particularly in New York, Boston, Washington, D.C., and in Miami—and who have received very little attention in the clinical and research literature. Although they share some similarities with African American families, it would be a serious error to assume that all the issues presented in this book apply to a West Indian family as well. There is also a great deal of cultural diversity among these families, many of whom originated from different Caribbean islands in the West Indies. By the second generation, many of these families lose their accents, and mental health clinicians assume that they are African American. African families who have immigrated to this country since World War II constitute another group of Black families that have been virtually ignored in the literature. As Chapter 8 has also shown, there are also a growing number of individuals and families who identify as biracial or multiracial. Once again, although a comprehensive discussion of these topics is beyond the scope of this book, more research and clinical case material is needed to document the issues presented by these populations in treatment.

Throughout this process, I have reiterated my concern that the cultural and clinical material presented here not be taken as a set of stereotypes that must be rigidly applied to all African American families. I am acutely aware that this material can be misinterpreted or misused in this way. Rather, as I have stated throughout, it is my sincere hope that therapists will view this book as presenting a set of hypotheses that can be accepted or rejected by each therapist with each new African American family in treatment. This is in fact the strength of this model, providing as it does a new beginning point for each new therapeutic encounter. It can therefore be useful to the beginning therapist, while also providing a thoughtful, comprehensive summary for the experienced clinician.

The course of writing this book has forced me to examine these issues at a very deep, personal level and to take full ownership of my own beliefs. I truly hope that it will enable others to begin this process for themselves, for it is only then that we can really provide effective services to African Americans and to all of the families we treat. This aspect of exploring our own core beliefs, values, stereotypes, and family experiences as a prerequisite to our work with African American families is a very important contribution of this book. These were some of the most difficult sections to write and required a very special level of "soul searching" on my part. I recommend that process highly. It is liberating; it opens up the many parts of ourselves that we need to be able to tap in order to be clinically effective. This liberation allows us to listen freely, use ourselves differently, and interact with others more openly and effectively.

Some readers, after completing this book, will wish for more comparisons with other ethnic groups. The process of clarifying the cultural and clinical issues for African American families was an enormous task. It was never my intent to provide this comparison and it is clearly beyond the scope of this book. McGoldrick et al. (1996) have provided some of these comparisons. However, there is a need for far more clinical literature and research exploring similarities and differences between ethnic groups. This will further our understanding of the ways in which we are different and the things that we all share in common.

The multisystems model presented in this book has major implications in terms of planning for ethnically diverse populations and for the development and implementation of public policy. It speaks to a clear approach to service delivery for African American and other minority populations and argues for a reallocation of resources in the direction of creating more agencies and reordering the priorities of existing ones in order to address these culture-specific needs.

This second edition has gone beyond the first with its inclusion of a chapter on public policy concerns (Chapter 12) and its discussions of welfare reform, the Adoption and Safe Families Act, kinship care, managed care, and affirmative action. It is clear throughout this book that public policy considerations must refocus on the mental health needs of poor African American and other ethnic minority populations and develop governmental strategies for changing our training and service delivery approaches. There must also be further exploration of the needs of African American families who are not at the poverty level but at other class levels. Although a more extensive exploration of this topic is beyond the scope of this book, it is urgently needed if change is to occur.

Finally, as I have stressed throughout, it is imperative that ethnicity, racial issues, and the treatment of African American families become an integral part of the curriculum of every training program in family therapy, psychology, and social work and in every other health, education, pastoral counseling, and mental health discipline. We must progress beyond the "one course model" and offer many more courses on African American and other ethnic minority clients and families. It is also essential that these racial and cultural issues be integrated throughout the entire curriculum. In terms of continuing education in all disciplines, clinicians must be required to take ongoing courses on these issues and to continue to update, expand, and renew their cultural competency throughout their careers.

In the past I have described the work on ethnicity and race as a pendulum within this field. As recently as 45 years ago it was not viewed as a relevant area of study. This book illustrates the swing of the pendulum to a very specific, in-depth focus on African American families. It is my hope that the areas presented here will assume a central focus in training and receive full acceptance as a major part of our training approaches. The pendulum will then reach its center and our view of families will be more complete.

Over the years, when I have made presentations at conferences, I have met many well-meaning clinicians and practitioners of all disciplines—

including family therapists, psychiatrists, psychologists, social workers, nurses, physicians, teachers, educators, and pastoral counselors—who desperately wanted to learn to treat African American families more effectively. Many felt, however, that they did not have the tools to do so. A large number of these clinicians were burdened by heavy caseloads and lack of training and were prime candidates for burnout. I have written this book for the dedicated service providers who need tools with which to accomplish a much-needed job. It is intended as a curriculum resource for training programs in all mental health and educational disciplines and as a tool for teachers of family therapy. It is also a handbook for those on the "front line" of service delivery to all African American families. With this in mind, I have stressed clinical case examples and the need to conceptualize treatment as a multisystems approach. In my own personal experience, it is these skills that are most needed by and useful to those directly involved in this work. It is my hope that this book will generate clinical, theoretical, and research questions for years to come. There is definitely a need for more studies that demonstrate empirical rigor in the clinical and family therapy field, particularly those related to African American and other minority families. It would also be especially gratifying if graduate students interested in those issues were to find meaningful dissertation and thesis projects from the material presented here. This book is intended as a summary of what we currently know about the treatment of African American families. It is my hope that it is only a starting point that will inspire more discussion and debate in the clinical field.

References

Abimola, W. (1997). *Ifa will mend our broken world: Thoughts on Yoruba religion and culture in Africa and the Diaspora*. Roxbury, MA: Aim Books.

Adams, D. (1998). Family preservation: An adoption challenge. *Bridges, 4,* 4. (Retrieved from: *http://www.Aaicama.aphsa.org/publications/98Winter.*)

Akbar, N. (1984). *Chains and images of psychological slavery.* Chicago: Third World Press.

Akinyela, M. (in press). Towards a post-colonial therapy. *International Journal of Narrative Therapy.*

Allen, B. (1982, July). It ain't easy being pinky. *Essence,* pp. 67, 128.

Allen, W. R. (2001). The struggle continues. Race, equity and affirmative action in U.S. higher education. In L. A. Daniels (Ed.), *The state of Black America 2001* (pp. 87–100). New York: National Urban League.

Allwood, S. (2001). *Afrocentricity: History and application.* Unpublished paper, Rutgers University, Piscataway, NJ.

Amen, R. U. N. (1990). *Metu Neter: Vol. 1. The Great Oracle of Tehuti and the Egyptian system of spiritual cultivation.* Brooklyn, NY: Khamit.

Anderson, C. (1994). *Black labor, White wealth.* Edgewood, MD: Duncan & Duncan.

Anderson, E. (2002). *Race, gender, and affirmative action.* (Retrieved from: *http://www-personal.umich.edu~eanderson/biblio.htm,* pp. 1–47.)

Ani, M. (1994). *Yurugu: An African-centered critique of European cultural thought and behavior.* Trenton, NJ: Africa World Press.

Aponte, H. (1976). The family–school interview: An ecostructural approach. *Family Process, 15*(3), 303–311.

Aponte, H. (1994). *Bread and spirit: Therapy with the new poor.* New York: Norton.

Aponte, H., & Van Deusen, J. (1981). Structural family therapy. In A. Gurman & D. Kniskern (Eds.), *Handbook of family therapy.* New York: Brunner/Mazel.

Asante, M. K. (1988). *Afrocentricity.* Trenton, NJ: Africa World Press.

Asante, M. K. (1990). *Kemet, Afrocentricity, and knowledge.* Trenton, NJ: Africa World Press.

Association for Children of New Jersey (ACNJ). (1999). *Working—but still poor in New Jersey.* (Retrieved from: *http://www.acnj.org/main.asp?uri=1005&ci=34.*)

Association for Children of New Jersey (ACNJ). (2002). *Working poor families.* (Retrieved from: *http://www.acjn.org/main.asp?uri=1003&di=93.htm&dt=o&chi=2.*)

Austad, C., & Berman, W. (1995). Managed health care and the evolution of psychotherapy. In C. Austad & W. Berman (Eds.), *Psychotherapy in managed health care: The optimal use of time and resources* (pp. 3–18). Washington, DC: American Psychological Association.

Azibo, D. A. (1996). *African psychology in historical perspective and related commentary.* Trenton, NJ: Africa World Press.

Bagarozzi, D. A. (1980). Family therapy and the Black middle class: A neglected area of study. *Journal of Marital and Family Therapy, 6*(2), 159–166.

Barkley, R. A. (2000). *Taking charge of ADHD: The complete, authoritative guide for parents* (rev. ed.). New York: Guilford Press.

Beatty, A. C. (2002). Priming "bitch" schemas with violent and gender-oppositional female rap lyrics: A theoretical overview of effects on tolerance for aggression against women. *African American Research Perspectives, 8*(1), 131–141.

Berg, I. K. (1994). *Family based services: A solution-focused approach.* New York: Norton.

Bergin, A. E., & Jensen, J. P. (1990). Religiosity of psychotherapists: A national survey. *Psychotherapy, 27,* 3–7.

Berrick, J., & Barth, R. P. (Eds.) (1994). Kinship foster care. *Children and Youth Service Review, 16*(2).

Billingsley, A. (1968). *Black families in White America.* Englewood Cliffs, NJ: Prentice-Hall.

Billingsley, A. (1992). *Climbing Jacob's ladder: The enduring legacy of African-American families.* New York: Simon & Schuster.

Billingsley, A. (Ed.) (1994). The Black church. *National Journal of Sociology, 8*(1–2).

Billingsley, A., & Giovannoni, J. M. (1970). *Children of the storm: Black children and American child welfare.* New York: Harcourt Brace Jovanovich.

Birdwhistell, R. L. (1970). *Kinesis and context: Essays on body motion communication.* Philadelphia: University of Pennsylvania Press.

Bowen, M. (1976). Theory in the practice of psychotherapy. In P. J. Guerin (Ed.), *Family therapy: Theory and practice* (pp. 42–90). New York: Gardner Press.

Bowen, M. (1978). *Family therapy in clinical practice.* New York: Jason Aronson.

Bowen, W. G., & Bok, D. (1998). *The shape of the river: Long-term consequences of considering race in college and university admissions.* Princeton: Princeton University Press.

Boyd-Franklin, N. (1983). Black family life styles: A lesson in survival. In A. Swerdlow & H. Lessinger, *Class, race, and sex: The dynamics of control.* Boston: G. K. Hall (with Barnard College Women's Center).

Boyd-Franklin, N. (1987). The contribution of family therapy models to the treatment of Black families. *Psychotherapy, 24,* 621–629.

Boyd-Franklin, N. (1989). *Black families in therapy: A multisystems approach.* New York: Guilford Press.

Boyd-Franklin, N., Aleman, J., Steiner, G., Drelich, E., & Norford, B. (1995). Family systems interventions and family therapy. In N. Boyd-Franklin, G. Steiner, & M. Boland (Eds.), *Children, families and HIV/AIDS: Psychosocial and therapeutic issues* (pp. 115–126). New York: Guilford Press.

Boyd-Franklin, N., & Bry, B. H. (2000). *Reaching out in family therapy: Home-based, school, and community interventions.* New York: Guilford Press.

Boyd-Franklin, N., & Franklin, A. J. (1998). African American couples in therapy. In M.

McGoldrick (Ed.), *Re-visioning family therapy: Race, culture, and gender in clinical practice* (pp. 268–281). New York: Guilford Press.

Boyd-Franklin, N., Franklin, A. J., & Toussaint, P. (2001). *Boys into men: Raising our African American teenage sons.* New York: Plume.

Boyd-Franklin, N., & Lockwood, T. W. (1999). Spirituality and religion: Implications for psychotherapy with African American clients and families. In F. Walsh (Ed.), *Spiritual resources in family therapy* (pp. 90–103). New York: Guilford Press.

Boyd-Franklin, N., Steiner, G., & Boland, M. (Eds.). (1995). *Children, families and AIDS/HIV: Psychosocial and therapeutic issues.* New York: Guilford Press.

Brice-Baker, J. (1996). Jamaican families. In M. McGoldrick, J. Giordano, & J. K. Pearce (Eds.), *Ethnicity and family therapy* (2nd ed., pp. 85–96). New York: Guilford Press.

Brisbane, F. L., & Womble, M. (1985–1986). Treatment of Black alcoholics. *Alcoholism Treatment Quarterly, 2*(3–4).

Broman, C. L. (1996). Coping with personal problems. In H. W. Neighbors & J. S. Jackson (Eds.), *Mental health in Black America* (pp. 117–129). Thousand Oaks, CA: Sage.

Bronfenbrenner, V. (1977). Toward an experimental ecology of human development. *American Psychologist, 45,* 513–530.

Brown, P. M. (1990). Biracial identity and social marginality. *Child and Adolescent Social Work, 7,* 319–337.

Buckley, T., & Carter, R. (in press). Biracial (Black/White) women: A qualitative study of racial attitudes and beliefs and their implications for therapy. In A. R. Gillem & C. A. Thompson (Eds.), *Biracial women in therapy: Between the rock of gender and the hard place of race.* New York: Haworth Press.

Budge, W. (1991). *Egyptian religion: Egyptian ideas of the future life.* New York: Carol.

Burton, L. M. (1992). Black grandparents rearing children of drug-addicted parents. *Gerontologist, 32*(6), 744–751.

Burton, L. M. (1995). Family structure and nonmarital fertility: Perspectives for ethnographic research. In *Report to Congress on Out-of-Wedlock Childbearing.* Washington, DC: National Center for Health Statistics.

Buxenbaum, K. U. (1996). *Racial identity development and its relationship to physical appearance and self-esteem in adults with one Black and one White biological parent.* Unpublished doctoral dissertation, Rutgers University, Piscataway, NJ.

Carter, E., & McGoldrick, M. (1999). *The expanded family life cycle: Individual, family, and social perspectives* (3rd ed.). Boston: Allyn & Bacon.

Carter, E., & McGoldrick-Orfanidis, M. (1994). Family therapy with one person and the family therapist's own family. In P. Guerin (Ed.), *Family therapy: Theory and practice* (pp. 193–219). Lake Worth, FL: Gardner Press.

Carter, R. T. (1995). *The influence of race and racial identity in psychotherapy: Toward a racially inclusive model.* New York: Wiley.

Cauce, A. M., Hiraga, Y., Graves, D., Gonzales, N., Ryan-Finn, K., & Grove, K. (1996). African American mothers and their daughters: Closeness, conflict and control. In B. J. R. Leadbeater & N. Way (Eds.), *Urban girls resisting stereotypes, creating identities* (pp. 100–116). New York: New York University Press.

Chaisson, R. E., Keruly, J. C., & Moore, R. D. (1995). Race, sex, drug use, and progression of human immunodeficiency virus disease. *New England Journal of Medicine, 333*(12), 751–756.

Chambless, D., Sanderson, W., Shoham, V., Bennett-Johnson, S., Pope, K., & Crits-

Chistoph, P. (1996). An update on empirically validated therapies. *Clinical Psychologist, 49,* 5–18.

Chatters, L. M., Taylor, R. J., & Lincoln, K. D. (1999). African American religious participation: A multi-sample comparison. *Journal for the Scientific Study of Religion, 38,* 132–145.

Children's Defense Fund. (2000, December 14). *Families struggling to make it in the workforce: A post welfare report* [Press Release]. (Retrieved from: *www.childrensdefense.org/release001214.htm.*)

Clark, K., & Clark, M. (1939). The development of self and the emergence of racial identification in Negro preschool children. *Journal of Social Psychology, 10,* 591–599.

Cohen, C. (1999). *The boundaries of Blackness: AIDS and the breakdown of Black politics.* Chicago: University of Chicago Press.

Collins, S. M. (1997). *Black corporate executives: The making and breaking of a Black middle class.* Philadelphia: Temple University Press.

Colon, F. (1980). In E. A. Carter & M. McGoldrick (Eds.), *The family life cycle: A framework for family therapy.* New York: Gardner Press.

Comer, J., & Poussaint, A. (1992). *Raising Black children.* New York: Plume.

Coner-Edwards, A. F., & Spurlock, J. (Eds.). (1988). *Black families in crisis: The middle class.* New York: Brunner/Mazel.

Constantine, M. G., Lewis, E. L., Conner, L. C., & Sanchez, D. (2000). Addressing spiritual and religious issues in counseling African Americans: Implications for counselor training and practice. *Counseling and Values, 45*(1), 28–39.

Cose, E. (1993). *The rage of the privileged class.* New York: HarperCollins.

Cose, E. (2003, March 3). The Black gender gap. *Newsweek,* pp. 47–55.

Cross, T. (Ed.). (2003). *The case for race-sensitive admissions in American higher education: A symposium of articles and commentary published in the* Journal of Blacks in Higher Education. New York: Author.

Cross, T., & Slater, R. B. (2003). How bans on race-sensitive admissions severely cut Black enrollments at flagship state universities. *Journal of Blacks in Higher Education, 38.* (Retrieved from: *http://www.jbhe.com/features/38_race_sensitive.html,* pp. 1–7.)

Cross, W. E. (1978). The Thomas and Cross models of psychological nigrescence: A review. *Journal of Black Psychology, 5*(1), 13–31.

Cross, W. E. (1991). *Shades of black.* Philadelphia: Temple University Press.

Cross, W. E., Parham, T. A., & Helms, J. E. (1998). Nigrescence revisited: Theory and research. In R. Jones (Ed.), *African American identity development* (pp. 3–72). Hampton, VA: Cobb & Henry Press.

Cushman, P., & Gilford, P. (2000). Will managed care change our way of being? *American Psychologist, 55,* 985–996.

Dana, R. (1998). Problems with managed health care for multicultural populations. *Psychological Reports, 83,* 283–294.

Daniel, G. R. (1996). Black and White identity in the new millennium: Unsevering the ties that bind. In M. Root (Ed.), *The multiracial experience: Racial borders as the new frontier.* Thousand Oaks, CA: Sage.

Daniels, C. (2002a, July 22). The most powerful Black executives in America. *Fortune,* pp. 60–76.

Daniels, L. A. (Ed.). (2001). *The state of Black America 2001.* New York: National Urban League.

Daniels, L. A. (Ed.). (2002b). *The state of Black America 2002.* New York: National Urban League.

Davis, F. J. (1991). *Who is Black?: One nation's definition.* University Park: Pennsylvania State University Press.

DeLeon, P., & VandenBos, G. (1995). Psychotherapy in managed health care: Integrating federal policy with clinical practice. In C. Austad & W. Berman (Eds.), *Psychotherapy in managed health care: The optimal use of time and resources* (pp. 251–263). Washington, DC: American Psychological Association.

de Veaux, A. (1982, July). Loving the dark in me. *Essence,* pp. 67, 128.

DiNitto, D. M. (2000). *Social welfare: Politics and public policy* (5th ed.). Boston: Allyn & Bacon.

Diop, C. A. (1974). *The African origin of civilization: Myth or reality?* Chicago: Lawrence Hill Books.

Du Bois, W. E. B. (1903). *The souls of Black folk.* Chicago: McClurg.

Duncan, G. J., Harris, K. M., & Boisjoly, J. (2000). Time limits and welfare reform: New estimates of the number and characteristics of affected families. *Social Science Review, 74*(1), 55–75.

Edwards, H. (1968). Black Muslim and Negro Christian family relationships. *Journal of Marriage and the Family, 30,* 604–611.

Epston, D., & White, M. (1992). *Experience, contradiction, narrative, and imagination: Selected papers of David Epston and Michael White, 1989–1991.* Adelaide, South Australia: Dulwich Centre Publications.

Falicov, C. (1988). Learning to think culturally in family therapy training. In H. Little, D. Breunlin, & D. Schwartz (Eds.), *Handbook of family therapy training and supervision* (pp. 335–357). New York: Guilford Press.

Feagin, J. R., & Sikes, M. P. (1994). *Living with racism: The Black middle-class experience.* Boston: Beacon Press.

Fick, A., Osofsky, J., & Lewis, M. (1997). Perceptions of violence: Children, parents and police officers. In J. Osofsky (Ed.), *Children in a violent society* (pp. 261–276). New York: Guilford Press.

Field, L. D. (1996). Piecing together the puzzle: Self-concept and group identity in biracial Black/White youth. In M. Root (Ed.), *The multiracial experience: Racial borders as the new frontier* (pp. 211–226). Thousand Oaks, CA: Sage.

Finegold, K., & Staveteig, S. (2002). Race, ethnicity, and welfare reform. In A. Weil & K. Finegold (Eds.), *Welfare reform: The next act* (pp. 203–224). Washington, DC: Urban Institute Press.

Ford, D. Y. (1995). Desegregating gifted education: A need unmet. *Journal of Negro Education, 64*(1), 52–62.

Fordham, S., & Ogbu, J. U. (1986). Black students' school success: Coping with the "burden of acting White." *Urban Review, 18*(3), 176–206.

Foucault, M. (1965). *Madness and civilization: A history of insanity in the age of reason.* New York: Random House.

Foucault, M. (1975). *The birth of the clinic: An archeology of medical perception.* London: Tavistock.

Foucault, M. (1980). *Power/knowledge: Selected interviews and other writings.* New York: Pantheon Books.

Foucault, M. (1984). *The history of sexuality.* Middlesex, UK: Peregrine Books.

Frank, R., & VandenBos, G. (1994). Health reform: The 1993–1994 evolution. *American Psychologist, 49,* 851–854.

Franklin, A. J. (1992). Therapy with African-American men. *Families in Society: The Journal of Contemporary Human Services, 73*(6), 350–355.

Franklin, A. J. (1993, July–August). The invisibility syndrome. *Family Therapy Networker,* pp. 33–39.

Franklin, A. J. (1999). The invisibility syndrome and racial identity development in psychotherapy and counseling of African American men. *Counseling Psychologist, 27*(6), 761–693.

Franklin, A. J. (in press). *From brotherhood to manhood: How Black men rescue their dreams and relationships from the invisibility syndrome.* New York: Wiley.

Franklin, A. J., Boyd-Franklin, N., & Draper, C. (2002). A psychological and educational perspective on Black parenting. In H. McAdoo (Ed.), *Black children: Social, educational and parental environments* (2nd ed., pp. 119–140). Thousand Oaks, CA: Sage.

Franklin, A. J., Carter, R. T., & Grace, C. (1993). An integrative approach to psychotherapy with Black/African Americans: The relevance of race and culture. In G. Striker & J. Gold (Eds.), *Comprehensive handbook of psychotherapy integration* (pp. 465–479). New York: Plenum Press.

Franklin, J. H., & Moss, A. A. (2000). *From slavery to freedom: A history of African Americans.* New York: McGraw-Hill.

Frazier, E. F. (1963). *The Negro church in America.* New York: Schocken Books.

Freedman, J. (1996, Fall). AFTA voices on the annual meeting. *AFTA Newsletter,* pp. 30–32.

Freedman, J., & Combs, G. (1996). *Narrative therapy: The social construction of preferred realities.* New York: Norton.

Funderburg, L. (1994). *Black, White, other: Biracial Americans talk about race and identity.* New York: Morrow.

Gans, H. J. (1995). *The war against the poor: The underclass and antipoverty policy.* New York: Basic Books.

Gardere, J. (1999). *Smart parenting for African Americans: Helping your kids thrive in a difficult world.* Secaucus, NJ: Citadel Press.

Gardner, H. (1995). Cracking open the IQ box. In S. Fraser (Ed.), *The bell curve wars: Race, intelligence, and the future of America* (pp. 23–35). New York: Basic Books.

Gary, L. (Ed.). (1981). *Black men.* Beverly Hills, CA: Sage.

Gary, L., Beatty, L., Berry, G., & Price, M. (1983, December). *Stable Black families.* Washington, DC: Howard University Institute for Urban Affairs and Research.

Gergen, K. (1985). The social constructionist movement in modern psychology. *American Psychologist, 40,* 266–275.

Gergen, K. (1991a). *The saturated self.* New York: Basic Books.

Gergen, K. (1991b). The saturated family. *Family Therapy Networker, 15,* 26–35.

Gibbs, J. T. (1987). Identity and marginality: Issues in the treatment of biracial adolescents. *American Journal of Orthopsychiatry, 57*(2), 265–278.

Gibbs, J. T., & Hines, A. (1992). Negotiating ethnic identity: Issues for Black–White biracial adolescents. In M. P. P. Root (Ed.), *Racially mixed people in America* (pp. 223–238). Newbury Park, CA: Sage.

Giddings, P. (1983). *When and where I enter.* New York: Morrow.

Gil, E. (1994). *Play in family therapy.* New York: Guilford Press.

Gillem, A., Cohn, L., & Throne, C. (2001). Black identity in biracial Black/White people: A comparison of Jacqueline who refuses to be exclusively Black and Adolphus who wishes he were. *Cultural Diversity and Ethnic Minority Psychology, 7*(2), 182–196.

Gopaul-McNicol, S. (1993). *Working with West Indian families.* New York: Guilford Press.

Gould, S. J. (1995). Curveball. In S. Fraser (Ed.), *The bell curve wars: Race, intelligence, and the future of America* (pp. 11–22). New York: Basic Books.

Gould, S. J. (1996). *The mismeasure of man.* New York: Norton.

Graham, L. O. (1999). *Our kind of people: Inside America's Black upper class.* New York: HarperCollins.

Greene, B. (1994). African American women. In L. Comas-Diaz & B. Greene (Eds.), *Women of color: Integrating ethnic and gender identities in psychotherapy* (pp. 10–29). New York: Guilford Press.

Greene, B., White, J. C., & Whitten, L. (2000). Hair texture, length, and style as a metaphor in the African American mother–daughter relationship: Considerations in psychodynamic psychotherapy. In. L. Jackson & B. Greene (Eds.), *Psychotherapy with African American women: Innovations in psychodynamic perspectives and practice* (pp. 166–193). New York: Guilford Press.

Grier, W., & Cobbs, P. (1968). *Black rage.* New York: Basic Books.

Grimm, B. (1997). Adoption and Safe Families Act brings big changes in child welfare. *Youth Law News, 18*(6), 1–15.

Guerin, P. J., & Pendagast, E. G. (1976). Evaluation of the family system and the genogram. In P. Guerin (Ed.), *Family therapy: Theory and practice* (pp. 450–464). New York: Gardner Press.

Guerin, P. J., & Pendagast, E. G. (1994). Evaluation of the family system and the genogram. In P. Guerin (Ed.), *Family therapy: Theory and practice* (pp. 450–464). Lake Worth, FL: Gardner Press. (Reprint).

Hacker, A. (1992). *Two nations: Black and White, separate, hostile, unequal.* New York: Scribners.

Haley, A. (1977). *Roots: The saga of an American family.* New York: Doubleday.

Haley, J. (1973). *Uncommon therapy: The psychiatric techniques of Milton H. Erickson.* New York: Norton.

Haley, J. (1976). *Problem-solving therapy.* San Francisco: Jossey-Bass.

Hall, R. E. (1992). Bias among African Americans regarding skin color: Implications for social work practice. *Research on Social Work Practice, 2*(4), 479–486.

Hardy, K. V. (1989). The theoretical myth of sameness: A critical issue in family therapy training and treatment. *Journal of Psychotherapy and the Family, 6*(1–2), 17–33.

Harris, R. (1991, May 13). For youths, fear for lives is part of living. *Los Angeles Times,* pp. A1, A9.

Hartman, A. (1978). Diagrammatic assessment of family relationships. *Social Casework, 59,* 465–476.

Hartman, A., & Laird, J. (1983). *Family-centered social work practice.* New York: Free Press.

Harvey, A. R. (2001). Individual and family intervention skills with African Americans: An Africantric approach. In R. Fong & S. Furuto (Eds.), *Culturally competent practice: Skills, interventions and evaluations* (pp. 225–240). Needham Heights, MA: Allyn & Bacon.

Harvey, A. R., & Hill, R. B. (in press). Africentric youth and parent rites of passage program: Promoting resiliency among at-risk African American males. *Social Work.*

Harvey, A. R., & Rauch, J. B. (1997). A comprehensive Afrocentric rites of passage program for Black male adolescents. *Health and Social Work, 22*(1), 30–37.

Hatchett, S. J., Cochran, D. L., & Jackson, J. S. (1991). Family life. In J. S. Jackson (Ed.), *Life in Black America* (pp. 46–83). Newbury Park, CA: Sage.

Hatchett, S., Veroff, J., & Douvan, E. (1995). Marital instability among Black and White couples in early marriage. In M. B. Tucker & C. Mitchell-Kernan (Eds.), *The decline in marriage among African Americans* (pp. 177–218). New York: Russell Sage Foundation.

Helms, J. E. (1990). *Black and White racial identity: Theory, research, and practice.* Westport, CT: Greenwood Press.

Helms, J. E., & Cook, D. A. (1999). *Using race and culture in counseling and psychotherapy: Theory and process.* Boston: Allyn & Bacon.

Henggeler, S. W., & Borduin, C. M. (1990). *Family therapy and beyond: A multisystemic approach to treating the behavior problems of children and adolescents.* Pacific Grove, CA: Brooks/Cole.

Henggeler, S. W., Schoenwald, S. K., Borduin, C. M., Rowland, M. D., & Cunningham, P. B. (1998). *Multisystemic treatment of antisocial behavior in children and adolescents.* New York: Guilford Press.

Henry, D. L. (1999). Resilience in maltreated children: Implications for special needs adoption. Child Welfare. *Journal of the Child Welfare League of America, 78*(5), 519–540.

Herrnstein, R., & Murray, C. (1994). *The bell curve: Intelligence and class structure in American life.* New York: Free Press.

Hill, P. (1992). *Coming of age: African American male rites-of-passage.* Chicago: African American Images.

Hill, R. (1972). *The strengths of Black families.* New York: Emerson-Hall.

Hill, R. (1977). *Informal adoption among Black families.* Washington, DC: National Urban League Research Department.

Hill, R. (Ed.). (1993). *The research on the African-American family: A holistic perspective.* Westport, CT: Auburn House.

Hill, R. (1994). The role of the Black church in community and economic development activities. In A. Billingsley (Ed.), Special issue: The Black church, *National Journal of Sociology, 8,* 149–159.

Hill, R. (1999a). *The strengths of African American families: Twenty-five years later.* Lanham, MD: University Press of America.

Hill, R. (1999b, April). *Welfare-to-work legislation: Its impact on children and families.* Paper presented to the Delta Research and Educational Foundation Policy Forum, Washington, DC.

Hill-Collins, P. (1991). The meaning of motherhood in Black culture and Black mother–daughter relationships. In P. Bell-Scott, B. Guy-Sheftall, J. J. Royster, J. Sims-Wood, M. DeCosta-Willis, & L. Fultz (Eds.), *Double stitch: Black women write about mothers and daughters* (pp. 42–60). Boston: Beacon Press.

Hilliard, A., Payton-Stewart, L., & Williams, L. O. (1990). Infusion of African and African American content in the school curriculum. In *Proceedings of the First National Conference, October 1989.* Morristown, NJ: Aaron Press.

Hines, P. M. (1988). The family life cycle of poor Black families. In B. Carter & M. McGoldrick (Eds.), *The changing family cycle: A framework for family therapy* (2nd ed., pp. 513–544). New York: Gardner Press.

Hines, P. M. (1999). The family life cycle of African American families living in poverty. In E. Carter & M. McGoldrick (Eds.), *The expanded family life cycle: Individual, family and social perspectives* (3rd ed., pp. 327–345). Boston: Allyn & Bacon.

Hines, P. M., & Boyd-Franklin, N. (1996). African American families. In M. McGoldrick, J. Giordano, & J. K. Pearce (Eds.), *Ethnicity and family therapy* (pp. 66–84). New York: Guilford Press.

Hines, P. M., & Sutton, C. (1997). *Sankofa: A violence prevention and life skills curriculum.* Piscataway: University of Medicine and Dentistry of New Jersey.

Holcomb, P. A., & Martinson, K. (2002). Putting policy into practice: Five years of welfare reform. In A. Weil & K. Finegold (Eds.), *Welfare reform: The next act* (pp. 1–16). Washington, DC: Urban Institute.

Holman, A. (1985). *Family assessment: Tools for understanding and intervention.* Beverly Hills, CA: Sage.

Holzer, H. J. (2000). *Career advancement prospects and strategies for low-wage minority workers.* Washington, DC: Urban Institute.

Holzer, H. J., Stoll, M. A., & Wissoker, D. (2001). *Job performance and retention among welfare recipients* (Working Paper 231). Chicago: Joint Center for Poverty Research.

hooks, b. (1981). *Black women and feminism.* Boston: South End Press.

hooks, b. (1993). *Sisters of the yam: Black women and self-recovery.* Boston: South End Press.

Hopson, D., & Hopson, D. (1990). *Different and wonderful: Raising Black children in a race-conscious society.* New York: Prentice-Hall.

Hrabowski, F., Maton, K., & Greif, G. (1998). *Beating the odds: Raising academically successful African American males.* New York: Oxford University Press.

Hughes, D. A. (1999). Adopting children with attachment problems. Child Welfare. *Journal of the Child Welfare League of America, 78*(5), 541–560.

Hughes, D., & Chen, L. (1997). When and what parents tell children about race: An examination of race-related socialization among African American families. *Applied Developmental Science, 1*(4), 200–214.

Hughes, D., & Chen, L. (1999). The nature of parents' race-related communications to children: A developmental perspective. In L. Balter & C. Tamis-LeMonda (Eds.), *Child psychology: A handbook of contemporary issues.* Philadelphia: Taylor & Francis.

Hughes, M., & Hertel, B. R. (1990). The significance of color remains: A study of life chances, mate selection, and ethnic consciousness among Black Americans. *Social Forces, 68*(4), 1105–1120.

Hunt, P. (1987). Black clients: Implications for supervision of trainees. *Psychotherapy, 24*(1), 114–119.

Hurtado, S., Milem, J., Clayton-Pederson, A., & Allen, W. R. (1999). *Enacting diverse learning environments: Improving the climate for racial/ethnic diversity in higher education* (ASHE ERIC Higher Education Report, 26[8]). Washington, DC: George Washington University, Graduate School of Education and Human Development.

Jackson, G. (1980). The emergence of a Black perspective in counseling. In R. Jones (Ed.), *Black psychology* (2nd ed., pp. 294–313). New York: Harper & Row.

Jackson, L., & Greene, B. (2000). *Psychotherapy with African American women: Innovations in psychodynamic perspectives and practice.* New York: Guilford Press.

Jackson, S. (2002). How are the children post-ASFA? *Black Administrators in Child Welfare News, 7*(2), 1, 5.

Jackson-Lowman, H. (1998). Sankofa: A Black mental health imperative for the 21st century. In R. Jones (Ed.), *African American mental health: Theory, research, and intervention* (pp. 51–70). Hampton, VA: Cobb & Henry Press.

Jencks, C., & Peterson, P. E. (Eds.). (1991). *The urban underclass.* Washington, DC: Brookings Institute.

Jensen, A. (1969). How much can we boost IQ and school achievement? *Harvard Educational Review, 39,* 1–123.

Jensen, A. R. (1985). The nature of Black–White difference on various psychometric tests: Spearman's hypothesis. *Behavioral and Brain Sciences, 8,* 193–258.

Jones, J. (1997). *Prejudice and racism* (2nd ed.). New York: McGraw-Hill.

Jones, R. (1998a). *African American mental health: Theory, research, and intervention.* Hampton, VA: Cobb & Henry Press.

Jones, R. (1998b). *African American identity development.* Hampton, VA: Cobb & Henry Press.

Jones, R. (in press). *Black psychology* (4th ed.). Hampton, VA.: Cobb & Henry Press.

Kagan, R., & Schlossberg, S. (1989). *Families in perpetual crisis.* New York: Norton.

Kaiser Family Foundation and UCLA Center for Health Policy Research. (2000). *Racial and ethnic disparities in access to health insurance and health care.* Menlo Park, CA: Kaiser Family Foundation.

Kambon, K. K. (1998). *African/Black psychology in the American context: An African-centered approach.* Tallahassee, FL: Nubian Nation Publications.

Kardiner, A., & Ovesey, L. (1951). *The mark of oppression.* Cleveland: World Publishing.

Karenga, M. (1997). *Kwanzaa: A celebration of family, community, and culture.* Philadelphia, PA: University of Sankore Press.

Kelly, S. (2003). African American couples: Their importance to the stability of African American families, and their mental health issues. In J. S. Mio & G. Y. Iwamasa (Eds.), *Culturally diverse mental health: The challenges of research and resistance* (pp. 141–157). New York: Taylor & Francis.

Kiecolt, K. J., & Fossett, M. A. (1995). Mate availability and marriage among African Americans: Aggregate and individual-level analyses. In M. B. Tucker & C. Mitchell-Kernan (Eds.), *The decline in marriage among African Americans* (pp. 121–135). New York: Russell Sage Foundation.

Kliman, J., & Trimble, D. (1983). Network therapy. In B. Wolman & G. Stricker (Eds.), *Handbook of family and marital therapy.* New York: Plenum Press.

Knox, D. H. (1985). Spirituality: A tool in the assessment and treatment of Black alcoholics and their families. *Alcoholism Treatment Quarterly, 2*(3–4), 31–44.

Kunjufu, J. (1985). *Countering the conspiracy to destroy Black boys.* Chicago: African American Images.

Kunjufu, J. (1988). *To be popular or smart: The Black peer group.* Chicago: African American Images.

Landry, B. (1987). *The new Black middle class.* Berkeley and Los Angeles: University of California Press.

La Roche, M., & Turner, C. (1997). Self-orientation and depression level among Dominicans in the United States. *Hispanic Journal of Behavioral Sciences, 19,* 479–488.

La Roche, M. J., & Turner, C. (2002). At the crossroads: Managed mental health care, the ethics code and ethnic minorities. *Cultural Diversity and Ethnic Minority Psychology, 8*(3), 187–198.

Lawson, E., & Thompson, A. (1994). The historical and social correlates of African

American divorce: Review of the literature and implications for research. *Western Journal of Black Studies, 18*(2) 91–103.

Le Prohn, N. (1994). The role of the kinship foster parent. *Children and Youth Services Review, 16*(2), 107–122.

Levin, J. S., Taylor, R. J., & Chatters, L. M. (1994). Race and gender differences in religiosity among older adults: Findings from four national surveys. *Journal of Gerontology: Social Sciences, 49*(Suppl.), S137–S145.

Lewis, J., & Looney, J. (1983). *The long struggle: Well-functioning working-class Black families.* New York: Brunner/Mazel.

Lewis, M. (1999). The hair combing task: A new paradigm for research on African American mother–child interaction. *American Journal of Orthopsychiatry, 69,* 1–11.

Lewis, M., & Osofsky, J. (1997). Violent cities, violent streets: Children draw their neighborhoods. In J. Osofsky (Ed.), *Children in a violent society* (pp. 277–299). New York: Guilford Press.

Lincoln, C. E. (1996). *Black Muslims in America.* Trenton, NJ: Africa World Press.

Lincoln, C. E. (1999). *Race, religion, and the continuing American dilemma.* New York: Hill & Wang.

Lincoln, C. E., & Mamiya, L. H. (1990). *The Black church in the African American experience.* Durham, NC: Duke University Press.

Lindblad-Goldberg, M., & Dukes, J. (1985). Social support in Black, low-income, single-parent families: Normative and dysfunctional patterns. *American Journal of Orthopsychiatry, 55,* 42–58.

Lindblad-Goldberg, M., Dukes, J., & Lasley, J. (1988). Stress in Black, low-income, single-parent families: Normative and dysfunctional patterns. *American Journal of Orthopsychiatry, 58*(1), 104–120.

Logan, S. L. (Ed.). (2001). *The Black family: Strengths, self-help, and positive change* (2nd ed.). Boulder, CO: Westview Press.

Mack, D. (1974). The power relationship in Black families and White families. *Journal of Personality and Social Psychology, 39*(3), 409–413.

Madanes, C. (1981). *Strategic family therapy.* San Francisco: Jossey-Bass.

Majors, R., & Billson, J. M. (1992). *Cool pose: The dilemmas of Black manhood in America.* New York: Lexington Books.

Marks, B., Settles, I., Cooke, D., Morgan, L., & Sellers, R. M. (in press). African American racial identity: A review of contemporary models and measures. In R. Jones (Ed.), *Black psychology* (4th ed.). Hampton, VA: Cobb & Henry Press.

Mayfield, W. (1972). Mental health in the black community. *Social Work, 17,* 106–110.

Mbiti, J. S. (1970). *African religions and philosophy.* Garden City, NY: Anchor Books.

Mbiti, J. S. (1990). *African religions and philosophy* (2nd ed.). Portsmouth, NH: Heinemann Press.

Mbiti, J. S. (1992). *Introduction to African religion* (2nd ed.). Portsmouth, NH: Heinemann Press.

McAdoo, H. P. (1978). Factors related to stability in upwardly mobile Black families. *Journal of Marriage and the Family, 40*(4), 761–776.

McAdoo, H. P. (Ed.). (1981). *Black families.* Beverly Hills, CA: Sage.

McAdoo, H. P. (Ed.). (1996). *Black families* (3rd ed.). Thousand Oaks, CA: Sage.

McAdoo, H. P. (Ed.). (2002). *Black children: Social, educational and parental environments* (2nd ed.). Thousand Oaks, CA: Sage.

McAdoo, H. P., & McAdoo, J. L. (Eds.). (1985). *Black children: Social, educational and parental environments.* Beverly Hills, CA: Sage.

McGoldrick, M. (1982). Normal families: An ethnic perspective. In F. Walsh (Ed.), *Normal family processes* (pp. 399–424). New York: Guilford Press.

McGoldrick, M. (1998). *Re-visioning family therapy: Race, culture, and gender in clinical practice.* New York: Guilford Press.

McGoldrick, M., & Carter, B. (1999). Remarried families. In B. Carter & M. McGoldrick (Eds.), *The expanded family life cycle: Individual family and social perspectives* (3rd ed., pp. 417–435). Boston: Allyn & Bacon.

McGoldrick, M., & Gerson, R. (1985). *Genograms in family assessment.* New York: Norton.

McGoldrick, M., Giordano, J., & Pearce, J. (Eds.). (1996). *Ethnicity and family therapy* (2nd ed.). New York: Guilford Press.

McLanahan, S. S., & Casper, L. (1995). Growing diversity and inequality in the American family. In R. Farley (Ed.), *State of the union: America in the 1990's—Social trends* (Vol. 2, pp. 1–45). New York: Russell Sage Foundation.

McQueen, A. (1971, Spring). *Incipient, social mobility among poor Black urban families.* Paper presented at Howard University Research Seminar, Washington, DC.

Middleton, R., & Putney, S. (1970). Dominance in decisions in the family: Race and class differences. In C. V. Willie (Ed.), *The family life of Black people* (pp. 16–22). Columbus, OH: Merrill.

Mikesell, R., Lusterman, D. D., & McDaniel, S. (Eds.). (2000). *Casebook for integrating family therapy: An ecosystemic approach.* Washington, DC: American Psychological Association.

Miller, I. (1996). Managed care is harmful to outpatient mental health services: A call for accountability. *Professional Psychology: Research and Practice, 29,* 31–36.

Minuchin, S. (1974). *Families and family therapy.* Cambridge, MA: Harvard University Press.

Minuchin, S., & Fishman, C. (1981). *Family therapy techniques.* Cambridge, MA: Harvard University Press.

Minuchin, S., Montalvo, B., Guerney, B. G. Jr., Rosman, B. L., & Schumer, F. (1967). *Families of the slums.* New York: Basic Books.

Mitchell, H., & Lewter, N. (1986). *Soul theology: The heart of American Black culture.* San Francisco: Harper & Row.

Moynihan, D. P. (1965). *The Negro family: The case for national action.* Washington, DC: U.S. Department of Labor.

Murphy, M., DeBernardo, C., & Shoemaker, W. (1998). Impact of managed care on independent practice and professional ethics: A survey of independent practitioners. *Professional Psychology: Research and Practice, 29,* 43–51.

National Center for Education Statistics. (1995). *1993 National household education survey public use data.* Washington, DC: U.S. Department of Education.

Neal, A. M., & Wilson, M. L. (1989). The role of skin color and features in the Black community: Implications for Black women and therapy. *Clinical Psychology Review, 9,* 323–333.

Neimark, P. J. (1993). *The way of Orisa: Empowering your life through the ancient African religion of Ifa.* New York: HarperCollins.

Nichols, M. P., & Schwartz, R. (1998). *Family therapy: Concepts and methods.* Boston: Allyn & Bacon.

Nisbett, R. (1995). Race, IQ, and scientism. In S. Fraser (Ed.), *The bell curve wars: Race, intelligence, and the future of America* (pp. 36–57). New York: Basic Books.

Nobles, W. (in press). African philosophy: Foundation of Black psychology. In R. Jones (Ed.), *Black psychology* (4th ed.). Hampton, VA: Cobb & Henry Press.

Oliver, M., & Shapiro, T. (1995). *Black wealth/White wealth.* New York: Routledge.

Orbuch, T. L., Veroff, J., & Hunter, A. G. (1999). Black couples, White couples: The early years of marriage. In E. M. Hetherington (Ed.), *Coping with divorce, single parenting, and remarriage: A risk and resiliency perspective* (pp. 23–43). Mahwah, NJ: Erlbaum.

Osofsky, J. (1997). *Children in a violent society.* New York: Guilford Press.

Papp, P. (1981). Paradoxes. In S. Minuchin, & C. Fishman (Eds.), *Family therapy techniques.* Cambridge, MA: Harvard University Press.

Parham, T. A. (1992). Cycles of psychological nigrescence. *Counseling Psychologist, 17*(2), 187–226.

Parham, T., & Helms, J. (1981). The influence of Black students' racial identity attitudes on preferences for counselor's race. *Journal of Counseling Psychology, 32*(2), 431–440.

Parker, S., & Kleiner, R. (1966). Characteristics of Negro mothers and single headed households. *Journal of Marriage and the Family, 28,* 507–513.

Parnell, M., & Vanderkloot, J. (1989). Ghetto children. In L. Combrinck Graham (Ed.), *Children in family contexts: Perspectives on treatment.* New York: Guilford Press.

Pattillo-McCoy, M. (1999). *Black picket fences: Privilege and peril among the Black middle class.* Chicago: University of Chicago Press.

Pattison, E. M. (1977). A theoretical-empirical base for social system therapy. In E. F. Foulks et al. (Eds.), *Current perspectives in cultural psychiatry.* New York: Spectrum.

Patton, J. M. (1992). Assessment and identification of African American learners with gifts and talents. *Exceptional Children, 59*(2), 150–159.

Perkins, K. R. (1996). The influence of television images on Black females' self perceptions of physical attractiveness. *Journal of Black Psychology, 22*(4), 453–469.

Peters, M. F. (1981). Parenting in Black families with young children: A historical perspective. In H. McAdoo (Ed.), *Black families* (pp. 211–224). Beverly Hills, CA: Sage.

Phelps, R., Kohout, J., & Eisman, E. (1998). *Professional Psychology: Research and Practice, 29,* 31–36.

Pinderhughes, E. (1982). Afro-American families and the victim system. In M. McGoldrick, J. K. Pearce, & J. Giordano (Eds.), *Ethnicity and family therapy* (pp. 108–122). New York: Guilford Press.

Pinderhughes, E. (1989). *Understanding race, ethnicity and power: The key to efficacy in clinical practice.* New York: Free Press.

Poston, W. S. C. (1990). The biracial identity development model: A needed addition. *Journal of Counseling and Development, 69,* 152–155.

Poussaint, A. (1993). African American couples. *Ebony,* pp. 88–89.

Prothrow-Stith, D., & Weissman, M. (1991). *Deadly consequences: How violence is destroying our teenage population and a plan to begin solving the problem.* New York: HarperCollins.

Report to the Congress on Kinship Foster Care. (2000). *U.S. Department of Health and Human Services Administration for Children and Families, Administration on Children, Youth and Families, Children's Bureau.* (Retrieved from: *aspe.hhs.gov/hsp/kinr2000.*)

Richards, D. M. (1980). *Let the circle be unbroken: The implications of African spirituality in the Diaspora.* Lawrenceville, NJ: Red Sea Press.

Rockeymoore, M. (2002). African Americans confront a pandemic: Assessing community impact, organization, and advocacy in the second decade of AIDS. In L. A. Daniels (Ed.), *The state of Black America 2002* (pp. 123–146). New York: National Urban League.

Root, M. P. (Ed.). (1992). *Racially mixed people in America.* Newbury Park, CA: Sage.

Root, M. P. (Ed.). (1996). *The multiracial experience: Racial borders as the new frontier* Thousand Oakes, CA: Sage.

Russell, K., Wilson, M., & Hall, R. (1993). *The color complex: The politics of skin color among African Americans.* New York: Doubleday.

Russo, C. J., & Talbert-Johnson, C. (1997). The overrepresentation of African American children in special education: The resegregation of educational programming? *Education and Urban Society, 29*(2), 136–148.

Sampson, R. J. (1995). Unemployment and imbalanced sex ratios: Race-specific consequences for family structure and crime. In M. B. Tucker & C. Mitchell-Kernan (Eds.), *The decline in marriage among African Americans* (pp. 229–254). New York: Russell Sage Foundation.

Sanchez-Hucles, J. (2000). *The first session with African Americans: A step-by-step guide.* San Francisco: Jossey-Bass.

Satterfield, M. (2002, August). *Kinship adoption.* Paper presented at the Kinship Adoption Symposium [sponsored by the Child Welfare League of America, Washington, DC.].

Scanzoni, J. (1971). *The Black family in modern society.* Boston: Allyn & Bacon.

Scheflen, A. E. (1973). *Communicational structure: Analysis of a psychotherapy transaction.* Bloomington: Indiana University Press.

Seligman, M., & Levant, R. (1998). Managed care policies rely on inadequate science. *Professional Psychology: Research and Practice, 29,* 211–212.

Selvini-Palazzoli, M., Boscolo, L., Cecchin, G., & Prata, G. (1978). *Paradox and counterparadox.* New York: Jason Aronson.

Serwatka, T. S., Deering, S., & Grant, P. (1995). Disproportionate representation of African Americans in emotionally handicapped classes. *Journal of Black Studies, 25*(4), 492–506.

Shockley, W. (1987). Jensen's data on Spearman's hypothesis: No artifact. *Behavioral and Brain Sciences, 10,* 512.

Smith, A. (1997). *Navigating the deep river: Spirituality in African American families.* Cleveland, OH: United Church Press.

Smith, R. (1988). *Kinship and class in the West Indies.* New York: Cambridge University Press.

Solomon, B. (1976). *Black empowerment: Social work in oppressed communities.* New York: Columbia University Press.

Speck, R., & Attneave, C. (1973). *Family networks.* New York: Vintage Books.

Springer, A. (2003). *Update on affirmative action in higher education: A current legal overview.* American Association of University Professors. (Retrieved from: http://www.aaup.org/Issues/AffirmativeAction/aalegal.htm, pp. 1–16.)

Stack, C. (1974). *All our kin: Strategies for survival in a Black community.* New York: Harper & Row.

Staples, R., & Johnson, L. (1993). *Black families at the crossroads: Challenges and prospects.* San Francisco: Jossey-Bass.

Steinberg, S. (1995). *Turning back: The retreat from racial justice in American thought and policy.* Boston: Beacon Press.

Stevenson, H. C. (1993). Validation of the scale of racial socialization for African American adolescents. *Psych Discourse.* Washington, DC: Association of Black Psychologists.

Stevenson, H. C. (1998). Theoretical considerations in measuring racial identity and socialization: Extending the self further. In R. Jones (Ed.), *African American identity development: Theory, research and intervention* (pp. 227–263). Hampton, VA: Cobb & Henry Press.

Stevenson, H. C., & Davis, G. Y. (in press). Racial socialization. In R. Jones (Ed.), *Black psychology* (4th ed.). Hampton, VA: Cobb & Henry Press.

Stevenson, H. C., Davis, G. Y., & Abdul-Kabir, S. (2002). *Stickin' to, watchin' over, and getting' with: African American parent's guide to discipline.* San Francisco: Jossey-Bass.

Stockard, R. L., & Tucker, M. B. (2001). Young African American men and women: Separate paths? In L. Daniels (Ed.), *The state of Black America 2001* (pp. 143–160). New York: National Urban League.

Sue, D. W., & Sue, D. (1999). *Counseling the culturally different.* New York: Wiley.

Tatum, J., Moseley, S., Boyd-Franklin, N., & Herzog, E. (1995). A home based family systems approach to the treatment of African American teenage parents and their families. *Zero to Three: Journal of the National Center for Clinical Infant Programs, 15*(4), 18–25.

Taylor, R. J., Chatters, L. M., Jayakody, R., & Levin, J. S. (1996). Black and White differences in religious participation: A multisample comparison. *Journal for the Scientific Study of Religion, 35,* 403–410.

Taylor, R. J., Jackson, J. S., & Chatters, L. M. (1997). *Family life in Black America.* Thousand Oaks, CA: Sage.

Taylor, R. J., Tucker, M. B., Chatters, L. M., & Jayakody, R. (1997). Recent demographic trends in African American family structure. In R. J. Taylor, J. S. Jackson, & L. M. Chatters (Eds.), *Family life in Black America* (pp. 14–62). Thousand Oaks, CA: Sage.

Testa, M., & Krogh, M. (1995). The effect of employment on marriage among Black males in inner-city Chicago. In M. B. Tucker & C. Mitchell-Kernan (Eds.), *The decline in marriage among African Americans* (pp. 59–95). New York: Russell Sage Foundation.

Thompson, C. (1987). Racism or neuroticism?: An entangled dilemma for the Black middle-class patient. *Journal of the American Academy of Psychoanalysis, 15*(3), 395–405.

Tizard, B., & Phoenix, A. (1993). *Black, White or mixed?: Race and racism in the lives of young people of mixed parentage.* New York: Routledge.

Triandis, H. (1994). Theoretical and methodological approaches to the study of collectivism and individualism. In U. Kim, H. Triandis, C. Kagitcibasi, S. Choi, & G. Yoon (Eds.), *Individualism and collectivism* (pp. 41–51). Thousand Oaks, CA: Sage.

Tucker, J. (2000). *The role of skin color, hair texture, facial features, and body shape, size and weight on the self-esteem and body satisfaction of professional African American women: An exploratory study.* Unpublished doctoral dissertation, Rutgers University, Piscataway, NJ.

Tucker, M. B., & Mitchell-Kernan, C. (Eds.). (1995). *The decline in marriage among African Americans.* New York: Russell Sage Foundation.

Tucker, W. (1994). *The science and politics of racial research.* Chicago: University of Illinois Press.

U.S. Bureau of the Census. (2000, September). The Black population in the United States: March 1999. *Current Population Reports* (Series P20-530). Washington, DC: U.S. Government Printing Office.

U.S. Bureau of the Census. (2001a, June). America's families and living arrangements: 2000. *Current Population Reports* (Series P20-537). Washington, DC: U.S. Government Printing Office.

U.S. Bureau of the Census. (2001b, August). The Black population: 2000. *Census 2000 Brief* (Series C2KBR/01-5). Washington, DC: U.S. Government Printing Office.

U.S. Bureau of the Census. (2001c, September). Poverty in the United States: 2000. *Current Population Reports* (Series P60-214). Washington, DC: U.S. Government Printing Office.

U.S. Bureau of the Census. (2002, September). Money and income in the United States: 2001. *Current Population Reports* (Series P60-218), Appendix A, Table A-1, pp. 15–16. Washington, DC: U.S. Government Printing Office.

U.S. Bureau of Labor Statistics. (2003, January). *Employment and earnings, 50*(1).

U.S. Department of Health and Human Services, Administration for Children and Families, Administration on Children, Youth and Families, and the Children's Bureau. (2000). *Report to the Congress on kinship foster care.* (Retrieved from: *www:aspe.hhs.gov/hsp/kinr2c00/.*)

U.S. Department of Health and Human Services, Substance Abuse and Mental Health Services Administration, Center for Mental Health Services, National Institutes of Health and National Institute of Mental Health. (1999). *Mental health: A report of the Surgeon General.* Rockville, MD: U.S. Government Printing Office.

Van Sertima, I. (1976). *They came before Columbus: The African presence in ancient America.* New York: Random House.

Vega, W., & Rumbaut, R. (1991). Ethnic minorities and mental health. *Annual Revision of Sociology, 17,* 354–383.

Visher, E., & Visher, J. (1979). *Stepfamilies: A guide to working with stepparents and stepchildren.* New York: Brunner/Mazel.

Visher, E., & Visher, J. (1990). Dynamics of successful stepfamilies. *Journal of Divorce and Remarriage, 14,* 3–12.

Walker, A. (1982, July). Embracing the dark and the light. *Essence,* pp. 67, 128. (Reprinted from *Black Scholar,* March–April, 1973.)

Walsh, F., & McGoldrick, M. (1991). *Living beyond loss: Death in the family.* New York: Norton.

Wardle, F. (1987, January). Are you sensitive to interracial children's special identity needs? *Young Children,* pp. 53–59.

Wardle, F. (1991). Interracial children and their families: How school social workers should respond. *Social Work in Education, 13*(4), 209–272.

Warfield-Coppock, N. (1992). The rites of passage movement: A resurgence of African-centered practices for socializing African American youth. *Journal of Negro Education, 61*(4), 471–482.

Watkins, C. M. (2001). A tale of two classes: The socio-economic divide among Black Americans under 35. In L. Daniels (Ed.), *The state of Black America 2001* (pp. 67–86). New York: National Urban League.

Weil, A., & Finegold, K. (Eds.). (2002). *Welfare reform: The next act.* Washington, DC: Urban Institute Press.

Welsing, F. C. (1991). *The Isis papers: The keys to the colors.* Chicago: Third World Press.

White, J. (1972). Towards a Black psychology. In R. Jones (Ed.), *Black psychology.* New York: Harper & Row.

White, J. (1984). *The psychology of Blacks: An Afro-American perspective.* Englewood Cliffs, NJ: Prentice-Hall.

White, J. (in press). Towards a Black psychology. In. R. Jones (Ed.), *Black psychology* (4th ed.). Hampton, VA: Cobb & Henry Press.

White, J., & Cones, J. (1999). *Black men emerging: Facing the past and seizing a future in America.* New York: Routledge.

White, J., & Parham, T. (1994). *The psychology of Blacks.* Englewood Cliffs, NJ: Prentice-Hall.

White, M. (1989). *Selected papers.* Adelaide, Australia: Dulwich Centre Publications.

White, M. (1995). *Re-authoring lives: Interviews and essays.* Adelaide, Australia: Dulwich Centre Publications.

White, M., & Epston, D. (1990). *Narrative means to a therapeutic end.* New York: Norton.

Wilds, D. J. (2000). *Minorities in higher education 1999–2000: Seventeenth annual status report.* Washington, DC: American Council on Education.

Williams, L. (1987, July 14). For the Black professional: The obstacles remain. *New York Times,* p. A16.

Willie, C. V. (1974). The black family and social class. *American Journal of Orthopsychiatry, 44,* 50–60.

Willie, C. V., & Greenblatt, S. L. (1978). Four classic studies of power relationships in Black families: A review and look to the future. *Journal of Marriage and the Family, 40*(4), 691–696.

Wilson, D., & Chipungu, S. (Eds.). (1996). Kinship care. *Child Welfare, 75*(5).

Wilson, H. (1998). Does affirmative action for Blacks harm Whites?: Some evidence from the higher education arena. *Western Journal of Black Studies, 22*(4), 218.

Wilson, W. J. (1980). *The declining significance of race* (2nd ed.). Chicago: University of Chicago Press.

Wilson, W. J. (1987). *The truly disadvantaged: The inner city, the underclass and public policy.* Chicago: University of Chicago Press.

Wilson, W. J. (1996). *When work disappears: The world of the new urban poor.* New York: Knopf.

Wimberly, E. P. (1997). *Counseling African American marriages and families.* Louisville, KY: Westminster John Knox Press.

Wyatt, G. (1997). *Stolen women: Reclaiming our sexuality, taking back our lives.* New York: Wiley.

Author Index

Subject Index